To my wife, Pauline
For her exceptional love and encouragement

To my father
For instilling a thirst for excellence in his children

To my mother
For having enough love for all of us

Contents

Preface

Students in an increasing number of disciplines are finding it necessary to gain some understanding of the nervous system. This book is written to present the essential features of nervous system physiology to students who would like to develop a background in the area. A conscious and purposeful effort has been made throughout the text to develop those concepts judged basic to an understanding of the topics suggested by each chapter title. This book is not intended to be an all-inclusive presentation of the much wider field of neuroscience. The material selected and the level of complexity presented reflect the author's view of those concepts of neurophysiology which students might reasonably be expected to learn in a single initial course. Accordingly, it should satisfy the needs of an introductory course for students in physiology, medicine, biology, psychology, pharmacology, nursing, neuroscience, and other allied health fields.

The order in which information is presented within each chapter has been carefully planned so that students build on the material as they encounter it in their reading. Attention has also been given to sequencing the chapters so that concepts developed in one chapter are fundamental to an understanding of the central ideas of the next. The illustrations in the text have all been drawn specifically to enhance understanding of these essential features. As a further aid to learning, review questions are included after each chapter to allow students to test their comprehension of the material presented.

The author has been offering the content of these chapters as an introductory course in neurophysiology to upper-level undergraduate and beginning graduate students for several years. He has been encouraged by positive feedback from many of these same students in later years when they encounter more sophisticated aspects of the material in advanced training programs. A sincere appreciation is expressed to all of these students for their many contributions to the development of this text.

Parts of the manuscript have been read by several colleagues, notably, Dr. Harold D. Swanson of the Drake biology faculty and Dr. Richard J. Morrow of the Drake College of Pharmacy. The author would like to thank them for their helpful comments and suggestions concerning revisions of the text. A deeply felt sense of gratitude is expressed to Mr. Roger K. Menken, who did the illustrations.

Donald B. Stratton

Neuroembryology and Nervous System Organization

So many aspects of human neuroanatomy and neurophysiology refer to early development that even casually interested students sooner or later find out they must come to grips with the underlying embryology. This chapter is designed (1) to present only those neuroembryological concepts that are necessary for the study of neurophysiology and (2) to review the major structures and systems involved in nervous system organization and classification. It is not intended to be an exhaustive (or exhausting) treatment of the field.

The basic units of nervous tissue are its cells. These include *neurons,* which are the excitable impulse-conducting cells, as well as several types of nonexcitable cells. The latter include the *neuroglial* and *ependymal cells* of the central nervous system (CNS) and the *Schwann cells* of the peripheral nervous system (PNS).

A PRELIMINARY OVERVIEW OF NEUROEMBRYOLOGY

Many students of neurophysiology find themselves somewhat baffled by terminology and classification systems. Many of the terms and systems are based on embryological origins, and the student who has avoided or not been exposed to embryology will encounter some difficulty. One major effort of this chapter is to

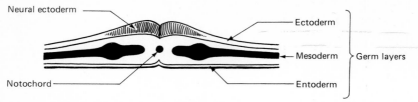

Figure 1-1   The developing embryo with a cross section showing the germ layers.

present just enough embryology to explain the origins of the various components of nervous tissue. The student should also come to appreciate the reasons
behind many of the classification schemes for nerve fibers, receptors, and the
various functional divisions of the nervous system.

The developing embryo is characterized by three germ layers, which give
rise to the various specialized systems of the body. These are the *ectoderm,* the
mesoderm, and the *entoderm* (Fig. 1-1). The ectoderm is of particular interest
to the neuroscientist because it gives rise to the nervous system as well as the
epidermis with all of its sensory receptors. The mesoderm gives rise to connective tissue as well as the skeletal, muscular, circulatory, and urogenital systems
and glands. From the entoderm arise the digestive and respiratory epithelia.
The three germ layers and the tissues which develop from them are summarized in Fig. 1-2.

About the seventeenth day following fertilization, the notochord induces
the ectoderm in the middorsal region to differentiate. That is, it thickens, forms
a neural groove, and becomes the *neural ectoderm.* During the next 4 days the
neural ectoderm begins to separate from the remaining ectoderm (called the
surface ectoderm) and begins to invaginate, converting the neural groove to a
neural tube with two parallel-running *neural crests.* This process is called

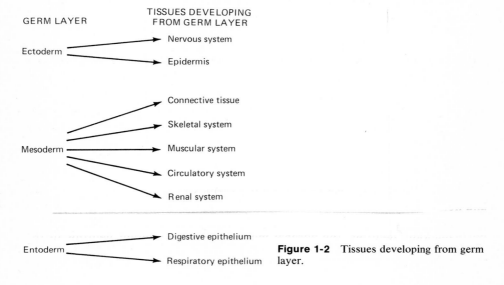

Figure 1-2   Tissues developing from germ
layer.

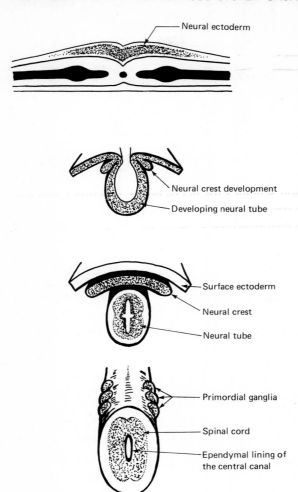

Figure 1-3 The process of neurolation in which the neural ectoderm gives rise to the neural crests and neural tube.

neurolation (Fig. 1-3). Soon after formation of the neural tube, the neural crests subdivide into *primordial ganglia*. Each of these ganglia corresponds to a primitive *somite* or body segment.

Structures of Neural Crest Origin

The neural crest gives rise to *neuroblasts* (cells which later become neurons) and nonneuroblastic cells which later become the Schwann cells of the peripheral nervous system. Neuroblasts eventually give rise to the autonomic postganglionic neurons, the adrenal medulla, and the afferent neurons of the cranial and spinal ganglia (Fig. 1-4).

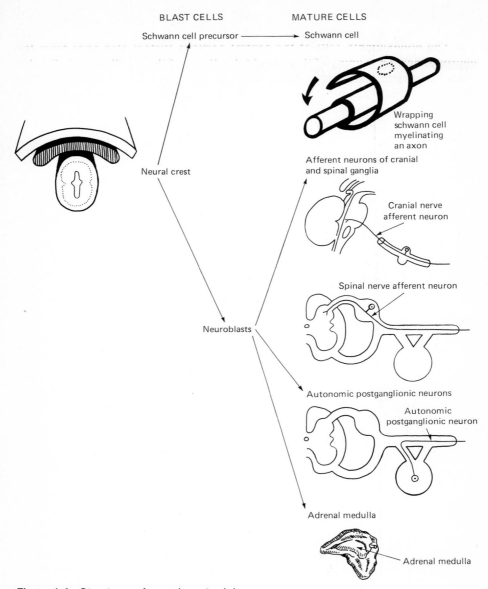

Figure 1-4   Structures of neural crest origin.

Structures of Neural Tube Origin

The neural tube becomes the brain and spinal cord of the central nervous system. The neuroepithelial cell lining of the neural tube gives rise to neuroblasts from which arise all CNS neurons with the exception of those in the mesencephalic nucleus of cranial nerve V, which are probably of neural crest origin.

Certainly the motor neurons of the cranial, spinal, and preganglionic autonomic nerves arise from neuroblasts of neural tube origin.

The nonexcitable cells of the central nervous system also arise from the neuroepithelial cell lining of the neural tube. Some of these cells remain fixed in position and become the single layer of epithelial cells which later line the ventricles of the brain and the central canal of the spinal cord. This lining is the *ependyma* and it separates the cerebrospinal fluid (CSF) of the ventricles and central canal from the excitable tissue of the brain and spinal cord. Other cells *(glioblasts)* migrate through the neural tube and give rise to the neuroglial cells of the CNS. The structures which arise from neural tube origin are illustrated in Fig. 1-5.

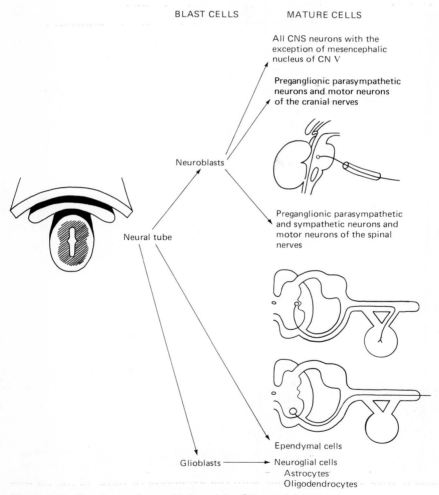

BLAST CELLS   MATURE CELLS

All CNS neurons with the exception of mesencephalic nucleus of CN V

Preganglionic parasympathetic neurons and motor neurons of the cranial nerves

Neuroblasts

Neural tube

Preganglionic parasympathetic and sympathetic neurons and motor neurons of the spinal nerves

Ependymal cells

Glioblasts ⟶ Neuroglial cells
Astrocytes
Oligodendrocytes

Figure 1-5 Structures of neural tube origin. CN, cranial nerve.

Development of the Brain

The cephalic end of the neural tube, which is larger than the posterior end from the very beginning of its embryological development, gives rise to the brain. The brain includes the cerebral hemispheres, the brainstem, and the cerebellum. The embryo, which is essentially a disk during its early stage, begins to undergo *flexion,* a process of curving during which time it is transformed into a tube (Fig. 1-6). It is eventually joined to its extraembryonic membranes only by a thin stalk, the umbilical cord. Flexion results from the rapid growth of the dorsal aspects of the embryo and is characterized by a relatively rapid growth and development of its cephalic (front) end into the brain.

The *notochord,* a midline structure, is apparently responsible for inducing the development of the brain and spinal cord. The notochord itself is mesodermal tissue and eventually gives rise to the vertebral column and cranium, which enclose and protect the brain and spinal cord.

Examination of the 28-day embryo shows that the lumen of the neural tube

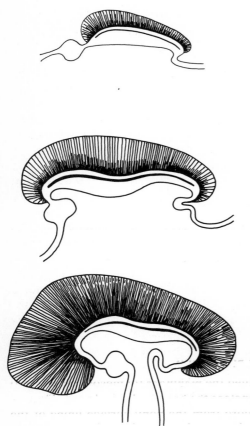

Figure 1-6 The embryo undergoing flexion, during which time it is transformed into a tube which is eventually joined to its extraembryonic membranes only by a thin stalk, the umbilical cord.

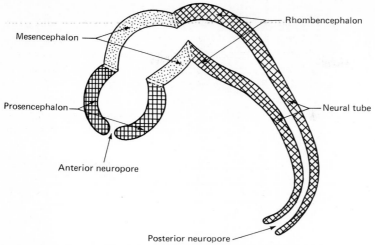

Figure 1-7 Sagittal section of the developing embryo showing the three early embryonic enlargements of the brain, the prosencephalon (forebrain), mesencephalon (midbrain), and rhombencephalon (hindbrain).

is large in the cephalic end and relatively narrow in the rest of the tube. The large cephalic lumen becomes the *ventricular system* of the brain, while the remaining narrow lumen becomes the *central canal* of the spinal cord. The ventricular system and the central canal are continuous with each other and are filled with CSF. The cephalic neural tube itself becomes brain tissue proper.

Early on, three easily identifiable enlargements can be seen in the embryonic brain. These are the *prosencephalon* (forebrain), the *mesencephalon* (midbrain), and the *rhombencephalon* (hindbrain). These are illustrated in Fig. 1-7. The neural tube is initially open at the anterior pole of the prosencephalon (anterior neuropore) and also at the posterior end of the neural tube (posterior neuropore). These pores later close.

With subsequent development, the prosencephalon differentiates into the *telencephalon* (endbrain), which is entirely represented by the two cerebral hemispheres, and the *diencephalon* (betweenbrain), composed of the thalamus, hypothalamus, subthalamus, and epithalamus. The mesencephalon also continues to develop but it undergoes no further subdivision. The rhombencephalon gives rise to the *metencephalon* (afterbrain), which includes the pons and cerebellum, as well as the *myelencephalon* (marrowbrain), which becomes the medulla oblongata (Fig. 1-8).

Meningeal Coverings of the Brain and Spinal Cord

As the embryo develops, coverings called the *meninges* (of mesodermal origin) develop along with it and completely enclose the brain and spinal cord. The meninges separate the brain and spinal cord from the bony surface lining of the cranium and vertebral canal. Soft meninges or leptomeninges include the *pia*

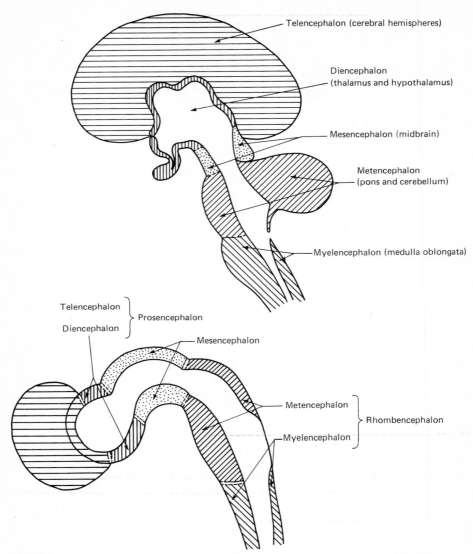

Figure 1-8 Sagittal section of the developing brain showing how the prosencephalon, mesencephalon, and rhombencephalon give rise to later structures.

mater, an extremely thin membrane which is in direct and intimate contact with the brain and spinal cord, and the *arachnoid membrane,* connected to the pia by strands or webs. The *dura mater* (hard meninges) is a tough covering which separates the soft meninges from the bony cranial vault and the vertebral canal. The leptomeninges may be derived from the neural crest, while the hard meninges develop from ordinary mesenchyme. The meninges are illustrated in Fig. 1-9. In addition to providing protection to the brain and spinal cord, the menin-

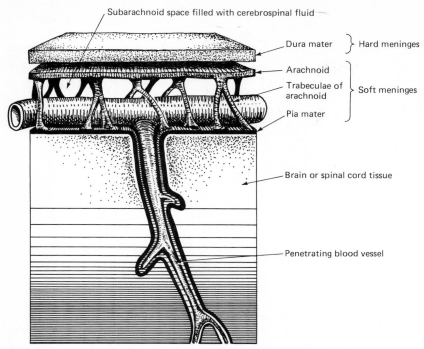

Subarachnoid space filled with cerebrospinal fluid

Dura mater } Hard meninges

Arachnoid

Trabeculae of arachnoid } Soft meninges

Pia mater

Brain or spinal cord tissue

Penetrating blood vessel

Figure 1-9 The relationship between the various meningeal layers and central nervous system tissue.

ges serve to accompany blood vessels to and from CNS tissue as well as to channel CSF around the exterior surfaces of the brain and spinal cord.

The Ventricular System and the Cerebrospinal Fluid

The brain's ventricular system develops right along with the brain itself. The ventricles represent the full development of the lumen of the cephalic end of the neural tube. They are filled with CSF, interconnected, and continuous with the central canal of the spinal cord. As the telencephalon develops in a lateral and caudal direction, forming the hemispheres, the lumen of the telencephalic neural tube develops along with them, forming two *lateral ventricles,* one within each hemisphere. The CSF of the two lateral ventricles eventually becomes separated by a thin membrane, the *septum pellucidum.*

As the diencephalon develops, the neural tube lumen expands in the midsagittal plane into a broad, flat *third ventricle.* The CSF in the lateral ventricles communicates with that in the third ventricle through the *foramina of Monro.* The medial walls of the diencephalon are completely bathed by the CSF of the third ventricle, which flows around the interthalamic adhesion into the *cerebral aqueduct* (Fig. 1-10).

The cerebral aqueduct is a narrow channel through the midbrain. The CSF of the third ventricle flows through this channel into the *fourth ventricle,*

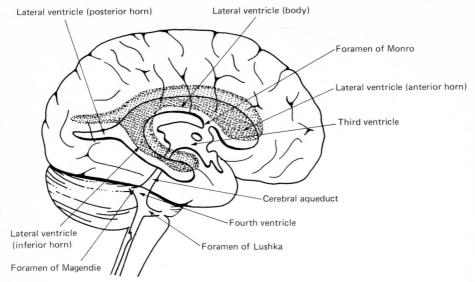

Lateral ventricle (posterior horn)

Lateral ventricle (body)

Foramen of Monro

Lateral ventricle (anterior horn)

Third ventricle

Cerebral aqueduct

Fourth ventricle

Lateral ventricle (inferior horn)

Foramen of Lushka

Foramen of Magendie

Figure 1-10 The ventricular system of the brain. A lateral view.

located posterior to the pons and anterior to the cerebellum. A small amount of the CSF from the fourth ventricle flows into the central canal of the spinal cord, but the greatest bulk of it flows into the subarachnoid spaces of the meninges through three openings in the fourth ventricle. Two of these openings, the *foramina of Luschka,* are located in the anterior lateral extensions of the fourth ventricle around the brainstem inferior to the pons. The other is the *foramen of Magendie,* a posterior opening in the inferior medullary velum below the cerebellum.

Cerebrospinal Fluid Formation and Circulation

A convoluted network of blood vessels traveling in the pia projects into the ventricular system at several points. These blood vessels are covered with ependyma since the entire ventricular system is lined with ependyma. The vascular protrusions with their coverings of specialized ependymal cells are the *choroid plexuses* of the ventricular system (Fig. 1-11).

The choroid plexus is located in the medial walls of the lateral ventricles, the roof of the third ventricle, and the roof and anterior lateral extensions of the fourth ventricle.

Cerebrospinal fluid is a clear and colorless liquid. It is actively secreted by the choroid plexus into the ventricular system at several points, but it is not a simple ultrafiltrate of the plasma from which it is formed. The CSF formed by the choroid plexus of the lateral ventricles flows through the foramina of Monro into the third ventricle, where it joins that produced by the choroid plexus of the third ventricle. As previously noted, it then leaves the third ventricle through the cerebral aqueduct to enter the fourth ventricle, where, most of it

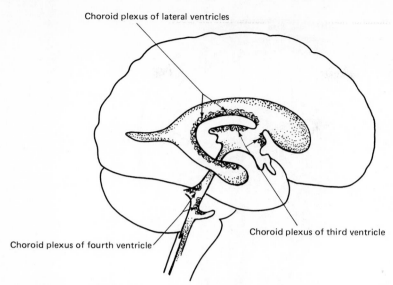

Choroid plexus of lateral ventricles

Choroid plexus of third ventricle

Choroid plexus of fourth ventricle

Figure 1-11   The ventricular system of the brain showing the position of choroid plexus.

flows out through the foramina of Luschka and Magendie into the subarachnoid spaces of the meningeal system (Fig. 1-12). Through this system CSF flows over and around the entire brain and spinal cord.

Because CSF is constantly being formed by the choroid plexus (about 500 mL per day) and entering the ventriculomeningeal system, it is apparent that it must also be removed from the system at the same rate in order to maintain the constant value of 150 mL which is common in the adult. Small elevations of the

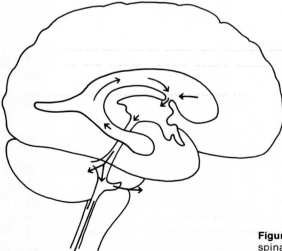

Figure 1-12   Circulation of the cerebro-spinal fluid in the ventricular system of the brain.

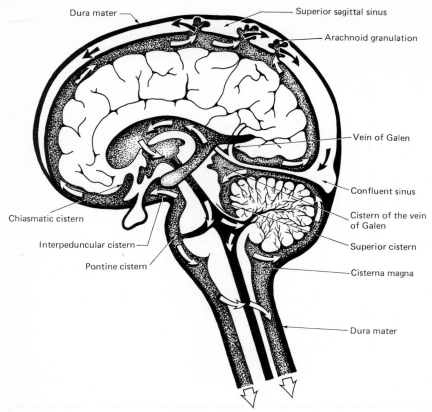

Figure 1-13 The ventriculomeningeal system. Cerebrospinal fluid is seen to flow from its origin in the ventricular system to its ultimate return to the circulatory system in the superior sagittal sinus.

arachnoid *(arachnoid granulations)* into the superior sagittal and transverse sinuses apparently function as one-way valves allowing CSF to be reabsorbed back into the venous blood (Fig. 1-13).

CSF tends to accumulate in certain large subarachnoid areas of the brain and spinal cord. These are called *cisterns* in the brain (Fig. 1-13). The *cisterna magna,* just below the cerebellum, is the largest of these. Others include the *pontine cistern,* anterolateral to the pontomedullary border, the *interpeduncular cistern,* anterior to the midbrain and inferior to the diencephalon, the *chiasmatic cistern* surrounding the optic chiasm, the *superior cistern,* between the cerebellum and the inferior colliculi of the posterior midbrain, and the *cistern of the vein of Galen,* posterior to the diencephalon.

The subarachnoid space is relatively large below the level of the second lumbar vertebra and contains a relatively large amount of CSF. Because this is

Table 1-1   Plasma and CSF Concentrations

	Cerebrospinal fluid	Plasma
Na$^+$	147 meq/kg H_2O	150 meq/kg H_2O
K$^+$	2.9 meq/kg H_2O	4.6 meq/kg H_2O
Cl$^-$	113 meq/kg H_2O	106 meq/kg H_2O
Osmolality	289 mosmol/kg H_2O	289 mosmol/kg H_2O
Protein	20 mg/100 mL	6000 mg/100 mL
Glucose	64 mg/100 mL	100 mg/100 mL
pH	7.307	7.397

below the termination of the spinal cord, a needle can be safely passed into the subarachnoid space in this region to withdraw a CSF sample or to make an injection. Less commonly the cisterna magna is used for this purpose.

Cerebrospinal Fluid Composition

The chemical composition of CSF is similar to plasma. This is not surprising since it is actively secreted by the choroid plexus. The principal difference is that plasma contains about 300 times as much protein as CSF. A brief summary of plasma and CSF concentrations is given in Table 1-1.

THE NEURON

The functional unit of the nervous system is the *neuron,* a term coined by Waldeyer in 1891. Neurons are the excitable cells of nervous tissue which conduct impulses. They arise from the neuroblasts of neural tube and neural crest origin. The complex nervous systems of vertebrates, especially humans, represent remarkably coordinated networks of these fundamental units. Thus it is not surprising to find great diversity in the form and function of individual neurons. Consequently, neurons are classified according to a number of different criteria: (1) morphology or appearance, (2) anatomical location, (3) whether they are sensory or motor, (4) conduction velocity, (5) fiber diameter, and (6) whether they are myelinated or not.

Morphological Classification

Neurons are single cells composed of a *perikaryon* or cell body (soma) and a variable number of *neurites* (processes) extending out from it. Adult neurons are classified as monopolar, bipolar, or multipolar according to whether the perikaryon has one, two, or many neurites (Fig. 1-14).

Monopolar Neurons   Monopolar neurons have only one prominent neurite extending from the perikaryon, which then branches into two long processes, one central (directed toward the CNS) and one peripheral (directed away from the CNS). Most neurons of this type are sensory and are exclusively located in the peripheral nervous system. The dorsal root ganglion cells of the spinal

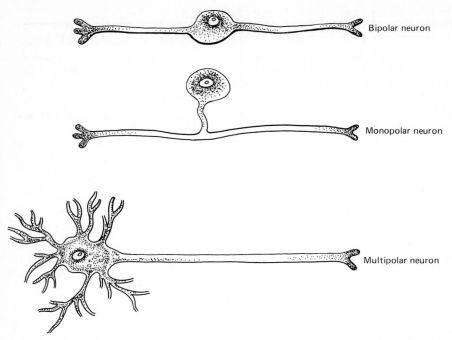

Figure 1-14   Schematic illustration of a bipolar, monopolar, and multipolar neuron.

nerves are monopolar neurons. They relay information from receptors sensitive to touch, pressure, pain, temperature, and stretch, as well as body position and movement.

Bipolar Neurons   Bipolar neurons have two prominent neurites extending from the perikaryon. One conducts impulses toward and one away from the soma. Bipolar neurons are found in the retina, the cochlear and vestibular ganglia, the olfactory epithelium, and in some parts of the central nervous system.

Multipolar Neurons   These are by far the most common type of neuron. They populate both the central and peripheral nervous systems and are characterized by several short, highly branched processes called *dendrites* and a single, long process extending out from the soma called an *axon*. A slight enlargement at the point where the axon leaves the soma, called the *axon hillock,* is often observed.

Considerable confusion exists regarding the proper use of the terms *dendrite* and *axon*. A workable definition is that dendrites are the processes which are specialized to receive stimuli from other cells, while the axon is specialized to conduct impulses. This applies quite adequately to multipolar neurons, but the terms are arbitrary and confusing when applied to monopolar and bipolar neurons. Both the central and peripheral processes of the latter two types conduct impulses. Some neuroscientists refer to both as axons while others call the central process an axon and the peripheral process a dendrite.

A system proposed by Bodian describes that portion of the neuron which is specialized to receive stimuli from other neurons or receptors as the *dendritic zone*. He further describes that portion which is specialized to conduct impulses (essentially the rest of the neuron) as the *axon*. Accordingly, the soma is included in the dendritic zone of multipolar neuron because a considerable number of synapses (contacts) from other neurons converge on it. However, no synaptic contacts are made with the somas of monopolar and bipolar neurons. In fact, only a very limited part of one of the processes of these latter two types actually receives synaptic contacts from other neurons or receptors. Thus this limited area represents the dendritic zone of monopolar and bipolar neurons. Impulses generated here are then conducted over the rest of the neuron, including the soma. In Bodian's system all of this impulse-conducting portion is the axon. The dendritic zones and axons of the three types of neurons are illustrated in Fig. 1-15.

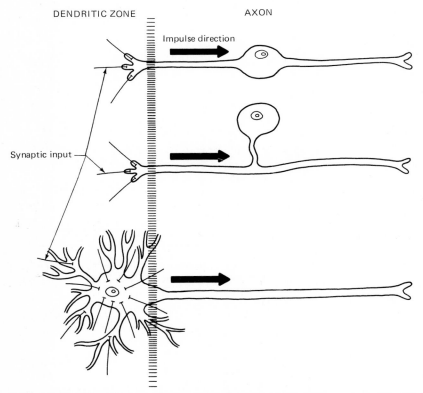

Figure 1-15 Classification of neuronal regions according to the system of Bodian. That portion of the neuron which is specialized to receive stimuli from other neurons or receptors is the dendritic zone. That portion which is specialized to conduct impulses (essentially the rest of the neuron) is the axon.

Classification of Nerve Fibers by Group and Type

A neuron is *a*fferent *to* a particular site if it conducts impulses toward it and *ef*-ferent *from* that site if it conducts impulses away. For example, a neuron which conducts impulses from the thalamus to the cerebral cortex is efferent from the thalamus and afferent to the cerebral cortex.

An efferent neuron which directly innervates a muscle or a gland and causes it to respond in some way is called a *motor neuron*. An afferent neuron which responds to changes in the external or internal environment and gives rise to conscious sensation is termed a *sensory neuron*. The latter is a strict definition of the term *sensory*. Not all afferent neurons give rise to conscious sensation, and thus not all afferent neurons are sensory. Nevertheless, the two terms (*sensory* and *afferent*) are often used interchangeably.

Historically, mammalian PNS nerve fibers can be classified by group or type because of an observed correlation between conduction velocity and fiber diameter. The group system classifies afferent fibers only, while the type system classifies both. The two systems are codified in Table 1-2.

Nerves and Nerve Fiber Tracts

The long process which extends out from the soma of the nerve cell is also called a nerve *fiber*. These fibers are distributed throughout the peripheral nervous system in anatomically distinct structures called *nerves*. It is important to note that nerves exist only in the peripheral nervous system. There are no nerves within the brain or spinal cord itself. Instead, nerve fibers are distributed throughout the central nervous system in reasonably distinct anatomical groupings called nerve fiber *tracts*. Thus it is appropriate to speak of a spinal or cranial nerve since it is part of the peripheral nervous system but not to speak of a nerve within the brain or spinal cord. Tract is the appropriate terminology here. An example is the anterior spinothalamic tract, which is composed of a group of fibers which conduct impulses from the spinal cord to the thalamus, a route entirely within the CNS.

Schwann Cells

The *Schwann cells* are the nonexcitable cells of the peripheral nervous system. By definition they do not conduct impulses. Recall that Schwann cells are derived from Schwann cell precursors of the primitive neural crests. They develop in close association with all of the neuroblasts of the peripheral nervous system. In some cases this association is so close that the Schwann cells wrap many times around the axon of a developing neuron, laying down layer after layer of myelin and producing a *myelinated neuron*. In other cases, the association is not characterized by wrapping Schwann cells and the neuron remains *nonmyelinated*.

Myelinated Neurons   In those neurons destined to become myelinated, a Schwann cell begins to wrap around a given length of axon in a spiral fashion.

Table 1-2 Group and Type Classification of Mammalian Nerve Fibers

Group	Type	Fiber diameter, μm	Conduction velocity, m/s	Description
	A	13–22	70–120	Alpha motor neurons to skeletal muscles
Ia	A	13–22	70–120	Primary afferents from muscle spindles
Ib	A	13–22	70–120	Afferents from Golgi tendon organs
II	A	8–13	40–70	Secondary afferents from muscle spindles, afferents from touch and pressure receptors
	A	4–8	15–40	Gamma motor neurons to muscle spindles
III	A	1–5	5–15	Afferents from touch, pressure, pain, and temperature receptors
	B	0.1–3	0.3–14	Preganglionic autonomic fibers
	C	0.1–3	0.2–2	Postganglionic autonomic fibers
IV	C	0.1–3	0.2–2	Afferents from pain and temperature receptors

In doing so, the Schwann cell extrudes its cytoplasm as its two membranes press together. In this manner it lays down layer after layer of its own membrane, forming a laminated sheath of highly lipid material called *myelin*. Several Schwann cells myelinate a single axon in this manner, each on a different section of its length.

Because of the tight packing and lamination of the myelin, the small volume of fluid in the periaxonal space immediately surrounding the axon (Figs. 1-16 and 17) is not readily interchangeable with the extracellular fluid of the nerve trunk. The *external* and *internal mesaxons* formed by the circling Schwann cell are not free conduits for fluid exchange. The mesaxon is the double membrane formed by the Schwann cell. Thus the axonal membrane is only in contact with a freely interchangeable fluid space at the *node of Ranvier*, where one Schwann cell meets another. The unique anatomical arrangement of Schwann cells around the axons of myelinated neurons endows them with a special pattern of impulse conduction called *saltatory conduction*. The entire Schwann cell is surrounded by a basement membrane, which together with the outer Schwann cell membrane comprises the *neurilemma*.

Nonmyelinated Neurons Postganglionic autonomic fibers as well as some of the very narrow diameter nerve fibers from pain and temperature receptors

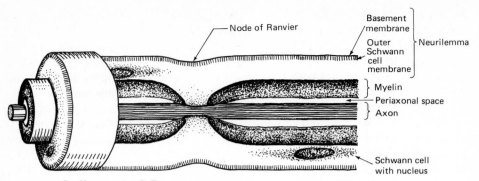

Figure 1-16   A close-up view of a myelinated neuron at a node of Ranvier.

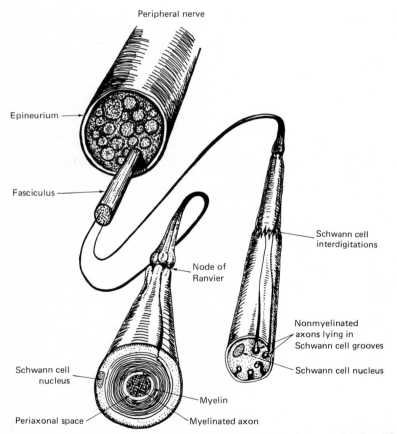

Figure 1-17   Exploded view of peripheral nerve, showing one myelinated nerve fiber and two nonmyelinated nerve fibers.

form a rather loose relationship with Schwann cells. These type C nerve fibers are usually found running in long, deep longitudinal depressions in Schwann cells (Fig. 1-17). A single Schwann cell may have depressions for several narrow fibers. In this case, unlike myelinated axons, the extracellular fluid of the nerve trunk is in contact with the axonal membrane via a gap in the mesaxon which is continuous with the periaxonal space. Thus the entire nonmyelinated axon is in constant contact with a freely interchangeable fluid space and the pattern of impulse conduction is therefore not saltatory as observed in myelinated axons. Even though Schwann cells are in intimate contact with these axons, they are not myelinated because they have not been wrapped by the cells. The characteristics of saltatory and nonsaltatory conduction will be explained in detail in Chap. 2. As Fig. 1-17 shows, Schwann cells form loose contacts with nonmyelinated axons and several of the cells interdigitate with each other enveloping the axon throughout its length.

Neuroglial Cells

Neuroglia ("neural glue") is a fine web of tissue which is composed of peculiar branched cells called *neuroglial cells*. They are located in the central nervous system only and fall into two categories: macroglia and microglia. *Macroglial cells* are derived from glioblasts of the neural tube and include small star-shaped cells called *astrocytes* as well as *oligodendrocytes,* which are the CNS equivalent of Schwann cells. *Microgliocytes* are small nonneural cells, possibly of mesodermal origin.

Neuroglial cells play a variety of roles in the CNS. Astrocytes appear to influence the transport of materials to the neurons of the central nervous system as well as to function to maintain an appropriate ionic environment for the neurons. Oligodendrocytes are responsible for myelinating the neurons of the central nervous system. However, unlike a single Schwann cell, which can only myelinate a single axon, each oligodendrocyte can myelinate the axons of several CNS neurons. As previously mentioned, microgliocytes are probably not of CNS origin at all. They are small cells of various forms with slender, branched processes which migrate into the CNS and act as phagocytes scavenging for waste products and breakdown components of CNS neurons.

Ependymal Cells

Recall that the ependyma is a single layer of epithelial cells lining the ventricles of the brain and the central canal of the spinal cord. They arise from the fixed neuroepithelial cells lining the neural tube. Later they differentiate into the ependymal linings of the central nervous system.

CENTRAL NERVOUS SYSTEM

Neuroscientists define the central nervous system as the brain and spinal cord. The brain is considered to include the cerebral hemispheres, brainstem, and cerebellum. The brainstem includes the diencephalon, midbrain, pons, and medulla oblongata.

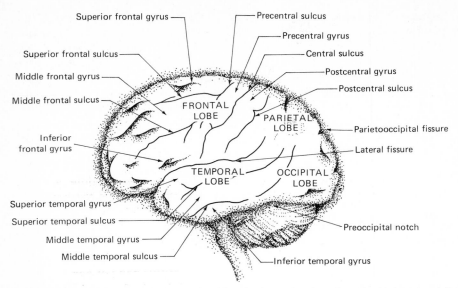

Figure 1-18 Lateral view of the cerebral hemisphere showing the principal gyri, sulci, fissures, and lobes.

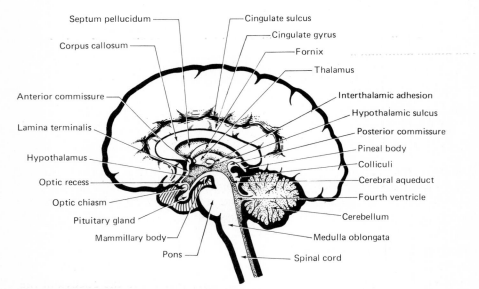

Figure 1-19 Median sagittal view of the brain.

The Brain

Several surface features of the brain are illustrated in Fig. 1-18. When the meningeal coverings are removed it is apparent that the cerebrum is divided into two equal hemispheres by a deep median, longitudinal fissure. It is also apparent that the surface of each hemisphere is very irregular with many ridges (gyri) separated by shallow grooves (sulci). A particularly deep sulcus is called a *fissure.* A central sulcus separates each hemisphere into a frontal (anterior) lobe and a parietal (posterior) lobe. A temporal lobe is separated from the frontal lobe in each hemisphere by a lateral fissure. The occipital lobe in each hemisphere is marked off by the parietooccipital fissure and the preoccipital notch.

Additional features of the anterior lobe are the superior, middle, and inferior frontal gyri and sulci. Just anterior to the central sulcus is the precentral sulcus and gyrus, while just posterior to it in the parietal lobe is the postcentral gyrus and sulcus. Each temporal lobe is characterized by a superior, middle, and inferior temporal gyrus and sulcus.

Several additional brain features can be seen in the median sagittal section illustrated in Fig. 1-19. The cingulate gyrus is a primitive band of cortical tissue circling the corpus callosum. The latter is a thick band of commissural (connecting) fibers between the two cerebral hemispheres. The septum pellucidum is a thin membrane separating the cerebrospinal fluid of the two lateral hemispheres. It can be seen between the fornix and the anterior portion of the corpus callosum.

The medial surfaces of the thalamus and hypothalamus form the lateral walls of the third ventricle, which is continuous with the lateral ventricles above through the foramina of Monro and with the fourth ventricle below through the cerebral aqueduct. The anterior and posterior commissures, like the corpus callosum, are bands of fibers which connect the two hemispheres. The pineal body and colliculi are prominent features of the posterior brainstem, while the optic chiasm, pituitary gland, and mammillary bodies are prominent anterior features.

The Spinal Cord

The spinal cord is the caudal extension of the brainstem into the vertebral canal. It is essentially a long, narrow structure with a cervical and lumbar enlargement. The *cervical enlargement* is due to the great number of afferent and efferent spinal nerve fibers from this region which innervate the arms. The *lumbar enlargement* represents a similar innervation of the leg musculature.

Several prominent sulci are noticeable in a posterior view of the cord (Fig. 1-20). These include a single posterior median sulcus with posterior intermediate and posterior lateral sulci on either side of it. An anterior view shows an anterior median fissure with an anterior lateral sulcus on either side. A long, thin extension of the spinal cord, the *filum terminale,* extends to the coccyx at the tip of the sacrum.

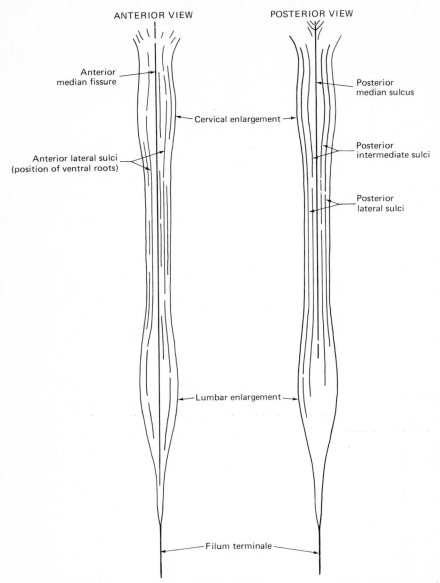

Figure 1-20 Anterior and posterior views of the spinal cord illustrating the principal sulci, fissures, and enlargements.

A cross section of the spinal cord at any level will show the characteristic butterfly-shaped pattern of gray matter surrounded by white matter. In Fig. 1-21 notice that the relative amount of gray matter to white matter varies from one level of the cord to another.

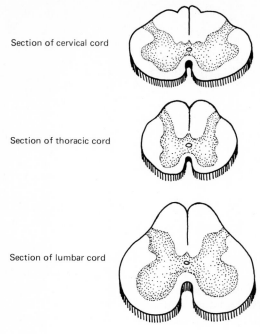

Section of cervical cord

Section of thoracic cord

Section of lumbar cord

Figure 1-21 Cross sections of the spinal cord at midcervical, midthoracic, and midlumbar levels. Notice that the relative ratio and position of gray matter to white matter varies at different levels of the cord.

Spinal Cord White Matter

The spinal cord white matter is divided into three large regions called *funiculi*. The *posterior funiculus* is bounded by the posterior median and posterior lateral sulci (Fig. 1-22). The *lateral funiculus* is that region of white matter between the posterior lateral and anterior lateral sulci. The *anterior funiculus* is bounded by the anterior lateral sulcus and the anterior median fissure. The white matter on both sides of the cord is continuous through the anterior white commissure.

Ascending and Descending Tracts in the Spinal Cord White Matter

The spinal cord white matter is composed of millions of ascending and descending fibers. The ascending fibers conduct impulses up the cord while descending fibers conduct impulses downward. Most of these fibers have also been myelinated by oligodendrocytes, and it is their resulting myelin sheaths which give the white matter its characteristic color.

Most of the spinal cord fibers are grouped together in functional units called *tracts*. The descending tracts typically become smaller as they pass downward through the cord. This is caused by fibers continually leaving the tracts as they reach their specific destinations. Ascending tracts, on the other

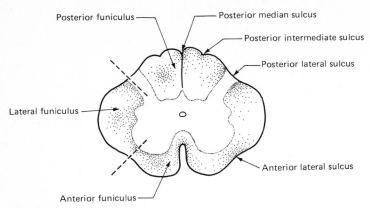

Posterior funiculus ——   —— Posterior median sulcus

——— Posterior intermediate sulcus

——— Posterior lateral sulcus

Lateral funiculus ——

——— Anterior lateral sulcus

Anterior funiculus ——

Figure 1-22 A composite cross section of the spinal cord (not any specific cord level) illustrating the three general divisions of the white matter: the posterior, lateral, and anterior funiculi. Also shown are the sulci which partially separate the white matter.

hand, become larger as they pass up the cord and are continually joined by new incoming fibers at increasingly higher levels. With this in mind, be aware that the composite drawing of the spinal cord in Fig. 1-23 shows the principal tracts in their "general" positions and are depicted in their "average" size. Later chapters will expand on the functional significance of the tracts. They are simply presented here for reference.

The principal ascending tracts are shown to the right while the principal descending tracts are shown to the left in Fig. 1-23. Of course this arrangement is only for illustration as both ascending and descending tracts are actually located on both sides of the cord. If this illustration looks prohibitively complex, take heart in the knowledge that it will reappear in a variety of forms

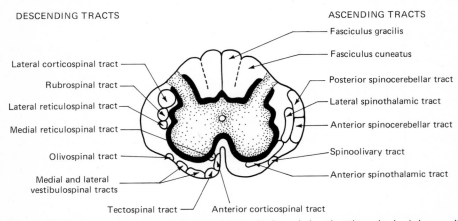

DESCENDING TRACTS   ASCENDING TRACTS

——— Fasciculus gracilis

——— Fasciculus cuneatus

Lateral corticospinal tract ——

Rubrospinal tract ——   ——— Posterior spinocerebellar tract

Lateral reticulospinal tract ——   ——— Lateral spinothalamic tract

Medial reticulospinal tract ——   ——— Anterior spinocerebellar tract

Olivospinal tract ——   ——— Spinoolivary tract

Medial and lateral   ——— Anterior spinothalamic tract
vestibulospinal tracts

Tectospinal tract ——   Anterior corticospinal tract

Figure 1-23 A composite cross section of the spinal cord showing the principal descending tracts to the left and the principal ascending tracts to the right. Of course this separation is only for purposes of illustration as both ascending and descending tracts are actually located on both sides.

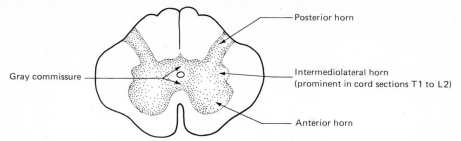

Posterior horn

Gray commissure

Intermediolateral horn
(prominent in cord sections T1 to L2)

Anterior horn

Figure 1-24   A composite cross section of the spinal cord illustrating the general divisions of the gray matter.

in later chapters with each tract associated with a functional role. The addition of a functional component as well as an examination of the clinical signs associated with selective destruction of the various tracts will make it easier to comprehend the anatomical distribution of the tracts illustrated in Fig. 1-23.

Spinal Cord Gray Matter

The gray matter in each half of the cord is subdivided into a posterior, intermediolateral, and anterior horn. The gray commissure connects the gray matter on each side of the cord around the central canal (Fig. 1-24).

Recognize that Fig. 1-24 is also a composite. Comparison with Fig. 1-21 will help to clarify what a composite is. Because the anterior horn contains the cell bodies of motor neurons to the skeletal muscles, it is considerably larger in the cervical and lumbar enlargements where the cord gives rise to the spinal nerves innervating the arms and legs. Also, because most of the sensory fibers of spinal nerves terminate in the posterior horn, it is not surprising to find a larger horn in the cervical and lumbar regions than in the thoracic cord.

An intermediolateral horn, which gives rise to preganglionic sympathetic neurons, is found only in cross sections of the cord between T1 and L2. A similar region giving rise to preganglionic parasympathetic neurons is located in the intermediate gray matter of sacral cord segments 2 to 4. However, unlike segents T1 through L2, it does not extend as a noticeable lateral "horn."

Laminar Architecture of the Gray Matter

A convenient way to subdivide the gray matter of the spinal cord is according to the general cytoarchitecture found in its various regions. These cell regions, or *laminae*, are illustrated in Fig. 1-25. It should be noted that this scheme is based on the spinal cord of the cat. Nevertheless, the system is being applied with due caution to humans.

Laminae I, II, III, and IV are thought to be the principal sensory receiving areas for afferent input to the cord. Laminae V and VI deal with proprioceptive input (dealing with body position and movement) as well as input from the cerebral cortex and other higher centers. Lamina VII has connections with many higher centers. Lamina VIII receives input from the opposite side of the cord

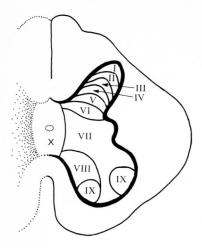

Figure 1-25 A composite half cross section of the spinal cord showing the gray matter subdivided into histologically distinguishable laminae according to the system of Rexed. Each lamina is designated by a specific Roman numeral.

as well as having numerous connections with higher brain centers. Lamina IX is the region of alpha and gamma motor neurons to skeletal muscles. Lamina X is probably a commissural area. It cannot be overstressed that the suspected roles assigned to the laminae above represent a considerable oversimplification. Nevertheless, it gives a basis for understanding synaptic relays as they relate to ascending and descending tracts in the cord and afferent input and efferent output with spinal nerves. These relationships will be examined in later chapters.

PERIPHERAL NERVOUS SYSTEM

The peripheral nervous system is composed of 12 pairs of cranial nerves and 31 pairs of spinal nerves. It represents an extension of the central nervous system into the far reaches of the body. Each spinal nerve contains both afferent and efferent fibers while cranial nerves, on the other hand, are more diverse. Some are afferent only, some are efferent only, and some are mixed (both afferent and efferent).

Spinal Nerves

Each pair of spinal nerves extends laterally from the cord at regular intervals from cervical to coccygeal regions. The spinal nerves leave the vertebral canal via regular openings in the vertebral column called *intervertebral foramina* (Fig. 1-27). Each spinal nerve is named according to the intervertebral foramina through which it exits. Notice in Fig. 1-26 that there is one spinal nerve pair for each vertebra with the exception of the cervical region, where there are seven cervical vertebrae but eight cervical nerve pairs.

Each spinal nerve communicates with the spinal cord via two short roots, one posterior (dorsal) and one anterior (ventral). The anterior and posterior roots of the spinal nerves lie entirely within the vertebral canal. They join and

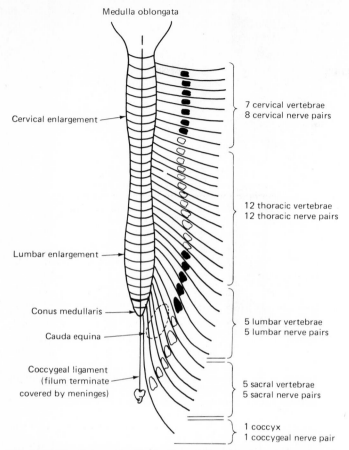

Figure 1-26   Schematic illustration of the spinal cord showing the relationship between the vertebrae and the emergence of the spinal nerves.

form the spinal nerve just before it exits the vertebral canal through the inter-vertebral foramen.

At the point where spinal nerves T1 through L2 leave their respective foramina, two short arms *(rami communicantes)* connect the spinal nerve with a *sympathetic ganglion* lying adjacent to the body of the vertebra (Fig. 1-27). A ganglion is a group of cell bodies located outside of the CNS. These 14 ganglia are connected to each other to form a vertical *sympathetic chain*. Three additional ganglia, the superior, middle, and inferior cervical, join the chain superiorly while another three to five ganglia in the lumbar region join it inferiorly. Thus 20 to 22 ganglia make up the sympathetic chain on each side of the cord. The three cervical ganglia and the last three to five ganglia in the chain communicate with spinal nerves via only one ramus while the ganglia associated with spinal nerves T1 through L2 communicate through two. The sympathetic ganglia and the autonomic nervous system will be explained in Chap. 14.

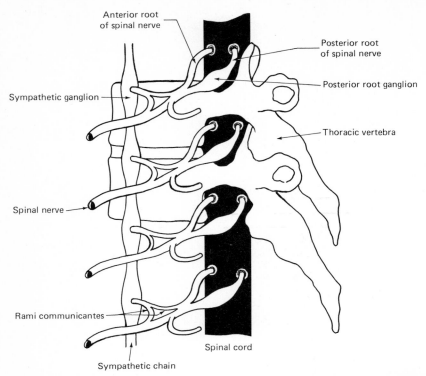

Figure 1-27   The origin of the spinal nerves on the left side of the spinal cord in the region of the thoracic vertebrae. Also illustrated is a portion of the left sympathetic chain showing how the rami communicantes connect the sympathetic ganglia to the spinal nerves.

Cranial Nerves

There are 12 pairs of cranial nerves communicating directly with the brain. They are analogous with the 31 pairs of spinal nerves which communicate with the spinal cord. They include the following:

I	Olfactory	VII	Facial
II	Optic	VIII	Vestibulocochlear
III	Oculomotor	IX	Glossopharyngeal
IV	Trochlear	X	Vagus
V	Trigeminal	XI	Accessory
VI	Abducens	XII	Hypoglossal

Cranial Nerve Emergence and the Brainstem

The cranial nerves and their relationship to the brainstem are shown in Fig. 1-28. The *olfactory nerves* (I) enter through the cribiform plate of the ethmoid bone as 20 to 30 fila (threadlike structures) to contact the olfactory bulb. The

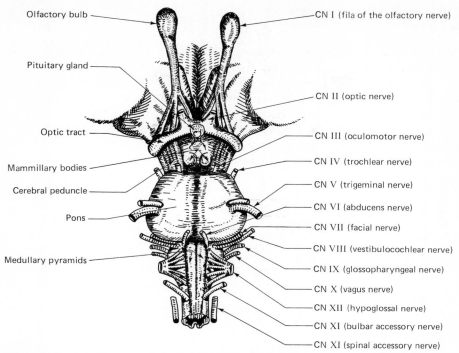

Olfactory bulb

CN I (fila of the olfactory nerve)

Pituitary gland

CN II (optic nerve)

Optic tract

CN III (oculomotor nerve)

CN IV (trochlear nerve)

Mammillary bodies

CN V (trigeminal nerve)

Cerebral peduncle

CN VI (abducens nerve)

Pons

CN VII (facial nerve)

CN VIII (vestibulocochlear nerve)

Medullary pyramids

CN IX (glossopharyngeal nerve)

CN X (vagus nerve)

CN XII (hypoglossal nerve)

CN XI (bulbar accessory nerve)

CN XI (spinal accessory nerve)

Figure 1-28 Anterior view of the brainstem illustrating the general location of the cranial nerves. Other prominent features of the anterior brainstem are also pictured.

optic nerves (**II**) cross anterior to the pituitary gland in the optic chiasm and continue around the cerebral peduncles of the midbrain as the optic tracts. The *oculomotor nerves* (**III**) originate in the midbrain and emerge anteriorly close together at the superior border of the pons. The *trochlear nerves* (**IV**) emerge from the posterior surface of the midbrain just below the inferior colliculi. From here they wrap around the cerebral peduncles to appear anteriorly at the superior border of the pons. The *trigeminal nerves* (**V**) arise from the anteriolateral surface of the pons. The *abducens nerves* (**VI**) originate in the pons and emerge close together at the anterior inferior border of the pons. The *facial nerves* (**VII**), originating in the pons, and the *vestibulocochlear nerves* (**VIII**), which originate in the upper medulla, emerge laterally at the pontomedullary border.

Emerging from the lateral medulla posterior to the olive (a rounded elevation lateral to the pyramids in the medulla oblongata) in order from superior to inferior are the *glossopharyngeal nerves* (**IX**), *vagus nerves* (**X**), and *bulbar accessory nerves* (**XI**). Appearing with them but originating in the spinal accessory nuclei of the upper cervical cord are the spinal portions of the accessory nerves, the *spinal accessory nerves* (**XI**). Finally, arising from the lateral medulla anterior to the olive are the *hypoglossal nerves* (**XII**).

CLASSIFICATION OF SPINAL
AND CRANIAL NERVE FIBERS

Spinal nerve fibers are either *afferent* or *efferent* with respect to the spinal cord (Table 1-3). The spinal efferent fibers are either *somatic* (innervating skeletal muscles derived from mesodermal somites) or *visceral* (innervating cardiac muscle, smooth muscle, or glands). Similarly, spinal afferent fibers are also classified as either somatic or visceral. All are called *general* fibers.

Cranial nerve fibers are classified in the same manner as spinal nerve fibers (Table 1-3). However, there is also a *special* classification. Nerve fibers classified as special innervate the special sense organs involved in hearing, seeing,

Table 1-3 Classification of Spinal and Cranial Nerve Fibers

I *Spinal nerve fiber classification*
   A *General afferent fibers.* The afferent unipolar neurons of the posterior root of the spinal cord with cell bodies in the posterior root ganglia
      1 *General somatic afferent* (GSA). From exteroceptors responding to touch, pressure, pain, and temperature as well as from the proprioceptors of muscles, tendons, and joints
      2 *General visceral afferent* (GVA). From interoceptors of the viscera
   B *General efferent fibers.* The efferent multipolar neurons with cell bodies in the anterior and intermediolateral horns of the spinal cord gray matter
      1 *General somatic efferent* (GSE). The alpha and gamma motor neurons to somatic skeletal muscle and muscle spindles with cell bodies in the anterior horn of the spinal cord gray matter
      2 *General visceral efferent* (GVE). The autonomic fibers to cardiac muscle, smooth muscle, and glands
II *Cranial nerve fiber classification.* (See Figs. 9-13 to 9-15 to identify the fiber types in each cranial nerve.)
   A *General afferent fibers.* The afferent unipolar neurons with cell bodies in the craniospinal ganglia
      1 *General somatic afferent* (GSA). From exteroceptors responding to touch, pressure, pain, and temperature as well as from the proprioceptors of muscles, tendons, and joints
      2 *General visceral afferent* (GVA). From interoceptors of the viscera
   B *Special afferent fibers.* The afferent neurons from the special sense organs (eye, ear, nose, and tongue) and the vestibular system
      1 *Special somatic afferent* (SSA). Exteroceptors from the eye and ear as well as proprioceptors from the vestibular system
      2 *Special visceral afferent* (SVA). Exteroceptors from the olfactory epithelium and the taste buds
   C *General efferent fibers.* The efferent neurons originating in brainstem nuclei innervating somatic skeletal muscle as well as those innervating cardiac muscle, smooth muscle, and glands
      1 *General somatic efferent* (GSE). To somatic skeletal muscles
      2 *General visceral efferent* (GVE). The autonomic fibers to cardiac muscle, smooth muscle, and glands
   D *Special efferent fibers.* The efferent neurons originating in brainstem nuclei innervating branchiomeric skeletal muscle
      1 *Special visceral efferent* (SVE). To branchiomeric skeletal muscles

smelling, and tasting. In addition, special fibers innervate the vestibular system and those skeletal muscles derived from the mesoderm of the branchial arches (embryonic segments which give rise to structures in the ear and neck).

REVIEW QUESTIONS

1 The ectodermal germ layer gives rise to
   a   the nervous system
   b   the circulatory system
   c   the renal system
   d   the epidermis
   e   the muscular system
   f   the skeletal system
2 The neuroblasts of neural tube origin give rise to
   a   preganglionic autonomic neurons
   b   ependymal cells
   c   astrocytes
   d   postganglionic autonomic neurons
   e   Schwann cells
   f   the adrenal medulla
3 Regions of the brain included in the prosencephalon are
   a   metencephalon
   b   telencephalon
   c   thalamus
   d   diencephalon
   e   midbrain
   f   hypothalamus
4 The following is (are) true concerning the meningeal coverings of the brain and spinal cord:
   a   The pia mater is the innermost layer.
   b   The "hard meninges" include the pia mater.
   c   The arachnoid membrane is a webbed and stranded structure.
   d   The leptomeninges are derived from the neural crest.
   e   All of the above.
5 Cerebrospinal fluid
   a   is formed by the arachnoid granulations
   b   is characterized by a protein concentration which is only one three-hundredths of that in plasma
   c   flows out of the third ventricle into the fourth through the foramina of Monro
   d   is formed at the rate of 500 mL per day
   e   none of the above
6 The following is (are) true concerning the nonexcitable cells of the nervous system:
   a   Oligodendrocytes myelinate PNS nerve fibers.
   b   Ependymal cells line the ventricles and the central canal of the spinal cord.
   c   Astrocytes and oligodendrocytes are microglial cells.
   d   Ependymal cells arise from glioblasts.
   e   All of the above.

7 The spinal cord gray matter is often subdivided into laminae in which

   a laminae I to IV represent the principal sensory receiving areas for spinal nerve afferent fibers

   b lamina VIII is the region of alpha and gamma motor neurons

   c laminae V and VI are the principal sensory receiving areas for proprioceptive input to the cord

   d the laminae are characterized by differences in their cytoarchitecture

   e lamina X is probably a commissural area

8 All of the following statements about the peripheral nervous system are true, *except:*

   a There are 12 pairs of cranial nerves and 31 pairs of spinal nerves.

   b There are eight cervical vertebrae but seven cervical nerve pairs.

   c The anterior and posterior spinal nerve roots lie entirely within the vertebral canal.

   d Every sympathetic ganglion is connected to a spinal nerve by two rami communicantes.

   e Every spinal nerve contains both afferent and efferent fibers.

9 All of the following statements about the emergence of cranial nerves from the brainstem are true, *except:*

   a The oculomotor nerves (III) originate in the midbrain.

   b The trigeminal nerves (V) arise from the anterolateral surface of the pons.

   c The abducens nerves (VI) emerge close together at the superior anterior border of the pons.

   d The hypoglossal nerves (XII) emerge from the lateral medulla anterior to the olive.

   e The glossopharyngeal nerves (IX) emerge from the lateral medulla anterior to the olive.

10 The following is (are) true concerning cranial nerve fiber classification:

   a GVE fibers innervate cardiac muscle, smooth muscle, and glands.

   b GVA fibers innervate proprioceptors in muscles, tendons, and joints.

   c GSE fibers are autonomic.

   d GSA fibers innervate interoceptors of the viscera.

   e All of the above.

Membrane Potentials and the Nerve Impulse

The means by which nerves conduct impulses have been puzzling researchers for centuries. The electrical nature of the impulse was first suspected by Luigi Galvani in 1780, when he caused the leg of a frog to contract after stimulating it with an electric charge from the newly developed Leyden jar. In the nineteenth century, Emil Du Bois Reymond first demonstrated the action potential and later wrote, "If I do not greatly deceive myself, I have succeeded in realising (albeit under a slightly different aspect) the hundred years dream of physicists and physiologists, to wit, the identity of the nervous principle with electricity." Later, in 1902, Julius Bernstein postulated the "membrane theory" of the nerve impulse, when he proposed that the impulse is related to changes in the ion permeability of the membrane. Finally much of our present knowledge concerning the events associated with the action potential and the nerve impulse is based on the ingenious work with the giant axon of the squid performed by Hodgkin and Huxley in England and Curtis and Cole in the United States during the late 1940s and early 1950s.

A PRELIMINARY OVERVIEW OF NEURON ACTIVITY

Neurons are ideally suited to function as the information-carrying units of the nervous system. The length of their individual processes varies from a fraction

of a millimeter in the brain to axons over 1 m in length in the spinal cord and peripheral nerves. The information-carrying signal that travels along the neuron is
an electrical event called the *impulse*. All impulses which a neuron conducts
are nearly alike. Therefore the information which a neuron can transmit is determined by the firing pattern as well as the number of *impulses per second*
(IPS) it sends. Neurons can vary their impulse firing rates from 0 to just over
1000 IPS. Because neurons have such a wide range of firing rates and patterns
they can transmit considerably more information to the brain than they could if
all they had was a simple "on-off" system.

For those functions in which speed of action is biologically important,
neurons with high *conduction velocities* are often employed. Neurons with considerably slower conduction velocities are often found in neural circuits which
do not require such speed. Conduction velocity is an inherent property of the
neuron, increasing with fiber diameter and the degree of myelination. In
mammalian neurons, conduction velocities vary anywhere from 0.2 up to 120
m/s.

Nervous systems are incredibly complex networks of nerve cells in which
impulses traveling along one neuron initiate impulses in other neurons at
chemically responsive junctures called *synapses*. Chemicals called *neurotransmitters* are released at these synapses in response to the arrival of impulses at
the *presynaptic terminals* of the first neuron.

When impulses arrive at a sufficient number of these presynaptic terminals, enough neurotransmitter is released to stimulate the postsynaptic neuron
to its *excitation threshold*. When this happens there occurs on the membrane of
the postsynaptic neuron a rapid and reversible change called an *action potential*. Once initiated this action potential generates a small *local current* which
initiates a second action potential on the adjacent membrane segment. The
local current from this action potential will, in turn, initiate a third, and so on
down the entire length of the axon to the very ends of its terminal branches. Although the action potential is actually reinitiated by this series of events, we
generally speak as though its propagation is a continuous smooth process. This
series of propagated action potentials constitutes the *impulse*, and represents
the signal which forms the basis for the information which the nervous system
conducts. In this chapter we will examine those properties which make action
potentials and impulses possible.

BASIC ELECTRICITY AND THE NEURON

Most students who take courses in neurophysiology would like to learn as
much as they can about neurons but are often confused by the electrical properties of neural function. Nevertheless, when neurons conduct impulses, electrical currents flow through their membranes and it is therefore not possible to
understand the former without a working knowledge of the latter. Besides, electronic instruments are used to record action potentials and impulses, and
neurophysiologists commonly employ electrical terms and symbols in describ-

ing neuronal events. So it is actually well worth the student's time to review a few basic principles of electricity which are critical to the understanding of nerve cells.

Current

Current is carried in wires by electrons, but in biological systems such as the neuron it is carried by ions. The passage of 6×10^{18} electrons or monovalent ions past any cross section of a conductor represents an electric charge equal to one *coulomb* (C). *Current I* represents the rate of flow of electric charge. Its basic unit is the *ampere* (A), which represents the flow of one coulomb per second. Each mole of monovalent ion can transfer 96,500 C of electric charge, a value useful to the neurophysiologist called the *Faraday constant*. By convention in biological systems, current is pictured as flowing in the direction of the positive ions (Fig. 2-1).

Because of relatively high extracellular and low intracellular concentrations, current flow outside the nerve cell and inward through the membrane is primarily carried by Na$^+$ ions. Similarly, intracellular and outward currents are primarily carried by K$^+$ ions because of its relatively high intracellular and low extracellular concentrations.

Resistance and Conductance

All conducting media offer some degree of resistance to the passage of current whether carried by electrons or by ions. The unit of *resistance R* is the *ohm* (Ω). It represents the resistance of a conductor such that a constant current of one ampere requires a potential of one volt between its ends. All things being equal, current follows the path of least resistance in any circuit. Neurophysiologists also use a related value called *conductance g*. It represents the reciprocal of resistance. The unit of conductance is the *siemen* (S). However, the earlier term *mho* (ohm spelled backward) is commonly used in most of the classical literature. Because of this reciprocal relationship, all statements

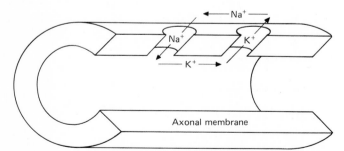

Figure 2-1 Opened view of the axon showing the direction of current flow through the membrane. The extracellular and inward current is carried primarily by Na$^+$ ions, while the intracellular and outward current is carried principally by K$^+$ ions. The thickness of the membrane is greatly exaggerated. Similarly, the Na$^+$ and K$^+$ "channels" are enlarged for clarity.

$$g = \frac{1}{R}$$

where g = conductance, S
R = resistance, Ω

concerning resistance are reciprocally related to conductance.

Neurophysiologists are often concerned with the total resistance in several resistive elements. Neuronal membranes behave in part as if they were composed of parallel resistive elements, while the extracellular and intracellular fluids surrounding the membrane behave like series resistors. Since electric currents flow through the membrane and both of these fluids during impulse conduction, it is important to be able to estimate the total resistance involved. Biologically, the important point to remember here is that the total resistance of series resistors is equal to their sum, but the total resistance of parallel resistors is equal to a value less than their sum. Figure 2-2 illustrates the series resistive nature of the axoplasm and extracellular fluid, while Fig. 2-3 pictures the axonal membrane in the form of parallel resistors.

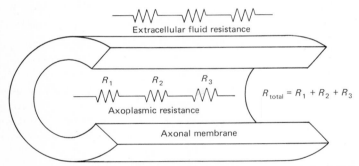

Figure 2-2 Both the axoplasm and extracellular fluid can be thought of as offering series resistance to the flow of current. The total resistance of resistors in series is equal to the sum of the individual resistors.

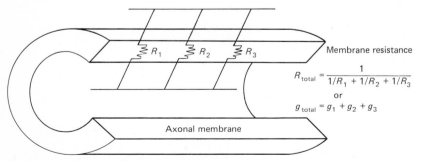

Figure 2-3 The axonal membrane is pictured as if it were composed, in part, of parallel resistors. The total resistance in parallel resistors is equal to the reciprocal of the sum of the reciprocals of the individual resistors. Since conductance g is the reciprocal of resistance, the total conductance is equal to the sum of the individual conductances.

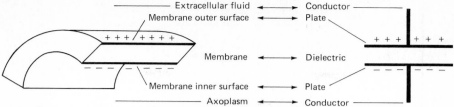

Figure 2-4 The similarity between the membrane and a capacitor. Both are charge-storing devices.

Capacitance

The neuronal membrane behaves in part as if it were composed of parallel capacitors. A capacitor is a charge-storing component consisting of two conductors separated by a dielectric (insulator). The membrane represents the dielectric while the extracellular fluid and the axoplasm represent the conductors (Fig. 2-4).

The unit of capacitance C is the *farad* (F). It represents the capacitance of a capacitor in which a charge of one coloumb produces a potential difference of one volt between the terminals (conductors). The relationship between capacitance (in farads) and the potential difference (in volts) produced by a given charge separation (in coulombs) is given by

$$C = \frac{Q}{V}$$

where C = capacitance, F
$\quad\quad Q$ = charge, C
$\quad\quad V$ = potential, V

By manipulation of the equation we can see that the charge that needs to be separated in order to produce a specific voltage is given by

$$Q = CV$$

Similarly, the potential developed by the transfer of a given charge across a capacitance is given by

$$V = \frac{Q}{C}$$

Neurophysiologists are generally concerned with the total capacitance in a section of membrane. Since the neuronal capacitance is only associated with the membrane, we need not concern ourselves with other aspects of the neuron. Because the membrane behaves as if it were in part composed of parallel capacitors, we are interested in the rules governing parallel capacitors (Fig. 2-5).

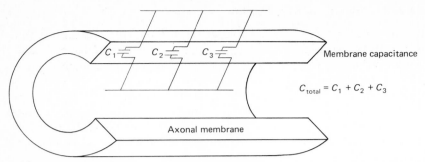

Figure 2-5 The axonal membrane is pictured as if it were composed, in part, of parallel capacitors. The total capacitance of capacitors in parallel is equal to the sum of the individual capacitors.

Electrical Potential and Ohm's Law

The unit of *potential E* is the *volt* (V). The difference in potential between two points is related to the work done in moving a point charge from the first point to the second. It is equal to the difference in the value of the potentials at the respective points. Biologically important voltages are usually quite small, in the order of millivolts (mV) or microvolts (μV).

In simple direct current (dc) wire circuits, the battery is an electronic component which represents a potential difference as well as a source of charge (electrons). In neurons, ions represent the charge while the chemical (concentration) gradient for a given ionic type represents the potential for that ion. The relationship between potential, current, and resistance is expressed by Ohm's law

$$I = \frac{E}{R}$$

where I = current, A
E = potential, V
R = resistance, Ω

In neuron studies we are often concerned with conductance. Consequently a useful form of the equation is

$$I = Eg$$

where g = conductance, S

The neurophysiology student should learn Ohm's law well because there are many equations which are derived from this basic relationship between current, potential, resistance, and conductance.

Resistance and Capacitance (RC) Circuits

Functionally a capacitor can do three things. It can become charged, it can store a charge, and it can discharge. When a capacitor is connected to a voltage source, current will flow and build up charges on one side of the capacitor while removing them from the other side in the process of completing the circuit.

Current will flow in the circuit only until the charge on the capacitor attains the same potential as the voltage source. At the point the capacitor is fully charged, current will no longer flow in the circuit. A resistor is usually pictured as being in series with the capacitor in such a circuit—hence, the name *resistance-capacitance (RC) circuit*.

If the voltage source is removed and the charged capacitor and resistor are connected in a closed loop, current will once again flow as charges are drawn off the capacitor through the resistor to equalize on both sides of the dielectric. Thus the capacitor is discharged and the potential removed. This current which flows only when the capacitor is being charged or discharged is called *capacitive current I_c*. It is proportional to the rate of change of voltage across the capacitor.

All physical systems require a certain amount of time to transmit given quantities of charge from input to output. This time in simple RC systems is characterized by the system *time constant τ*. It is mathematically equal to the product of the resistance (in ohms) and the capacitance (in farads). The resultant time constant is in seconds and represents the time required for the voltage to reach $1 - 1/e$ (63 percent) of its final value. The symbol e is the base of the natural logarithm ($2.71828\cdots$).

$$\tau = RC$$

where $\tau =$ time constant, s
$\quad R =$ resistance, Ω
$\quad C =$ capacitance, F

When a voltage source is suddenly applied across an uncharged RC circuit, there is a delay in the rise of the potential developed on the capacitor, which is accounted for by the time required to store charges (Fig. 2-6). The time constant represents the time in seconds it takes for the capacitor to produce a voltage 63 percent as high as its final value when it is fully charged. Similarly, when the capacitor is discharged, it takes just as long (i.e., one time constant) for the capacitor to lose 63 percent of its charge.

If you are a little confused at this point, don't be discouraged. Thinking of biological systems in electrical terms takes a little getting used to. Take heart, however, in knowing that the electrical principles summarized in the preceding few pages will be sufficient to carry you through an understanding of the complex workings of nerve cells as they conduct the electrical signals known as impulses.

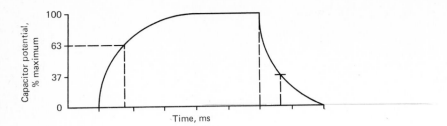

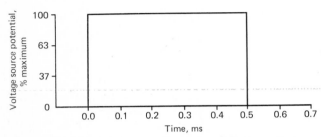

Figure 2-6 When a voltage source is suddenly applied across an uncharged RC circuit, there is a delay in the rise of the potential produced on the capacitor, as it stores charges. There is a similar delay in the discharge of the capacitor. The delay is characterized by the system time constant. One time constant is the time it takes to produce a voltage change equal to 63 percent of the final value.

THE RESTING MEMBRANE POTENTIAL

All cells exhibit an electrical potential across their membranes called a *membrane potential* (MP). However, nerve and muscle cells are somewhat unique in that this membrane potential can be reduced (depolarized) or increased (hyperpolarized) as a result of synaptic activity. This feature makes nerve and muscle cells excitable.

When a neuron is not being stimulated its membrane potential is relatively stable and is therefore referred to as a *resting membrane potential* (RMP). A typical RMP for mammalian nerve and muscle cells lies between 70 and 100 mV, with the intracellular fluid negative. For illustrative purposes consider a common average for a large mammalian nerve cell axon of −85 mV with the dendritic zone (soma and dendrites) being less polarized at approximately −70 mV.

Much of what we believe today concerning membrane potentials and action potentials is based on experiments with the giant axon of the squid. Such studies laid the groundwork for almost all of our present assumptions concerning nerve excitability. Accordingly, many of the examples included here will be based on action potentials and impulses in the squid axon.

When a squid or mammalian nerve axon is penetrated by a recording microelectrode and the internal potential compared to an external reference

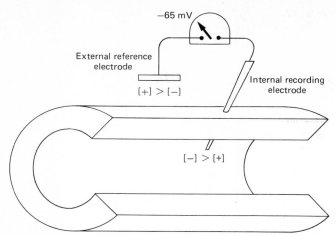

Figure 2-7   When a squid or mammalian nerve axon is penetrated by a recording microelectrode, the axoplasm is found to be negative with respect to the extracellular fluid. In this illustration, the axons from the squid and the membrane potential is found to be −65 mV. The obvious assumption which can be made is that there are slightly more negative than positive charges inside and slightly more positive than negative charges outside.

electrode, the axoplasm is found to be negative with respect to the outside. The magnitude of this potential is about −65 mV in the squid. The obvious assumption which can be made is that there are slightly more positive than negative charges outside, and slightly more negative than positive charges inside (Fig. 2-7).

How important is it for nerve cells to have a resting membrane potential? Quite simply, without it (1) they would not be excitable, (2) they could not produce action potentials, and (3) they could not conduct impulses. Thus because of its important role in the impulse conducting process, a good place to start our discussion is with the origin of the RMP itself.

Ionic Distribution and the Resting Membrane Potential

Julius Bernstein demonstrated in the early 1900s that ionic fluxes across the membrane were important to the impulse-conducting capabilities of neurons. He demonstrated that resting membranes were typically more permeable to K^+ ions than they were to Na^+ ions. Typical extracellular and intracellular concentrations of Na^+, K^+, and Cl^- in a large mammalian nerve cell axon and the giant axon of the squid are illustrated in Fig. 2-8.

Even a quick observation of the various concentrations in Fig. 2-8 shows us that Na^+ and Cl^- are much more concentrated extracellularly, while K^+ is much more concentrated intracellularly. The membrane which separates these two solutions in both the squid and mammalian cells is freely permeable to water but is much less permeable to the above-listed ions. Not depicted in Fig. 2-8 are the nonpermeable anions found within the intracellular fluid. These anions are composed primarily of large protein molecules. Because of the free

LARGE MAMMALIAN NERVE AXON GIANT AXON OF SQUID

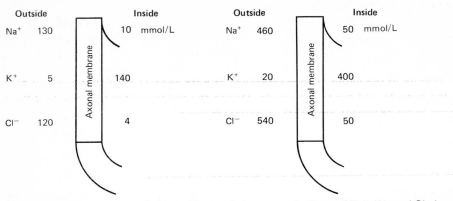

Figure 2-8 Typical extracellular and intracellular concentrations of Na+, K+, and Cl– ions in a large mammalian nerve axon and in the giant axon of the squid. Notice that in both cases, Na+ and Cl– are highly concentrated outside while K+ is highly concentrated inside.

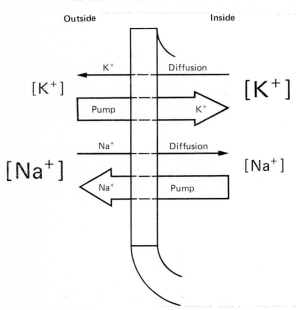

Figure 2-9 The membranes of both the mammalian and squid axons actively transport ("pump") Na+ ions outward and K+ ions inward. Hence, the tendency for ions to diffuse down their concentration (chemical) gradients is exactly balanced by the active transport of these same ions against their gradients.

permeability of the membrane to water, the inside and outside solutions have virtually the same osmolality.

Even though the membrane is not very permeable to either cation listed in Fig. 2-8, recall that Bernstein showed the resting membrane to be more permeable to K^+ than to Na^+. It was subsequently discovered that Cl^- permeates more readily than K^+ in the mammalian axon and less readily than K^+ in the giant axon of the squid. The membranes of both species actively transport Na^+ to the outside and K^+ to the inside. Hence the tendency for the ions to diffuse down their chemical gradients is counterbalanced by the Na^+ and K^+ active transport system (Na^+/K^+ "pump") transporting these ions against their chemical gradients (Fig. 2-9).

The Principles of Equimolality and Electrical Neutrality

When a cell is at rest it obeys two basic principles, the principle of equimolality and the principle of electrical neutrality. These two principles are summarized here.

1   *The principle of equimolality.* The concentrations of osmotically active particles on both sides of the cell membrane should be approximately equal.

2   *The principle of electrical neutrality.* The number of extracellular cations and anions should be approximately equal. Similarly, the number of intracellular cations and anions should be approximately equal.

Chemical analysis of the solutions on each side of the two types of nerve cells verifies that these two principles are essentially true. A second examination of the ionic distributions will show that the high extracellular concentration of Na^+ is primarily balanced by the high extracellular concentration of Cl^-, while the high intracellular K^+ concentration is primarily balanced by the high intracellular concentration of large nonpermeating anions we referred to earlier.

We have neglected to list other such ions as Mg^{2+}, Ca^{2+}, and several others which are also present in the solutions on either side. Their concentrations are small and otherwise unimportant in the events of the action potential and impulse. Nevertheless they help to contribute to the principles of equimolality and electrical neutrality.

You might well be wondering how it is possible to have a resting membrane potential if the solutions on both sides of the membrane are electrically neutral. The answer lies in the fact that the principle of electrical neutrality is only approximately true. As we have previously noted (Fig. 2-7) there are actually slightly more cationic than anionic charges outside and slightly more anionic than cationic charges inside. This slight imbalance, or violation of the principle of electrical neutrality, is sufficient to produce the potential difference across the resting membrane. As we will see later an imbalance of only a few picomoles (10^{-12} mol) is sufficient to produce the resting membrane potential.

Ionic Diffusion and the Resting Membrane Potential

A relatively simple experiment might be helpful in understanding how the resting membrane potential develops. If you were to place a highly concentrated salt solution on one side of a selectively permeable membrane and a less concentrated solution on the other side, the salt would diffuse through the membrane from the highly concentrated to the less concentrated side until it reached equilibrium.

Now if the membrane was more permeable to the cation of the salt than it was to the anion, positive charges would migrate to one side faster than negative charges and a *charge separation* would develop across the membrane with one side more positive than the other (Fig. 2-10). A sensitive voltmeter applied across the membrane would register a potential difference, and because this potential is caused by unequal diffusion rates it can properly be called a *diffusion potential*.

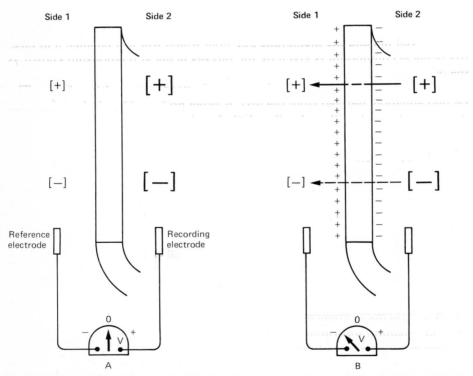

Figure 2-10   *A.* A highly concentrated salt solution is placed on one side of a selectively permeable membrane and a less concentrated solution placed on the other side. When the solutions are initially added there is no potential difference between the two sides as each is electrically neutral (has as many positive as negative charges). *B.* The membrane is more permeable to the cation of the salt than to the anion, causing positive charges to diffuse to side 1 faster than negative charges, producing a "charge separation." Consequently, side 2 becomes negative with respect to side 1.

The resting membrane potential which exists in both the mammalian and squid axons is thought to be primarily due to a diffusion potential caused by the charge separation which results as K^+ ions diffuse outward down their concentration gradient, leaving the large nonpermeating anions behind.

The Nernst Equation and the Equilibrium Potential

As K^+ ions diffuse outward following their chemical (concentration) gradient, the outside of the membrane becomes increasingly positive while the inside becomes more negative. This continual tendency for K^+ to diffuse outward is increasingly opposed by the buildup of an *electrical gradient* in the *opposite direction*, from outside to inside. That is, the increasing positivity on the outside opposes the further flow of positively charged K^+ outward, and the increasing negativity of the inside surface of the membrane tends to restrict the escape of K^+. When the electrical gradient has increased to a point where it is sufficient to stop the net outward flow of K^+, the ion is said to be at *electrochemical equilibrium*.

The relationship between the concentration gradient across the membrane of any given ion and the membrane potential which will just balance it at electrochemical equilibrium is given by the physiochemical relationship known as the *Nernst equation*. It represents the equilibrium potential for that particular ionic type. The Nernst equation is commonly used in one of two forms. The second equation, derived from the first, is often preferred by students because it is easier to work with and suffers little loss in accuracy.

$$E = \frac{RT}{zF} \ln \frac{C_1}{C_2} \tag{2-1}$$

$$E = 58 \log \frac{C_1}{C_2} \tag{2-2}$$

where E = equilibrium potential [expressed in volts in Eq. (2-1) and millivolts in Eq. (2-2)]

R = universal gas constant, 8.32 J mol^{-1} K^{-1}
T = absolute temperature, K
z = valence and charge of ion
F = Faraday constant, 96,500 C/mol
C_1/C_2 = chemical gradient
$\ln$ = natural logarithm
$\log$ = common logarithm

61 is used if preparation is at body temperature (37°C); 58 is used if preparation is at room temperature (20°C).

As a useful exercise let's calculate the equilibrium potential for K^+ ions in both the mammalian nerve cell and the giant axon of the squid. Further, let's calculate the equilibrium potential for the mammalian nerve cell at body temperature and for the squid axon at room temperature. Finally, to familiarize you with both equations, let's calculate the equilibrium potential first with Eq. (2-1) and then again with Eq. (2-2).

Large mammalian nerve cell

$$E_{K^+} = \frac{Rt}{zF} \ln \frac{C_1}{C_2}$$
$$= \frac{(8.32 \text{ J mol}^{-1} \text{ K}^{-1}) (310 \text{ K})}{(1) (96,500 \text{ C/mol})} \ln \frac{140}{5}$$
$$= 0.08906 \text{ J/C}$$
$$= 0.08906 \text{ V}$$
$$= 89.06 \text{ mV} \tag{2-1}$$

$$E_{K^+} = 61 \log \frac{C_1}{C_2}$$
$$= 61 \log \frac{140}{5}$$
$$= 88.28 \text{ mV} \tag{2-2}$$

Giant axon of the squid

$$E_{K^+} = \frac{RT}{zF} \ln \frac{C_1}{C_2}$$
$$= \frac{(8.32 \text{ J mol}^{-1} \text{ K}^{-1}) (293 \text{ K})}{(1) (96,500 \text{ C/mol})} \ln \frac{400}{20}$$
$$= 0.0757 \text{ J/C}$$
$$= 0.0757 \text{ V}$$
$$= 75.7 \text{ mV} \tag{2-1}$$

$$E_{K^+} = 58 \log \frac{C_1}{C_2}$$
$$= 58 \log \frac{400}{20}$$
$$= 75.5 \text{ mV} \tag{2-2}$$

Notice that the equilibrium potentials calculated are slightly different for each nerve cell depending on whether Eq. (2-1) or Eq. (2-2) is used. This is due to rounding errors in converting the quantity (RT/zF) ln to the quantity 61 log or 58 log. However, for all practical purposes, the error is quite small and can be ignored.

The Nernst equation is interpreted this way. In the squid axon, K^+ is 20 times more concentrated inside than outside and therefore has a chemical gradient directed outward. It would require an external positivity of about 76 mV (internal negativity equal to -76 mV) to just balance this gradient at electrochemical equilibrium and stop the net diffusion of K^+ outward. Since the RMP of the squid axon isn't quite this negative inside, there is a continual tendency for K^+ to diffuse outward. Now consider that a cation gradient from inside to outside and an anion gradient from outside to inside will be balanced at electrochemical equilibrium by internal negativity. Similarly, a cation gradient from outside to inside and an anion gradient from inside to outside will be balanced by internal positivity. (Read this again to make sure you have it.) Consequently, the following forms of the Nernst equation can theoretically predict both the magnitude and polarity of the *internal* potential:

$$E = -58 \log \frac{\text{cation}_i}{\text{cation}_o}$$

$$E = -58 \log \frac{\text{anion}_o}{\text{anion}_i}$$

Sodium and Potassium Equilibrium Potentials

As we have just seen, the equilibrium potential necessary to just balance a given chemical gradient can be theoretically predicted by the Nernst equation. The values for the mammalian nerve cell and the squid axon are listed below.

Large mammalian nerve cell

$E_{Na^+} = 68$ mV
$E_{K^+} = -88$ mV

Giant axon of the squid

$E_{Na^+} = 56$ mV
$E_{K^+} = -76$ mV

Remember that the RMP of the large mammalian nerve cell is -85 mV, while it is about -65 mV in the giant axon of the squid. Since the equilibrium potentials for K^+ and Na^+ listed above are not the same as the resting membrane potentials, it follows that neither K^+ nor Na^+ is really at electrochemical equilibrium in the large mammalian nerve cell nor in the giant axon of the squid. Any time that an ion is not in electrochemical equilibrium, net diffusion of that ion will occur and the chemical gradient will change unless some other factor such as membrane active transport acts to restore the gradient. Of course, in the nerve cells described here, the Na^+/K^+ pump does just that, and their respective chemical gradients are maintained.

Electrochemical Equilibrium and the Resting Membrane Potential

Neither Na^+ nor K^+ is in electrochemical equilibrium across the resting membrane of the mammalian neuron and the giant axon of the squid (Fig. 2-11).

For Na^+, notice that both the chemical and electrical gradients are directed inward. In order to be in equilbrium, the inside would need to be about $+68$ mV in the mammalian neuron, and about $+56$ mV in the squid. And we know by in-

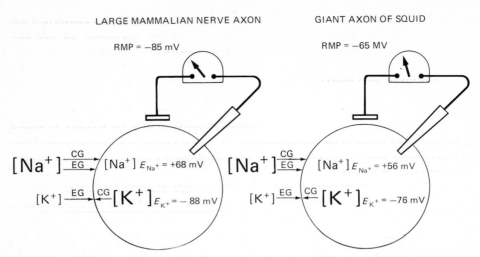

Figure 2-11   Both the chemical and electrical gradients for Na+ ions are directed inward and consequently these ions are not in electrochemical equilibrium. In order to be in equilibrium, the inside would need to be about 68 mV positive in the mammalian neuron and about 56 mV positive in the squid. In the case of K+ ions, the electrical gradient is directed inward while the chemical gradient is directed outward. The equilibrium potential for K+ ions in each species is slightly more negative than their experimentally measured resting membrane potentials. Therefore, K+ is almost, but not quite, at electrochemical equilibrium across the cell membrane. EG, electrical gradient; CG, chemical gradient; RMP, resting membrane potential; E_{Na^+}, sodium equilibrium potential; E_{K^+}, potassium equilibrium potential.

tracellular microelectrode recording that both interiors are actually negative in the resting membrane.

In the case of K+ ions, the electrical gradient is directed inward while the chemical gradient is directed outward because of relatively high intracellular K+ concentration. The inside would need to be about -88 mV in the mammalian neuron and about -76 mV in the squid in order for K+ to be in electrochemical equilibrium. Notice that the experimentally measured RMP is very close to these values in each case. That is, $E_{K^+} = -88$ mV compared to an RMP of -85 mV in the large mammalian nerve axon, and $E_{K^+} = -76$ mV compared to an RMP of -65 mV in the giant axon of the squid. It is apparent that K+ is almost in electrochemical equilibrium across the resting membrane of both cells. Nevertheless, the respective potassium equilibrium potentials are slightly more negative than their resting membrane potentials. Consequently, there is a continual tendecy for K+ ions to diffuse outward.

The Ionic Imbalance of Sodium and Potassium

You might be wondering at this point how the Na+/K+ "pump" fits into the picture. In our previous discussion we noted that both the electrical and chemical gradients for sodium are directed inward. In addition, while the membrane is not easily penetrated by Na+, some ions will nevertheless cross. Why then doesn't Na^+ simply diffuse down its two gradients and reach equilibrium on each side of the membrane? The answer lies in the capability of the cell membrane to actively transport (pump) Na^+ outward, against these two gradients.

Not all of this actively transported Na^+ stays outside, however, since a small amount leaks back inward because of the slight permeability of the membrane to this ion. One can readily appreciate, however, that the outward Na^+ transport and the inward Na^+ diffusion must match each other in effectiveness since there is no net change in the extracellular and intracellular concentrations of this ion during the time that the membrane is in the resting state.

As far as K^+ is concerned, remember that the chemical gradient is outward while the electrical gradient is inward. This inward electrical gradient coupled with the fact that the membrane actively transports K^+ to the inside accounts for the high intracellular K^+ concentration found in both cell types. Once again, not all of the actively transported K^+ which is pumped inward stays inside. Because of the outward-directed chemical gradient and the limited permeability of the membrane to this ion, some K^+ diffuses outward.

The membrane of the resting mammalian nerve axon is typically 100 times more permeable to K^+ than to Na^+, while in the squid axon a 25:1 ratio is observed. Nevertheless, the inward pumping and outward diffusion of K^+ must once again match each other since there is no net change in the inside and outside concentrations of this ion during the time the membrane is in the resting state.

The Goldman-Hodgkin-Katz Equation

You should keep in mind that in the resting membrane, none of the cations and anions in the solutions on either side of the membrane are at electrochemical equilibrium. Consequently, they are diffusing across the membrane with different diffusion rates and in different directions at all times in the resting membrane. Remember, the only time an ion won't diffuse is when (1) it is at electrochemical equilibrium or (2) the membrane is not permeable to it at all. Consequently a variety of charge separations are occurring simultaneously across the membrane, with each contributing to a greater or lesser extent to the experimentally measured resting membrane potential.

Hodgkin and Katz, using a formula developed earlier by Goldman, attempted to theoretically predict the resting membrane potential by considering the combined effects of all these ions including (1) the ionic charge, (2) the direction of the chemical gradient, and (3) the relative permeability of the membrane to each.

$$V_M = -58 \log \frac{[Na^+]_i P_{Na^+} + [K^+]_i P_{K^+} + [Cl^-]_o P_{Cl^-}}{[Na^+]_o P_{NA^+} + [K^+]_o P_{K^+} + [C^-]_i P_{Cl^-}}$$

where V_M = membrane potential, mV

P_{ion} = membrane permeability for a given ion

You should understand that the accuracy of this equation in predicting actual resting membrane potentials is dependent on the permeability factors for each ion which are only close approximations of their true values. Nevertheless, the predicted values are usually quite close to the measured RMPs.

Careful examination of this equation will show several things. First notice that the Goldman-Hodgkin-Katz equation is an extension of the Nernst equation. Since it considers the collective contributions of Na^+, K^+, and Cl^- chemical gradients as well as the relative permeability of the membrane to each, the integrated equilibrium potential which the equation predicts is at least theoretically a close approximation of the RMP itself. The theoretical prediction which this equation makes for the RMP of the large mammalian nerve cell at body temperature and the giant axon of the squid at room temperature is given below.

Large mammalian nerve cell

$$V_M = -61 \log \frac{10(0.01) + 140(l) + 120(2)}{130(0.01) + 5(1) + 4(2)}$$
$$= -87 \text{ mV}$$

Giant axon of the squid

$$V_M = -58 \log \frac{50(0.04) + 400(1) + 540(0.45)}{460(0.04) + 20(1) + 50(0.45)}$$
$$= -59 \text{ mV}$$

THE ACTION POTENTIAL AND THE IMPULSE

Earlier we noted that when a single area of axonal membrane is stimulated it becomes excited and undergoes a rapid and reversible electrical change called an *action potential*. And recall further that this action potential propagates as a continuous impulse down the entire length of the axon. Let's now examine the changes which occur in the neuron during the action potential.

The action potential results from a sudden change in the resting membrane potential (a condition necessary for impulse conduction). To illustrate this point, it is usually convenient in experimental laboratory conditions to stimulate the neuron at some point on its axon. You should recognize that this is not a normal situation. Neurons are rarely stimulated on their axons in vivo. Instead they are stimulated to produce action potentials in vivo via (1) generator potentials from sensory receptors, (2) neurotransmitters from presynaptic terminals at synapses, and (3) local currents. Nevertheless, an action potential is still an action potential no matter where or how it is produced and the axon is generally much more accessible in experimental situations than is the rest of the neuron.

By this time you should be aware that the resting membrane is a *polarized membrane*. That is, unlike charges are separated at the membrane with the inside negative and the outside positive. When the membrane is stimulated by an electronic stimulator in the laboratory, its resting membrane potential begins to decrease. That is, it becomes less negative and hence less polarized. If it is depolarized to a critical level known as the *excitation threshold,* an action potential will be produced at the point of stimulation. Once the membrane potential is depolarized to the excitation threshold, its Na$^+$ channels (routes through which Na$^+$ ions cross the membrane) suddenly open and a tremendous increase in Na$^+$ conductance g_{Na+} occurs with Na$^+$ ions now free to diffuse down both their chemical and electrical gradients. This is called *sodium activation.* You should note that conductance g is the electrical analog of permeability P. Thus it is also appropriate to say that there is a sudden and marked increase in sodium permeability on the part of the membrane when the excitation threshold is reached.

As the positively charged Na$^+$ ions suddenly diffuse inward the RMP is greatly disturbed at the local site of stimulation. Sufficient positively charged Na$^+$ is removed from the immediate membrane exterior surface and transferred to the immediate membrane interior surface to totally eliminate the internal negativity and replace it with positivity. Measurement now would record a reversed potential showing the interior now positive with respect to the exterior. We will see later that only a few picomoles of Na$^+$ actually need to diffuse inward to change the membrane potential by 125 mV, that is, from a RMP of -85 mV to a reversed potential of $+40$ mV in the large mammalian neuron or a RMP of -65 mV to a reversed potential of $+55$ mV in the giant axon of the squid.

This local reversed potential is not allowed to last. Even before the intracellular fluid reaches its maximum positivity, the local membrane channels for K$^+$ open, causing a great increase in membrane permeability to K$^+$ with a resulting increase in g_{K+} and carrying positive charges to the outside down their chemical and electrical gradients. At the same time there is a marked reduction in g_{Na+}. This coupled with the substantial increase in K$^+$ outflow is sufficient not only to eliminate the internal positivity caused by the Na$^+$ inflow, but also to actually restore the original resting membrane potential.

It is important to understand that the depolarization caused by the Na$^+$ inflow and the repolarization caused by the K$^+$ outflow occur locally. That is, they occur only on that section of axon which is initially stimulated. The entire action potential, including depolarization to the reversed potential and repolarization back to the resting membrane potential, happens very quickly, requiring no more than a few milliseconds.

The Action Potential Involves a Very Small Transfer of Ions

The capacitance of a typical nerve cell membrane has been estimated to be 1 μF/cm^2. Therefore the number of charges which need to be transferred across the membrane capacitor to change its potential by 125 mV is given by

$$Q = CV$$
$$= (10^{-6} \text{ F/cm}^2) (1.25 \times 10^{-1} \text{ V}) .$$
$$= 1.25 \times 10^{-7} \text{ C/cm}^2$$

Now the number of sodium ions which need to diffuse inward in order to transfer 1.25×10^{-7}C of charge from the extracellular fluid, through one square centimeter of membrane, to inside can be calculated from the Faraday constant.

$$\begin{array}{l} \text{Number of moles} \\ \text{transferred per} \\ \text{square centimeter} \end{array} = \begin{array}{l} \text{membrane charges transferred} \\ \text{per square centimeter} \end{array} \times \frac{1}{\text{Faraday constant}}$$

$$= (1.25 \times 10^{-7}\text{C/cm}^2)\ (1 \times 10^{-5}\ \text{mol/C})$$
$$= 1.25 \times 10^{-12}\ \text{mol/cm}^2$$
$$= 1.25\ \text{pmol/cm}^2$$

These few picomoles which diffuse inward during the depolarization of the membrane to the reversed potential stage are so insignificantly few in a large-diameter nerve fiber that they cause virtually no change in the measurable extracellular or intracellular sodium concentrations. Similarly, the outward diffusion of 1.25 pmol of K^+ per square centimeter is sufficient to repolarize the membrane back to the resting level, and yet this loss of intracellular K^+ is so insignificant as to leave virtually unchanged the extracellular and intracellular K^+ concentrations. Of course, the smaller the fiber the greater will be the change in the intracellular concentrations of these ions. But still the change would be insignificantly slight. In any event, the nerve cells are constantly being *recharged* by active transport outward of the few picomoles of Na^+ which diffuse inside during depolarization, and by actively transporting inward the few picomoles of K^+ which diffuse outward during depolarization. Recharging enables neurons to conduct virtually unlimited numbers of impulses without producing changes in the ionic concentrations which are vital for maintaining their excitability.

As a theoretical exercise you can calculate the small percentage of internal K^+ which needs to diffuse outward in order to repolarize the membrane by considering the axon to be a cylinder of uniform diameter. For example, consider a large mammalian nerve axon with a diameter of 20 μm (2×10^{-3} cm) and an intracellular concentration of K^+ equal to 140 mmol/L.

$$\begin{array}{l} \text{Percent of intracellular } K^+ \\ \text{diffusing out} \end{array} = \frac{\begin{array}{c}\text{number of moles of } K^+ \text{ diffusing} \\ \text{out through a given length of axon} \end{array}}{\begin{array}{c}\text{number of moles of } K^+ \text{ in axoplasm} \\ \text{for a given length of axon}\end{array}} \times 100$$

$$= \frac{[(\text{moles diffusing out})/(\text{cm}^2 \text{ of membrane})](\text{cm}^2 \text{ of membrane})}{(\text{mol/cm}^3 \text{ of axoplasm})(\text{cm}^3 \text{ of axoplasm})} \times 100$$

$$= \frac{(1.25 \times 10^{-12}\ \text{mol/cm}^2)\ [2\pi(1 \times 10^{-3}\ \text{cm})](\text{cm})}{(1.4 \times 10^{-4}\ \text{mol/cm}^3)\ [\pi(1 \times 10^{-3}\ \text{cm})^2](\text{cm})} \times 100$$

$$= \frac{7.9 \times 10^{-15}\ \text{mol}}{4.4 \times 10^{-10}\ \text{mol}} \times 100$$

$$= 1.8 \times 10^{-3}\ \text{percent}$$

During the remainder of our discussion on the events associated with the action potential we will examine exclusively the work done with the giant axon of the squid. You really lose nothing by abandoning for the moment the mammalian axon in favor of concentrating on the squid axon. In fact, quite to the contrary, you get a real feel for the work of Hodgkin and Huxley in developing the principles we accept so easily today.

Sodium and Potassium Conductance

Using a technique called the *voltage clamp*, Hodgkin and Huxley calculated the time course of sodium and potassium conductance, g_{Na+} and g_{K+}, as well as sodium and potassium current, I_{Na+} and I_{K+}, during an action potential. We will examine this technique later, but for the moment consider the calculated relationships with time during the action potential illustrated in Fig. 2-12.

The action potential pictured here underwent a sudden but reversible change in its membrane potential. Notice that the initial value of the RMP and the final value of the reversed potential are not indicated. Instead all we see is the magnitude of depolarization from the former to the latter. Notice that when the membrane potential has depolarized by about 10 mV (presumably to the excitation threshold) there is a sudden and large increase in g_{Na+} to about 30 mS/cm². This is responsible for the large and sudden change in the membrane potential. Notice further that this large increase in g_{Na+} is transient and the conductivity returns within a few milliseconds to practically zero. Meanwhile a slower increase in the g_{K+} to about 12 mS/cm², which started even before the membrane potential reached its maximum reversed potential, promotes the repolarization of the membrane. Consequently the membrane potential changes once again back to the resting level. In fact the membrane often

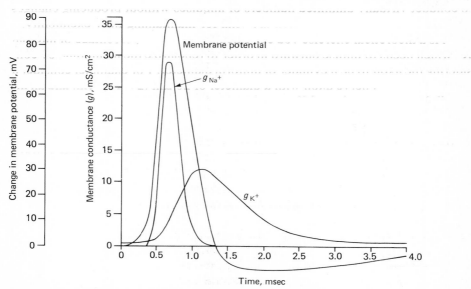

Figure 2-12 Illustration showing the changes in sodium conductance g_{Na+} and potassium conductance g_{K+} with time during a mathematically derived action potential. (*Drawn from Hodgkin and Huxley, 1952.*)

hyperpolarizes beyond the resting level by a few millivolts before gradually returning to the resting level after several milliseconds. This slow return to the resting level is called the *afterpotential*. The rapid rise and fall in membrane potential is called the *spike* or *spike potential*. However, the action potential includes both the spike potential and the afterpotential.

The Impulse

During the reversed potential the axoplasm immediately inside the stimulated area of membrane is temporarily made positive while the adjacent axoplasm is still negative. Similarly the extracellular fluid immediately outside the stimulated area is temporarily negative while the adjacent extracellular fluid is still positive. Thus charge gradients exist side by side and a small current begins to flow in a circuit through the membrane. The direction of this current is inward through the depolarized areas, laterally through the adjacent axoplasm, outward through the adjacent still-polarized membrane segment immediately adjacent to the depolarized area, laterally backward through the extracellular fluid, and inward once again through the depolarized area. The path of this local current is illustrated in Fig. 2-13.

As the local current flows outward through the adjacent still-polarized membrane, the membrane at this point begins to depolarize. Once it has depolarized to the excitation threshold, the sodium channels suddenly open and the resultant increase in g_{Na+} causes the now-familiar action potential to occur at that point on the membrane. Subsequently, as this new action potential develops, a new local current will flow from it to the next adjacent membrane segment, depolarizing it and propagating a continuous impulse down the axon.

Of course if the axon is stimulated at some point along its length the local current will spread in both directions away from the stimulus site and an impulse will travel in both directions. You should always keep in mind that this condition (impulse spread in both directions) occurs only in the laboratory preparations when neurons are stimulated along their axons. As we pointed out earlier, neurons are rarely stimulated on their axons in vivo. Instead they are stimulated in dendritic zones to produce action potentials via generator poten-

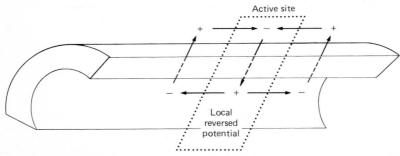

Figure 2-13 Path of the local current when the neuron is stimulated at some point (active site) along its axon.

tials from sensory receptors and neurotransmitters from presynaptic terminals at synapses. In axons, local currents traveling ahead of propagated action potentials are responsible. In all these naturally occurring stimulus situations, the local currents and hence the propagated action potentials travel in only one direction. This direction is toward the terminal branches of the axon.

Approximately 0.5 ms after the local area of membrane depolarizes, it starts to repolarize as a result of the progressive increase in g_{K+}. Thus the impulse which travels down an axon is followed about 0.5 ms later by a wave of repolarization as each succeeding membrane segment begins to repolarize.

Propagation of Action Potentials in Myelinated Neurons

Myelinated neurons propagate action potentials with the same kinds of ion movements as the nonmyelinated neurons just described. The fundamental difference is that the local current flows through the membrane only at the nodes of Ranvier. These nodes are the interruptions in the sheath which surrounds the axons of all myelinated neurons. Current flows through the membrane only at these nodes because they represent areas of relatively low electrical resistance, while the myelinated internodes offer relatively high resistance to current flow. Consequently, when a myelinated neuron is stimulated and an action potential is generated, the local current which flows through the adjacent axoplasm will pass out through the first node rather than through the next adjacent area of membrane. A comparison of the nature of local current flow in myelinated and nonmyelinated axons is illustrated in Fig. 2-14.

Nonmyelinated axon
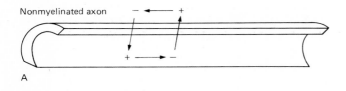
A

Myelinated axon
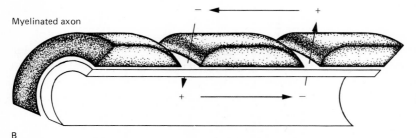
B

Figure 2-14 *A.* Nonmyelinated axon: local current spreads only short distance; slow conductance velocity. *B.* Myelinated axon: local current spreads large distance; high conduction velocity. In the nonmyelinated axon, the local current must depolarize each adjacent area of membrane, a relatively time-consuming process which imposes necessary restrictions on the conduction velocity. In the myelinated axon, only the nodes of Ranvier need to depolarize, allowing impulses to travel at greatly increased velocity.

In a nonmyelinated neuron the local current must depolarize each adjacent area of membrane—a relatively time-consuming process. Since the impulse proceeds only as rapidly as the spread of the local current, this need to depolarize each adjacent area of membrane imposes necessary restrictions on the conduction velocity. Myelinated neurons, on the other hand, have an advantage which enables them to conduct impulses with a much higher velocity. Since the local current does not need to depolarize each adjacent area of the membrane, impulses travel along the axon at a greatly accelerated velocity. This is called *saltatory conduction*.

Fiber Diameter and Conduction Velocity

Conduction velocity is roughly proportional to fiber diameter. The greater the diameter of the axon, the greater the conduction velocity. This is true because the larger the diameter, the greater the cross-sectional area of the axoplasm and hence the lower its electrical resistance. Thus a large local current will spread further along the axoplasm before flowing outward through the membrane to complete the circuit. Consequently a greater length of axonal membrane will be depolarized faster, and action potentials will be propagated at a greater velocity. If we think of a length of axon as having a uniform cross-sectional area, the internal axoplasmic resistance to current flow can be calculated using the same assumptions underlying resistance in a length of wire.

$$R_i = \frac{r_i}{\pi(\text{radius})^2}$$

where R_i = axoplasmic resistance per unit length of axon, Ω/cm
  r_i = axoplasmic resistivity, $\Omega \cdot \text{cm}$
 radius = radius of axon, cm

THE LOCAL CURRENT: A CLOSER EXAMINATION

An important point to consider is that one action potential cannot propagate a second without the contribution of the local current. Thus it is clear that the local current plays a crucial role in the impulse conduction process. Accordingly let's now give it its due by a closer examination.

Current flow in the axon has been likened to current flow in a large undersea cable. Both are composed of a long conducting core (the axoplasm in the neuron) surrounded by an insulator (the neuronal membrane) and immersed in a large-volume conductor (the neuronal extracellular fluid). The axon, however, behaves as a leaky cable in that current not only flows through the axoplasm but leaks out through the membrane as well. Since the same electrical rules apply to current flow in the cable and in the axon, neurophysiologists often speak of the *cable properties* of the axon.

The current which spreads with the impulse is an active current. The local current which we have been discussing is, by contrast, a passive current, and its

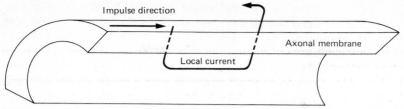

Figure 2-15 The local current travels a short distance in front of the impulse, depolarizing the membrane and producing an action potential. One can visualize the impulse traveling down the axonal membrane with the depolarizing local current moving just ahead of it.

spread depends only on electrical parameters of the conducting material such as the resistance and capacitance of a unit length of axon. These passive or cable properties of the axon determine the extent and magnitude of the local current.

The local current spreads only a very short distance through the axoplasm before flowing out through the membrane, partially depolarizing it, and producing an *electrotonic potential* (Fig. 2-19). Electrotonic potentials can be observed only when the degree of stimulation is subthreshold because once the excitation threshold is reached the small electrotonic potential is obliterated by the large potential changes associated with the much larger action potential.

The electrotonic potential is the difference between the subthreshold membrane potential at any given time and the resting membrane potential. As action potentials are propagated down the axon, local currents can be visualized as preceding them, depolarizing each newly encountered resting membrane segment and establishing electrotonic potentials which reach threshold and produce additional action potentials (Fig. 2-15).

Electrical Properties of the Membrane and Surrounding Fluids

It is often helpful to picture the membrane and surrounding fluids as an electrical circuit in order to understand the local current flow and the electrotonic potential which it produces. Students and researchers alike are indebted to the work of Hodgkin for our electrical models of the axon. He pictured the membrane as composed of an infinite number of electrotonic "patches" with

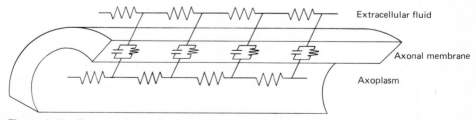

Figure 2-16 The membrane is pictured here as being composed of an infinite number of electronic "patches" with each patch composed of a resistance and capacitance in parallel, surrounded by intracellular and extracellular fluids, both offering series resistance to the flow of the local current.

each patch composed of a resistance and capacitance in parallel surrounded by intracellular and extracellular fluids, both offering series resistance to the flow of the local current (Fig. 2-16).

Ionic and Capacitive Current

Electrically, the membrane can be thought of as a resistance and capacitance in parallel. The membrane resistance R_M represents the difficulty encountered by ions in diffusing through their respective membrane channels, while the membrane capacitance C_M represents the charge which exists across the membrane at any time. Now remember that current flow in biological systems consists of moving charges carried by ions. Therefore both capacitive and ionic currents represent the flow of ionic charge. *Ionic current I_I* is the charge carried by ions as they flow through their respective ionic channels in the membrane. The difficulty they encounter in passing through these channels from one side of the membrane to the other is represented by the membrane resistance R_M. *Capacitive current I_C*, on the other hand, does not represent the actual flow of ions through the membrane. Its explanation is a little more subtle. If positive ions flow through the axoplasm to the inside of the membrane they will neutralize some of the negative ions already there. This will free some of the positive ions from the immediate membrane exterior to flow away since they are no longer held to the membrane capacitor. Thus positive ions have moved up to and away from the membrane. Thus current has, in effect, traveled outward through the membrane even though no actual ions have crossed from one side to the other. Remember that capacitive current I_C flows only while a capacitor is being charged or discharged. Ionic and capacitive currents are illustrated in Fig. 2-17.

The Nature of the Local Current

As we have said before, when the local membrane site undergoes an action potential, a local current flows which establishes an electrotonic potential on the

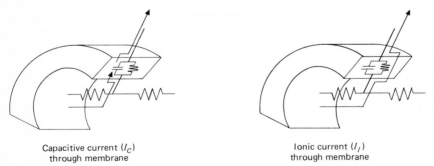

Capacitive current (I_C)
through membrane

Ionic current (I_I)
through membrane

Figure 2-17   A schematic illustration showing the difference between capacitive current I_C and ionic current I_I. Ionic current represents the charge carried by ions as they move through the membrane "channels." Capacitive current represents the removal of charge from one side of the membrane (outside in the above illustration) and the addition of like charge to the opposite side of the membrane (inside, in this case).

next adjacent area of membrane. When this electrotonic potential reaches the excitation threshold, g_{Na+} will suddenly increase and a second action potential will be generated, obliterating the electrotonic potential and the local current. Unfortunately for experimenters, action potentials propagate so quickly that there is not sufficient time to study the local current itself. However, if the membrane is stimulated to a subthreshold level and held there, the nature and time course of the local current can be studied.

A convenient way to do this is to penetrate an axon with a depolarizing microelectrode. In this way a steady but subthreshold level of depolarizing (positive) current can be released internally. By keeping the level of stimulation steady and subthreshold, and by recording the potential changes of the membrane at various distances from the stimulating site, one can examine the magnitude, distance, and time course of the local current spread. Consider the membrane circuit pictured in Fig. 2-18. A depolarizing microelectrode has been placed into the axoplasm at patch A while recording microelectrodes have been inserted at patches B, C, and D. Assume that a steady subthreshold depolarizing current is applied at patch A. A local current will now flow from the less negative region near the tip of the depolarizing microelectrode to the still polarized (more negative) regions of axoplasm at patches B, C, and D before flowing out through the membrane to complete the circuit.

From previous discussions we know that current flow through the membrane is both capacitive and ionic. Both kinds flow in the above circuit. When current is first applied to the axoplasm at patch A, most of it initially goes

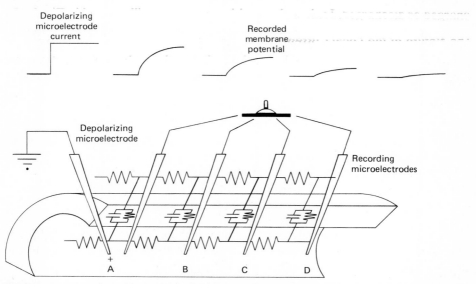

Figure 2-18 A steady subthreshold depolarizing current is applied at patch A. A local current spreads from the less negative region near the tip of the depolarizing microelectrode to the still polarized (more negative) regions of axoplasm at patches B, C, and D before passing out through the membrane, completing the circuit.

toward discharging the C_M at patch A. Hence I_C flows outward through the membrane at patch A. Initially no I_I flows outward through patch A because there is no net driving force across the membrane. But as the transmembrane potential is altered from its resting level (RMP) and an electrotonic potential is developed, a net driving force is built up across the membrane. Once the membrane capacitor at patch A has been charged up to the level of the steady depolarizing current at patch A, I_C stops and subsequent current flow outward through the membrane at patch A is purely ionic (I_I). Not all current from the depolarizing microelectrode becomes outward I_C and I_I at patch A. Some, progressively less, continues to flow through the internal axoplasmic resistance R_i to first become capacitive and then ionic current through membrane patches B, C, and D.

Because voltage drops (decreases) as current flows through increasingly distant lengths of axoplasmic resistance, the membrane capacitors at patches B, C, and D are progressively less completely discharged and exhibit smaller and smaller electrotonic potentials. This is illustrated by the progressively decreased voltage changes recorded by electrodes at patches B, C, and D. Remember that current follows the path of least resistance; therefore, most of the current flows out through the membrane at patch A with progressively less reaching and subsequently traversing more distant points on the membrane. At sufficiently great distances, beyond the reach of the local current, no electrotonic potential is established and the resting membrane potential remains undisturbed.

Axon Geometry and the Local Current

The electrotonic potential decreases exponentially with distance from the active (stimulated) site according to a value which is known as the *length constant* λ.

$$\lambda = \left(\frac{R_M}{R_i + R_e}\right)^{1/2}$$

where λ = length constant [the distance over which the electrotonic potential
    decreases to $1/e$ (37 percent) of its maximum value], cm
  R_M = membrane resistance per unit length of axon, $\Omega \cdot$cm
  R_i = axoplasmic resistance per unit length of axon, Ω/cm
  R_e = extracellular fluid resistance per unit length of axon, Ω/cm

Because of the relatively large volume of the extracellular fluid, its resistance to current flow is very small and can effectively be removed from the above equation, leaving the simple relationship below.

$$\lambda = \left(\frac{R_M}{R_i}\right)^{1/2}$$

Now don't lose sight of the fact that the length constant is a measure of how far the local current spreads along the axon in front of the action potential. Remember that action potentials give rise to local currents in vivo, while in the experimental situation just described, the depolarizing microelectrode gave rise to the local current. In any case, the longer the length constant the farther the local current will spread through the axon, producing progressively smaller electrotonic potentials before it dies out.

Let's now examine those factors which determine the values of R_M and R_i since these determine the value of the length constant. If we think of a length of axon as having a uniform cross-sectional area, we can calculate R_i as follows:

$$R_i = \frac{r_i}{\pi(\text{radius})^2}$$

where R_i = axoplasmic resistance per unit length of axon, Ω/cm
$\qquad r_i$ = axoplasmic resistivity, $\Omega \cdot \text{cm}$
$\quad$ radius = radius of axon, cm

The transverse resistance through the membrane for a given length of axon is

$$R_M = \frac{r_M}{2\pi(\text{radius})}$$

where R_M = membrane resistance per unit length of axon, $\Omega \cdot \text{cm}$
$\qquad r_M$ = specific membrane resistance, $\Omega \cdot \text{cm}^2$

Notice that increasing the radius of the axon decreases both the R_i and R_M, but there is a greater proportional decrease in R_i. Consequently the length constant increases with axon diameter. Now don't lose sight of the fact that a long length constant means that larger segments of adjacent membrane will be depolarized faster. Thus as we have already pointed out, the larger the axon diameter, the greater the impulse conduction velocity. Most of the aspects of the local current are illustrated in Fig. 2-19.

THE VOLTAGE CLAMP EXPERIMENTS OF HODGKIN AND HUXLEY

You should be thoroughly familiar now with the relationship between the local current and the action potential. You should also be aware that when the action potential is initiated, several membrane variables change rapidly as a function of time. These are potential, conductance, and current. Now remember that the Ohm's law relationship between them is expressed by

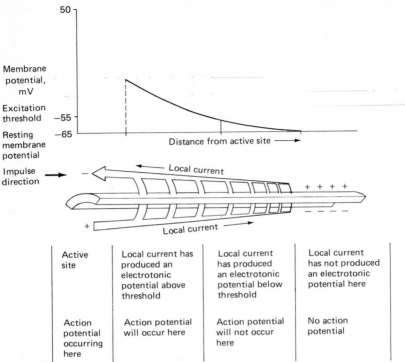

Figure 2-19   Several aspects of the local current as it spreads along the axon in front of the impulse.

$$g = \frac{I}{V}$$

where g = conductance, S
$\quad\;\;$ I = current, A
$\quad\;\;$ V = potential, V

Examination of this relationship shows that g varies as a function of I and V. Hodgkin and Huxley set out to determine the changes in membrane conductance g_M during the action potential. Their problem was that both the membrane current I_M and the membrane potential V_M are also changing constantly during the action potential. Now if one of these variables could be held constant during the action potential (i.e., V_M), measurement of I_M would enable them to calculate g_M at any instant. This is what the *voltage clamp technique* enabled them to do. A voltage clamp setup is diagrammatically illustrated in Fig. 2-20.

The system operates like this. The experimenter decides on a voltage he would like to produce across the membrane and then sets this "command volt-

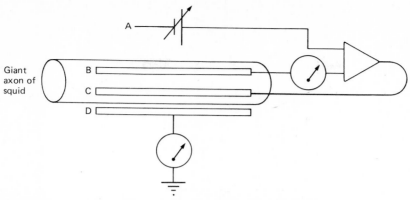

Figure 2-20 Diagrammatic illustration of a simple voltage clamp setup. *A.* Variable command voltage. *B.* Intracellular voltage-recording microelectrode. *C.* Intracellular current-passing microelectrode. *D.* Extracellular current-recording electrode.

age" on an external voltage source at A (V_A). The voltage recording microelectrode at B detects whatever voltage presently exists across the membrane (V_B) and sends this signal into the differential amplifier. The signal from the command voltage source is also transferred into the differential amplifier. Now a differential amplifier produces no output if the voltages on its two inputs are equal ($V_A = V_B$). But if they are not equal ($V_A \neq V_B$), the amplifier will send whatever current is necessary into the intracellular current-passing electrode at C in order to change the membrane voltage recorded by the recording microelectrode at B until it equals the command voltage. As soon as V_A equals V_B, the amplifier stops its output.

The differential amplifier effectively alters the voltage across the membrane by sending a current through the membrane from the current-passing electrode to the current-recording electrode at D. Remember that in the course of crossing a membrane, current discharges the membrane capacitor and hence the membrane voltage. This altered voltage is sent to the differential amplifier for comparison with the command voltage. Consequently the experimenter can "dial" any desired voltage across the membrane, and even more importantly, hold the membrane potential at that level.

Now let's examine an experimental situation. Suppose that the RMP of a giant squid axon is −65 mV and the experimenter wishes to "clamp" the voltage at −9 mV. The command voltage is first set at −9 mV. Within microseconds of applying the command voltage, the differential amplifier will pass sufficient current through the membrane to lower the RMP by 56 mV to the set level of −9 mV. Since the membrane potential has now greatly exceeded the excitation threshold, the Na$^+$ channels open, but because of the voltage clamp no actual change in membrane potential is observed. Nevertheless, Na$^+$ ions diffuse inward down their chemical gradient. As they do so, the differential

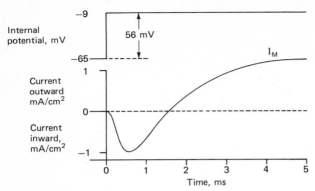

Figure 2-21 A plot of the data obtained by voltage clamping the membrane of the squid giant axon at −9 mV. This is a depolarization of 56 mV from the resting level of −65 mV. Notice that the membrane current I_M is first directed inward (presumably carried by Na+ ions) and then outward (presumably carried by K+ ions). (*Drawn from Hodgkin, 1958.*)

amplifier varies its current output proportionally to prevent the Na+ inflow from altering the condition which the amplifier is designed to preserve ($V_A = V_B$). Slightly later the K+ channels open and the differential amplifier once again varies its current output proportionally to prevent the K+ outflow from altering the clamped condition ($V_A = V_B$).

Remember that it only takes a few microseconds for the voltage clamp to fix the membrane potential at −9 mV once the command voltage is first applied. Therefore, any subsequent current changes detected by the current-detecting electrode (D) are in response to, and in the opposite direction from, any ionic currents crossing the membrane with Na+ inflow and K+ outflow.

The results obtained by Hodgkin and Huxley when they depolarized the membrane of the squid giant axon by 56 mV are pictured in Fig. 2-21. Notice that the membrane current I_M is first inward (presumably carried by Na+) and then outward (presumably carried by K+).

Sodium and Potassium Currents

When the squid giant axon is bathed by seawater, a solution similar to its extracellular fluid, and then stimulated to its excitation threshold, the I_M is first directed inward and then outward (Fig. 2-22). The contribution of Na+ to the I_M could conceivably be eliminated if the extracellular Na+ were reduced to the level of the axoplasm, as this would eliminate the chemical gradient which powers the inflow. Hodgkin and Huxley did this and obtained the results in Fig. 2-22. Notice that following the reduction of the extracellular Na+ to axoplasmic levels, the current flow following stimulation only has an outward component. This current is presumably due almost exclusively to K+ outflow and represents the potassium current I_{K+}. Accordingly, the sodium current I_{Na+} is calculated by subtracting the I_{K+} from the I_M. Presumably $I_M = I_{K+} - I_{Na+}$.

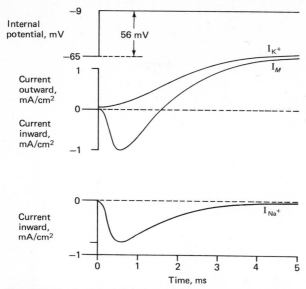

Figure 2-22 A plot of the data obtained by bathing the squid giant axon in a solution containing the same Na+ ion concentration as the axoplasm and voltage clamping the membrane at −9 mV. The resulting membrane current has an outward component only, and is due to K+ outflow. The contribution of sodium current to the normal membrane current can then be calculated by subtracting the potassium current from the membrane current. (*Drawn from Hodgkin, 1958.*)

Once they had recorded individual ionic currents against a fixed voltage, it was a simple matter using Ohm's law to mathematically calculate individual ionic conductances and then plot them as a function of time. They developed the following equations to do this and then plotted the results in Fig. 2-23.

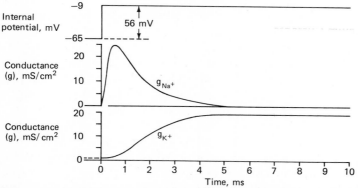

Figure 2-23 A time course of the changes in sodium and potassium conductance when the membrane of the squid giant axon is voltage clamped at −9 mV. (*Drawn from Hodgkin, 1958.*)

$$g_{ion} = \frac{I_{ion}}{V_M - E_{ion}}$$

$$g_{K+} = \frac{I_{K+}}{V_M - E_{K+}}$$

$$g_{Na+} = \frac{I_{Na+}}{V_M - E_{Na+}}$$

where g_{ion} = ionic conduction, $\mu mS/cm^2$
$\qquad I_{ion}$ = ionic current, mA/cm^2
$\qquad V_M$ = membrane potential, mV
$\qquad E_{ion}$ = ionic equilibrium potential, mV

Electrical Components of the Action Potential

We have learned by now that one action potential propagates a second by means of the local current. Further, we know that the local current depolarizes the adjacent membrane to the excitation threshold at which point rapid but reversible changes occur in g_{Na+}, I_{Na+}, and I_{K+}, resulting in the familiar action potential. Figure 2-24 illustrates the time course of all these events occurring at a single finite location as they were calculated by Hodgkin and Huxley for the data they collected with the voltage clamp experiments.

Now let's examine the various electrical changes which occur in one single axon location as the impulse arrives at this location, passes over it, and then proceeds down the length of the axon. Using Fig. 2-24 we will summarize the changes during eight instantaneous time segments beginning with the resting membrane before the arrival of the impulse.

A   The membrane is in the resting state since the approaching impulse has not yet reached this point on the axon. g_{K+} is greater than g_{Na+} and I_M is small.

B   The approaching impulse is closing in on the local axon section and the local current traveling in front of it is starting to depolarize the membrane and causing an initial outward I_C. g_{K+} is still greater than g_{Na+}. The I_C accounts for all of the I_M at this time.

C   The outward I_C caused by the local current has depolarized the membrane by about $10\,mV$ to the excitation threshold. Na^+ channels are opening so that inward Na^+ and outward K^+ diffusion is equal. Thus I_{Na+} and I_{K+} are temporarily equal and opposite. This is an unstable condition and the membrane is at threshold.

D   The g_{Na+} is now considerably greater than g_{K+} and the inward I_{Na+} now exceeds the outward I_{K+} and is responsible for the overall inward direction of the I_I. The I_I is discharging the membrane capacitor as it flows inward depolarizing the membrane.

E   The membrane is at the peak of its depolarization, having established its maximum reversed potential. The g_{Na+} and I_{Na+} have begun to decrease

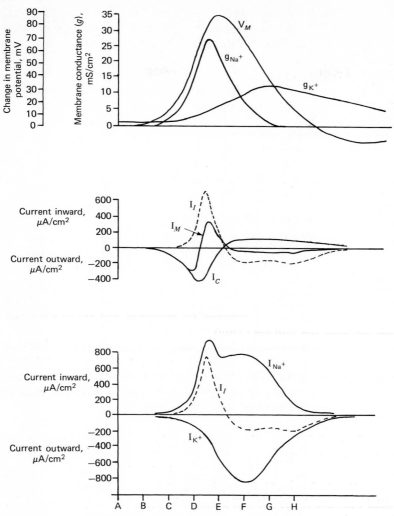

Figure 2-24 A calculated time course of the components of membrane current during a propagated action potential. (*Drawn from Hodgkin and Huxley, 1952.*)

while the g_{K+} and I_{K+} have begun to increase. The I_{Na+} and I_{K+} are equal and opposite.

F   The g_{Na+} has decreased to where it equals the increasing g_{K+}. But now the outward I_{K+} exceeds the inward I_{Na+} and thus the I_I is directed outward. This is countered by an opposite but less than equal inwardly directed I_C. Hence the I_M is now directed outward.

G The g_{K+} now greatly exceeds the g_{Na+} and the I_{K+} still exceeds the I_{Na+}. Thus the I_I is still directed outward. Since the outward I_I still slightly exceeds the inward I_C, the I_M is small, but still directed outward. The membrane continues to repolarize.

H The g_{K+} and I_{K+} are still greater than their resting levels, while the g_{Na+} is now even lower than its resting level. Hence the membrane potential V_M is driven toward the potassium equilibrium potential E_{K+} producing the hyperpolarized afterpotential.

REVIEW QUESTIONS

1 All of the following statements concerning electricity are true, *except:*
   a The Faraday constant is equal to 96,500 C of electric charge transferred per mole of monovalent ion.
   b Conductance is the reciprocal of resistance.
   c The unit of conductance is the ohm.
   d Current is equal to the product of voltage and conductance.
2 The following is (are) true concerning the resting membrane potential in the squid axon and the mammalian neuron:
   a Sodium ions are in electrochemical equilibrium across the resting membrane.
   b Increasing extracellular potassium causes the RMP to decrease.
   c Both the chemical and electrical gradients for sodium ions are directed inward in the resting membrane.
   d The potassium equilibrium potential is slightly more negative than the resting membrane potential.
3 All of the following statements concerning the action potential are true, *except:*
   a The local current depolarizes the membrane to the excitation threshold.
   b The buildup of internal positivity helps retard sodium inflow during the reversed stage of the action potential.
   c Repolarization of the membrane is a function of potassium inflow.
   d Repolarization of the membrane is primarily a function of the sodium pump pumping sodium out of the cell.
4 The number of charges which need to be transferred across the cell membrane in order to change its potential by 95 mV is
   a 0.095×10^{-8} C/cm²
   b 9.5×10^{-8} C/cm²
   c 1.05×10^{-5} C/cm²
   d 9.5×10^{4} C/cm²
5 Impulse conduction in myelinated axons is
   a typically slower than in nonmyelinated axons
   b saltatory
   c not characterized by propagated action potentials
   d typically retrograde
   e none of the above
6 The local current which travels ahead of the impulse
   a increases with fiber diameter
   b establishes an electrotonic potential
   c is carried primarily by sodium ions in the intracellular fluid

    d causes an initial outward ionic current I_I through the membrane segments it en-
        counters, rather than a capacitive current I_C

7 The length constant of the electrotonic potential
    a decreases as the fiber radius decreases
    b increases with an axoplasmic resistance increase
    c is the distance over which the electrotonic potential decreases to 37 percent of
        its maximum value
    d is typically large in axons with high conduction velocities

8 The following is (are) true of neuron studies involving the voltage clamp apparatus:
    a No action potential (voltage change) is associated with ionic fluxes caused by
        stimulation.
    b Ionic flow across the membrane is prevented.
    c The voltage across the membrane is held constant while conductance and cur-
        rent flow change.
    d Current flow can be recorded and conductance can be calculated.

9 The magnitude of the equilibrium potential calculated by the Nernst equation
    a decreases as the temperature increases
    b increases as the chemical gradient of the ionic type involved increases
    c is higher for divalent than for monovalent ions
    d is zero if the concentrations of the ionic type involved are equal on both sides of
        the membrane

10 All of the following statements are true about the action potential at the height of its
    reversed stage, *except:*
    a The sodium and potassium currents are equal and opposite.
    b Sodium conductance has begun to decrease.
    c Potassium conductance has begun to increase.
    d The membrane interior is negative with respect to the membrane exterior.

Chapter 3

The Synapse

Impulse conduction in a single axon is fascinating to behold but, taken by itself, functionally limited. The full potential of the impulse is appreciated only by the functional changes it produces in a postsynaptic cell. In this chapter we will examine the events which occur at these functional contacts known as *synapses.*

A PRELIMINARY OVERVIEW

Neurons make functional contact with other neurons as well as with the cells of skeletal muscle, cardiac muscle, smooth muscle, and glands. The contacts neurons make with these cells are called *synapses,* a term meaning "connection" coined by the English physiologist Sherrington. The "connection" is actually an extracellular fluid-filled *synaptic cleft* separating the nerve cell membrane from the postsynaptic cell membrane (Fig. 3-1). This narrow cleft is typically 20 nm wide, a span sufficiently great to bring to an abrupt halt the transmission of impulses.

The signal must bridge this cleft in order to influence the postsynaptic cell. This is effectively produced at chemical synapses by the release of chemical *neurotransmitters* from the presynaptic terminal, which diffuse within microseconds across the cleft to specific *receptor sites* on the postsynaptic cell membrane. The neurotransmitter–receptor site interaction then causes specific ion channels to open on the postsynaptic membrane, triggering ionic fluxes which either depolarize or hyperpolarize the membrane. *Excitatory synapses depolarize postsynaptic membranes while inhibitory synapses hyperpolarize them.*

Depolarization of muscle cell membranes leads to contraction while depolarization of a postsynaptic neuron leads to the propagation of impulses on its axon. Conversely the hyperpolarization of a muscle cell membrane prevents contraction, while hyperpolarization of postsynaptic neurons prevents impulse conduction.

In order to allow presynaptic terminals to effectively control postsynaptic cells, it is necessary to quickly inactivate the released neurotransmitters after they have activated receptor sites, otherwise the postsynaptic cells will continue to be stimulated or inhibited longer than desired. Only by having the postsynaptic response occur immediately following firing of the presynaptic terminal, and not for prolonged periods afterwards, can the presynaptic neuron maintain this control. Thus the postsynaptic cell can be driven to continual action by repetitive firing of the presynaptic neuron or brought to an abrupt halt by the termination of presynaptic input.

Released neurotransmitters are rendered inactive by any or all of three means. At some synapses the transmitters are rapidly and actively reabsorbed by the presynaptic neuron for possible release a second time, a process called *reuptake.* A second means of inactivation is by the enzymatic degradation of the neurotransmitters by hydrolyzing enzymes which are present in the synaptic cleft or on the postsynaptic membrane. Still a third means of inactivation is for the transmitters to diffuse out of the synaptic cleft and away from the receptor sites.

While the term *synapse* is often used to describe all functionally active neuron contact with receptor cells, certain additional terms are in common use. For example, the neuron-neuron contact is called a *neuronal synapse,* while the neuron–skeletal muscle cell contact is called a *neuromuscular* or *myoneural junction.* The contacts made by nerve cells with cardiac muscle, smooth muscle, and gland cells are all *neuroeffector junctions.*

The particular physiological response produced in a receptor cell is determined by (1) the type of neurotransmitter released, (2) the quantity released, (3) the type of receptor site encountered, and (4) the particular function of the receptor cell. The neurotransmitter acetylcholine (ACh), for example, causes an increase in the contractility of the smooth muscle of the stomach, while norepinephrine (NE) produces decreased activity in this same muscle. Sufficient ACh is typically released from a single discharge at the neuromuscular junction to produce contraction of the skeletal muscle cell. In certain disease conditions, however, insufficient ACh is released to reach the excitation threshold of the cell and it does not contract. Furthermore, receptor cells may contain different types of receptor sites for the same neurotransmitter. For example, NE binds with alpha receptor sites on some vascular smooth muscle cells to produce vasoconstriction while binding with beta receptor sites on others to produce vasodilation. Ultimately, of course, the response capability of a receptor cell is determined by its function in the body. Muscle cells can either contract or relax, glandular cells can either secrete or not, and nerve cells can be made either to conduct impulses or not.

NEUROTRANSMITTERS

Certain synapses in invertebrates are electrically mediated rather than dependent on chemical transmission. The clefts at such synapses are usually narrower than those at chemical synapses. The electrical currents associated with the impulse at the presynaptic terminal spread across the cleft to directly stimulate the postsynaptic membrane electrically. However, in the overwhelming majority of mammalian and other vertebrate synapses the cleft is too wide for electrical transmission, and chemical transmission is required to bridge the gap.

There is strong evidence to implicate certain chemicals as neurotransmitters at synapses. Others, known as *putative* transmitters, are also suspected to act in this way, but the evidence supporting their participation is not as complete. It is generally agreed that for a substance to qualify as a neurotransmitter it must satisfy the following criteria:

1   The substance and the enzymes necessary for its synthesis are present in the neuron.
2   Impulses reaching the presynaptic terminals will release the substance.
3   Systems exist for the rapid inactivation of the substance.
4   Local application of the substance produces changes similar to those produced by synaptic release.
5   Drug-induced responses to both locally applied and synaptically released substances are similar.

Acetylcholine, norepinephrine, and dopamine (DA) are chemicals which have fulfilled all of these criteria. Nevertheless, several additional physiological chemicals have met some but not all of the criteria and are also suspected to function as neurotransmitters. ACh, NE, and DA have been identified in both the peripheral and central nervous systems while the others listed in Table 3-1 are thought to operate in the CNS only.

It is presently not known whether the enzymes necessary for the synthesis of the various neurotransmitters are themselves synthesized at neuronal endings since no ribosomes have been detected in axons even with the aid of the electron microscope. Nevertheless, the enzymes are found there. There is some evidence to suggest that they are synthesized in the soma and sent by axonal transport to the neuronal endings. However, it might also be that they are synthesized at some point along the axon by mechanisms as yet unknown. In any event neurotransmitters are most certainly synthesized in the neuronal

Table 3-1   Known and Suspected Neurotransmitters

Acetylcholine (ACh)
Norepinephrine (NE)
Dopamine (DA)
Prostaglandins
Serotonin
Histamine
Glycine
Aspartic acid
Glutamic acid
γ-Aminobutyric acid (GABA)

endings since the rate of axonal transport is much too slow to account for the rapid replenishment which is necessary to prevent synaptic fatigue (neurotransmitter depletion) even in a slowly firing neuron.

THE NEURONAL SYNAPSE

Much of our knowledge about synapses is based on observations of the spinal motor neuron. The neuronal synapse is composed of a presynaptic terminal (PST), a synaptic cleft, and a postsynaptic membrane. These synapses are often classified according to where they contact the receptor neuron. Accordingly we have axodendritic, axosomatic, and axoaxonic synapses depending on whether the PSTs contact a dendrite, soma, or axon. Axoaxonic synapses are rare, with dendritic and somatic contacts being the general rule. Often hundreds to thousands of axodendritic and axosomatic synapses will occur on a single motor neuron.

The arrival of an impulse at the presynaptic terminal causes the release of transmitter and its subsequent diffusion across the cleft where it activates postsynaptic receptor sites opening specific ion channels (Fig. 3-1). At an excitatory synapse, ionic fluxes through these channels tend to depolarize the membrane, while different patterns of ionic flux hyperpolarize the membrane at inhibitory synapses.

The Exitatory Synapse and the EPSP

Interaction with receptor sites at excitatory synapses opens Na^+ and K^+ channels, thereby increasing the permeability of the postsynaptic membrane to each of these ions. Consequently Na^+ tends to diffuse into the cell while K^+ diffuses outward, each following its own chemical gradient. However, the inward Na^+ current is greater than the outward K^+ current, causing the postsynaptic membrane to depolarize. Thus the postsynaptic membrane potential is no longer resting and is now called an *excitatory postsynaptic potential* (EPSP) (Fig. 3-2). The potential is called excitatory because the membrane potential is closer to the excitation threshold than it was in the resting state.

If the EPSP is produced by a single, not a repetitive, volley of transmis-

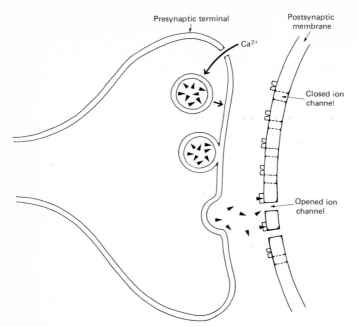

Figure 3-1 Schematic illustration of a typical synapse. The arrival of an impulse at the presynaptic terminal promotes the inflow of Ca²⁺ ions which trigger synaptic release of neurotransmitter. The inflow of Ca²⁺ causes the synaptic vesicles to migrate to the surface where the terminal membrane and vesicle membranes fuse, releasing neurotransmitter molecules into the cleft. The transmitters then diffuse across the cleft within microseconds and interact with specific receptor sites on the postsynaptic membrane, opening ion channels. The postsynaptic membrane is either depolarized or hyperpolarized depending on which channels the neurotransmitters open.

sions across the synapse, a small EPSP called a *local response* will be produced which will decay over a period of 15 ms or so to the resting state as the Na⁺ and K⁺ channels resume their normal permeabilities and neurotransmitter is inactivated. Recall that this normal permeability has K⁺ diffusing outward more readily than Na⁺ diffuses inward, thus repolarizing the membrane to the resting state.

The Inhibitory Synapse and the IPSP

An inhibitory synapse produces effects just opposite to those at the excitatory synapse. Here the action of the transmitters on the receptor sites is to open those ionic channels which hyperpolarize the postsynaptic membrane. Typically these are the K⁺ and Cl⁻ channels. Recall that the chemical gradients of these two ions are such that K⁺ diffuses outward while Cl⁻ diffuses in. This combination of ionic fluxes hyperpolarizes the membrane so that the internal potential becomes even more negative than the resting state. Consequently an *inhibitory postsynaptic potential* (IPSP) is established (Fig. 3-3). The potential is called inhibitory because the membrane potential is even farther from the excitation threshold than in the resting state.

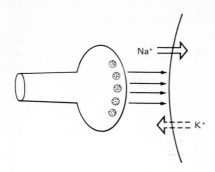

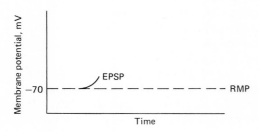

Figure 3-2 Schematic illustration of the excitatory synapse and the excitatory postsynaptic potential (EPSP). The interaction of neurotransmitters with receptor sites at an excitatory synapse opens Na⁺ and K⁺ channels. However, the inward flow of Na⁺ ions is much greater than the outward flow of K⁺ ions, resulting in a depolarization of the postsynaptic membrane from the resting membrane potential (RMP) to a less polarized EPSP. The potential is called excitatory because it is even closer to the excitation threshold than the RMP.

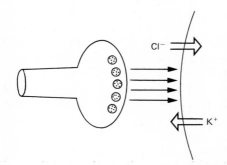

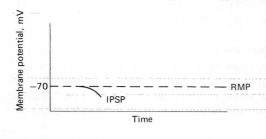

Figure 3-3 Schematic illustration of the inhibitory synapse and the inhibitory postsynaptic potential (IPSP). The interaction of neurotransmitters with receptor sites at an inhibitory synapse opens K⁺ and Cl⁻ channels. K⁺ then flows outward while Cl⁻ passes inward resulting in a hyperpolarization of the postsynaptic membrane from the resting membrane potential to a more polarized IPSP. The potential is called inhibitory because it is even farther from the excitation threshold than the RMP.

Electrotonic Current Spread From Dendrites to Axon Hillock

Before an action potential can develop in the receptor cell, the membrane must depolarize to the excitation threshold. In the spinal cord alpha motor neuron, this threshold is about -40 mV in the dendrites and soma but approximately -59 mV in the initial segment of the axon, the axon hillock. Since the resting membrane potential in all three regions is the same (approximately -70 mV), the axon hillock is easily the most excitable part of the neuron as it need depolarize only 11 mV in order to reach excitation to produce an action potential. Thus this is the point of impulse generation in the motor neuron.

Since the majority of synapses on the motor neuron are axo-dendritic and axo-somatic, one must ask the question, "How does depolarization at a distant excitatory synapse cause depolarization of the membrane in the axon hillock?" The answer lies in the spread of a depolarizing electrotonic current from each synapse as it depolarizes. An examination of the activity at a single synapse will serve to introduce the point. When the receptors at an excitatory synapse are activated by neurotransmitter and ion channels open which favor a net influx of positive charges, the postsynaptic membrane depolarizes slightly. It has been estimated that a single synapse firing once on the motor neuron releases enough neurotransmitter to establish an EPSP of approximately 100 to 200 μV. As this is obviously much too weak to reach excitation, no action potential is generated. Further, as we pointed earlier, this miniature EPSP will decay back to the resting membrane potential level within 15 ms if no additional firings occur at the synapse. Nevertheless, during the EPSP the interior of the postsynaptic membrane is temporarily less negative than the neuroplasm at a distance from the synapse. Accordingly, a passive electronic (local) current spreads from the less negative to the more negative region and out through the adjacent membrane as a depolarizing capacitive current. The length constant of this current is usually sufficient to reach from even the most distant dendrite to the soma and axon hillock. This means that while the strength of this outward-directed capacitive current decreases away from the synapse, there is still some left to help depolarize the axon hillock.

Now while the EPSP produced by a single synapse firing once is insufficient to produce a strong enough electrotonic current to depolarize the axon hillock to the excitation threshold, many separate synapses firing simultaneously, or even a single one firing repetitively at a very high rate, are sufficient to do so. The former pattern is *spatial summation* and the latter is *temporal summation*. Thus the membrane potential on the axon hillock can be depolarized to the excitation threshold and subsequently give rise to an action potential by either spatial or temporal summation of the synaptic EPSPs.

Spatial Summation of the Synaptic EPSPs

Spatial summation is the establishment of a summated EPSP by the simultaneous firing of many synapses distributed over the dendrites and soma. If enough of them fire at the same time, the local EPSPs will summate to produce an elec-

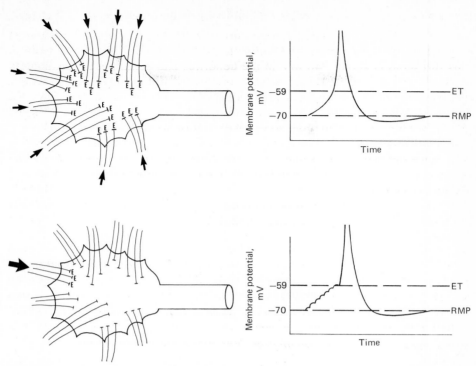

Figure 3-4 Spatial and temporal summation on the neuron. Spatial summation is illustrated in the top drawing. The axon hillock is depolarized to the excitation threshold by the simultaneous firing of several excitatory synapses spatially distributed over the membrane of the motor neuron. In the bottom illustration, the axon hillock is depolarized to the excitation threshold by the repetitive firing (at a high rate) of a very few excitatory synapses. In the top illustration all of the synapses fire simultaneously, but do it only once. However, in the bottom illustration only three are firing but at a very high rate, accounting for the stepwise depolarization which is observed.

trotonic current of sufficient strength to depolarize the axon hillock to the excitation threshold. In this way the synaptic potentials at distant dendritic sites contribute to the production of an action potential on the hillock through the instantaneous spread of the electrotonic current (Fig. 3-4). If an insufficient number of synapses fire simultaneously, the summated EPSPs will not reach the excitation threshold and a local response, but no action potential, will be seen. This local response is *graded* while the action potential is not. This means that the amplitude of the summated EPSPs varies directly with the number of synapses simultaneously firing. Thus, below the excitation threshold, increasing the number of presynaptic terminals firing will increase the amplitude of the potential while a decrease in the number firing will decrease it. On the other hand, if the number of PSTs firing is sufficient to reach the excitation threshold, a *nongraded* action potential will be generated. "Nongraded" means that the amplitude of the action potential will be the same any time enough synapses fire to reach threshold. Even if twice this number fire the amplitude will not change. Thus the action potential is an *all-or-none response.*

Once an action potential is generated on the hillock, it self-propagates down the length of the axon as explained in Chap. 2. That is, a local electrotonic current, initiated during the reversed stage of the action potential, travels through the axoplasm and out through the adjacent membrane as a depolarizing capacitive current bringing the adjacent membrane to the excitation threshold, establishing a second action potential, and so on. A little reflection will make it clear that the action potential, when it does occur, will start on the axon hillock rather than on the soma or dendrites. Even though the summated electrotonic current generated by simultaneously firing synapses depolarizes dendritic and somatic membranes on its way to the hillock, only 11 mV of depolarization are required for excitation here while approximately 30 mV are necessary on the less excitable dendrites and soma. Thus it is the first region to produce an action potential.

One should also be aware that the graded local response lasts longer than the increase in Na^+ *conductance* g_{Na+} which caused it, since restoration by K^+ outflow takes a little time. This is a significant feature because it allows the postsynaptic neuron an alternative to spatial summation by which it can produce an action potential and a propagated impulse. This alternative method is temporal summation.

Temporal Summation of Synaptic EPSPs

Temporal summation is the establishment of a summated EPSP by the repetitive firing at a high rate of a single excitatory synapse. Recall that the approximate 1 ms required for a single action potential imposes an upper limit of about a thousand impulses per second on a neuron's firing rate. Now since the EPSP from a single synaptic firing lasts up to 15 ms, it is apparent that if a single synapse fired repetitively at a high rate, the EPSPs would summate, producing a greater degree of depolarization than would be caused by a single firing. Thus the potentials are summed over time and the process is called *temporal summation.* If the depolarization produced by the temporal summation of the synaptic EPSPs is sufficient to reach excitation, an action potential is produced in the axon hillock. Because a single EPSP may start to decay before the next one summates, the rise to the excitation threshold can be pictured as a steplike progression (Fig. 3-4).

Synaptic Integration on the Neuron

A single motor neuron might receive presynaptic innervation from many hundreds or thousands of input neurons. Some of these synapses will be excitatory, while others will be inhibitory. We have previously described how excitatory synapses give rise to EPSPs while IPSPs are produced at inhibitory synapses. It should be apparent that the amplitude of the summated EPSP on the axon hillock will be decreased by the hyperpolarizing effect of several simultaneously firing synapses. Clearly then the state of the membrane potential on the soma and axon hillock of the motor neuron at any given time is determined by the number, type, and firing frequency of its incoming synapses. Only when this "integrated" potential exceeds the excitation threshold of the hillock will an action potential occur.

Thus several combinations of events exist that can produce an action potential in the motor neuron. These are (1) a single, or at least a very few, excitatory synapses firing simultaneously at a high rate with no inhibitory synapses firing simultaneously, (2) many excitatory synapses firing simultaneously at multiple locations on the neuron with no simultaneously firing inhibitory synapses, and (3) increasing the amplitude of the temporally or spatially summated EPSP in order to overcome the hyperpolarizing effect of inhibitory synapses firing simultaneously. In this latter case, if the inhibitory synapses considered by themselves could have produced an IPSP 3 mV more negative than resting (i.e., −73 mV), the summated EPSP produced by the excitatory synapses would need to be sufficiently increased to depolarize the hillock membrane by 14 mV rather than 11 mV in order to reach threshold and generate an action potential. A quantity of 3 mV is required to overcome the IPSP and another 11 mV to reach −59 mV, the excitation threshold.

The student must recognize that the membrane potential on the axon hillock is not a simple algebraic summation of the number of excitatory and inhibitory synapses firing at any given time. The relative position of the synapses on the dendritic tree of the motor neuron and the timing of their firing can have profound effects on this "integrated" potential. For example, if a single inhibitory synapse is located near the point where a dendrite joins the soma while a single excitatory synapse is located near the periphery of this same dendrite, and both are fired simultaneously, the IPSP will have a potent effect toward decreasing the EPSP, resulting in a seriously decreased EPSP on the axon hillock. If, however, the position of the two synapses is reversed with the excitatory synapse between the inhibitory synapse and the soma, the simultaneous firing of both does not cause much reduction in the hillock EPSP. Similarly, slight variations in the relative timing of the firings of the synapses can have significant effects on their ability to influence the hillock potential.

The Central State of the Neuron and Its Firing Rate

If all the synapses coverging on a single motor neuron were to fire just once with the overwhelming majority being excitatory, the neuron would depolarize to the excitation threshold of the axon hillock and a single impulse would be generated which would travel out along the axon to its terminals. However, if no synapses, either excitatory or inhibitory, were to fire, the membrane potential of the postsynaptic neuron would be considered truly resting (Fig. 3-5). It is possible, however, for several synapses to fire repetitively at a low enough rate and with sufficient timing to maintain a summated EPSP on the axon hillock several millivolts closer to the excitation threshold than the resting state. If this summated EPSP is 5 mV above the RMP, the neuron is said to have a *central excitatory state* (CES) of 5 mV. Recognize that a neuron which is maintaining a

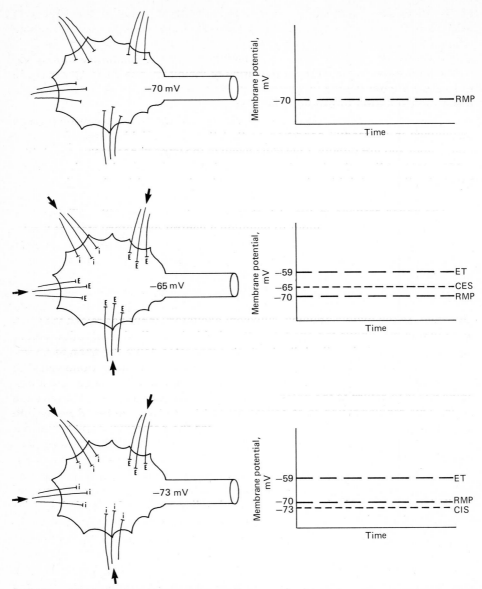

Figure 3-5 Schematic illustration of the central state (CS) of a motor neuron. In the top illustration, none of the 12 synpases is firing. Hence, the membrane potential over the soma and axon hillock is resting at −70 mV. In the middle illustration, 9 excitatory synapses and 3 inhibitory synpases are firing. The effect is integrated over the neuron, depolarizing the hillock membrane by 5mV to a central excitatory state (CES) of −65 mV. In the bottom illustration, 9 inhibitory and 3 excitatory synapses are firing, hyperpolarizing the hillock membrane by 3 mV to a central inhibitory state (CIS) of −73 mV.

central excitatory state of 5 mV is in a more excitable condition than if it were in the resting state since it need depolarize only 6 mV more to reach threshold (Fig. 3-5).

It is also possible for a neuron to maintain a *central inhibitory state* (CIS) by the appropriately timed repetitive firing of inhibitory synapses. Of course in this case a greater degree of subsequent excitatory input would be required to reach the excitation threshold (Fig. 3-5).

Thus, by a steady subthreshold repetitive excitatory input, neurons can be maintained in a "ready" condition so that they can quickly respond to additional input and fire rapidly. One can visualize the importance of this capability, for example, in the activation of escape mechanisms in animal muscle systems. Similarly, the excitability of a neuron can be decreased by the maintenance of a CIS.

The upper drawing in Fig. 3-6 shows a motor neuron with sufficient low level repetitive excitatory input to maintain a central excitatory state of 8 mV. That is, the membrane potential is being held at -62 mV, which is 8 mV above the resting state. Of course, the motor neuron does not generate an action potential and subsequent impulse, as the excitation threshold is not reached. It is merely in a more excitable state. The middle and lower drawings in Fig. 3-6 show the effect of maintaining a central excitatory state above the excitation threshold. In the middle drawing, sufficient excitatory input has raised the CES to 15 mV, 4 mV above the excitation threshold. Accordingly, an action potential will be generated on the hillock which propagates down the axon as an impulse. Now let's look more closely at this action potential. Following the depolarization phase in which the reversed potential is established, the membrane needs to return to the polarized resting state in order to be excitable once again. This repolarization is of course caused by a strong outward potassium current I_{K+} which drives the membrane toward the potassium equilibrium potential E_{K+}. However, following repolarization, the hillock membrane once again begins to depolarize because of the steady ongoing suprathreshold repetitive excitatory input which drives the CES back to 15 mV. Of course as soon as the threshold point is passed (at -59 mV), sodium conductance g_{Na+} dramatically increases, producing a strong inward sodium current I_{Na+} and giving rise to a second action potential. The neuron will continue to fire impulses at a steady rate as long as the same level of CES is maintained by the excitatory synaptic input.

Increasing the level of this input, and hence increasing the CES, will produce an increase in the neuron's firing rate. In the bottom drawing in Fig. 3-6 the CES is increased to 21 mV, maintaining the hillock membrane potential at -49 mV. Notice that the number of excitatory synapses firing onto the postsynaptic neuron has increased over that shown in the middle drawing, bringing about the increase in the CES. Notice also that the firing rate of the second neuron has correspondingly increased because of the increased CES. This increased firing rate is a direct result of an increase in the speed of depolarization following each action potential. Thus the firing rate of a continually stimulated

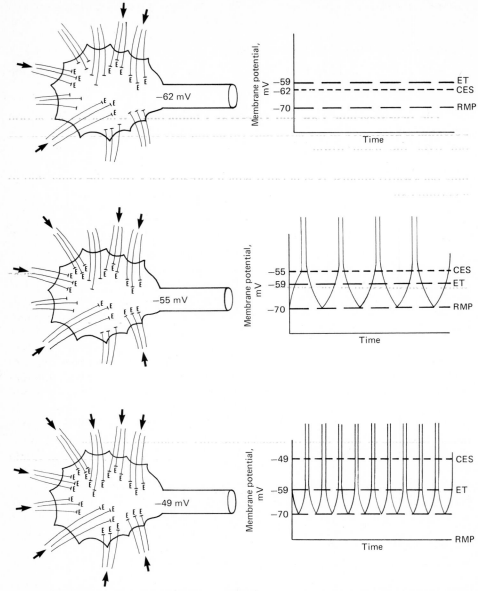

Figure 3-6 Schematic illustration showing the relationship between the central excitatory state and the firing rate of a motor neuron. In the top illustration, only 12 excitatory synapses are firing, which maintain the CES of the motor neuron at −62 mV (a value below the excitation threshold). Consequently, the motor neuron doesn't fire at all. In the middle illustration, 18 excitatory synapses are firing and the CES is maintained above the excitation threshold at −55 mV. Thus, the motor neuron continually depolarizes to the excitation threshold and fires repetitively. In the bottom illustration, the CES is maintained at −49 mV due to 27 synapses firing. The motor neuron depolarizes even more rapidly and thus discharges impulses at an even higher frequency.

neuron is a function of the degree to which this stimulation maintains a CES in excess of the neuron's excitation threshold.

Factors Affecting Synaptic Transmission

A number of factors have been identified which influence transmission at the synapse. These will be discussed here.

The Bell-Magendie Law and One-Way Conduction Whenever an action potential is generated in the axon hillock, an impulse is generated which travels out over the axon toward its terminal endings. This is described as an *orthodromic* (running forward) impulse. At the same time, an *antidromic* (running backward) impulse is generated which spreads back over the soma, and to a certain extent, out to the dendrites. The orthodromic impulse carries the potential for modulating activity in the postsynaptic neuron through synaptic transmission. That is, it causes transmitter release and subsequent excitation or inhibition of the postsynaptic membrane. On the other hand, the antidromic impulse has no such potential for modulation. There is no way for the postsynaptic membrane to communicate with the presynaptic terminal through "backward" transmission at the synapse. There are no vesicles releasing transmitter at the postsynaptic membrane. Thus transmission occurs in only one direction at the synapse, from the presynaptic terminal toward the postsynaptic membrane. This is the *Bell-Magendie law*.

Synaptic Delay The smallest nonmyelinated type C nerve fibers conduct impulses as slow as 0.2 m/s, whereas large myelinated type A fibers conduct impulses at velocities up to 120 m/s. However, regardless of the conduction velocity up to the synapse, the speed at which the postsynaptic cell is stimulated is limited by the time required for the events at the synapse, called *synaptic delay*. Because of their ease of access, the only synapses which have been extensively studied with regard to synaptic delay are those incorporated in spinal reflexes. As illustrated in Fig. 4-12 and explained in Chap. 4, the average synaptic delay time at these synapses is approximately 0.5 ms. This delay represents the time it takes to release and diffuse neurotransmitter across the synaptic cleft and for the receptor sites to become activated. The reader should be aware that the 0.5-ms time does not necessarily hold for all synapses, as we have no valid data for synaptic delay times in the brain, for example. However, it probably serves as a good first approximation.

Synaptic Fatigue If a presynaptic terminal fires and releases neurotransmitters faster than it can synthesize and store new transmitter, the synapse will soon be depleted of stored transmitter and stop functioning. This stoppage is called *synaptic fatigue*. It has been estimated that fatigue would occur within a few seconds if resynthesis were suddenly stopped and the synapses were fired at a high rate. There may be enough transmitter available for up to 10,000 transmissions by a single PST before it would become totally fatigued under these conditions. Nevertheless, recognize that under normal circumstances, synapses can fire as many as 1000 times per second for long periods of time and maintain a reuptake and resynthesis rate sufficient to prevent fatigue.

Ca^{2+} and Mg^{2+} Concentrations and Synaptic Transmission   Up to now we have implied that the arrival of an impulse at the presynaptic terminal is sufficient to release neurotransmitter from presynaptic vesicles in all circumstances. In fact, the amount of neurotransmitter released by the arrival of the impulse at the PST depends on the concentrations of Ca^{2+} and Mg^{2+} in the solution bathing the terminal. If the Ca^{2+} concentration is reduced or the Mg^{2+} concentration is increased, the amplitude of the synaptic potential is progressively reduced.

It is now well established that the release of neurotransmitter is dependent upon the entry of Ca^{2+} to the presynaptic terminal. When the normal sodium and potassium currents are blocked with tetradotoxin (TTX) and tetraethylammonium (TEA), respectively, there is a measurable inward current remaining in stimulated axon terminals that has been shown to be totally dependent on the concentration of external Ca^{2+}. These data indicate that Ca^{2+} enters the presynaptic terminals on the arrival of an impulse.

The inhibitory effect of Mg^{2+} on transmitter release appears to be due to its antagonistic effect on Ca^{2+} entry. It apparently competes with Ca^{2+} for membrane sites and thus interferes with the normal inward Ca^{2+} current. Thus it seems that the arrival of the impulse at the PST causes transmitter release indirectly by first moving Ca^{2+} into the terminal. Then, by some still unknown mechanism, this causes transmitter release. Evidence also suggests that the greatest part of the synaptic delay is taken up by the time required for Ca^{2+} entry and transmitter release.

In experiments that exploited the fact that transmitter release can be greatly reduced by manipulating the Ca^{2+} and Mg^{2+} concentrations, some significant features of the mechanisms of transmitter release were discovered. For example, at very low levels of transmitter release, the amplitude of the synaptic potential varies on repeated observations as a multiple of some irreducible unit size. It has been postulated that this unit amplitude results from the release of a "quantum" of neurotransmitter. It is likely that this quantum relates to the number of neurotransmitter molecules in a single synaptic vesicle. The "miniature potentials" produced by the release of a quantum of transmitter may be the building blocks upon which the normal synaptic potential is built when multiple vesicles release transmitter upon the arrival of an impulse at the PST when the concentrations of Ca^{2+} and Mg^{2+} are normal.

pH and Synaptic Transmission   Synaptic transmission is highly pH-dependent. Increasing the pH increases transmission while decreasing the pH decreases it. This is particularly apparent in brain synapses where alkalosis of 7.8 (normal, 7.4) increases excitability of neural pathways to the point of bringing on cerebral convulsions, while a decrease in pH to less than 7.0 decreases excitability to the point of coma. The latter is always seen in severe uremic or diabetic acidosis.

Drugs and Synaptic Transmission   A number of drugs are available which can alter transmission at the neuronal synapse. These will be discussed in more detail wherever appropriate later in the text. A few examples are caffeine (found in coffee) and theophylline (found in tea), which are known to increase synaptic excitability possibly by the mechanism of decreasing the threshold of excitation on the postsynaptic membrane. Strychnine is another. By its ability to interfere with the normal spinal inhibitory input to the alpha motor neurons, it produces hyperexcitability and muscular convulsions. Hexamethonium and mecamylamine can both block transmission at the synapses formed by the preganglionic and postganglionic neurons in the ganglia of the autonomic nervous system. In addition, a great number of agents are available which both stimulate or depress activity in the central nervous system. The mechanisms for their actions are largely unknown, including whether they directly stimulate or inhibit synaptic transmission or operate indirectly through metabolic changes in the neurons themselves.

THE NEUROMUSCULAR JUNCTION

In many respects the events at the neuromuscular junction (NMJ) and the neuronal synapse are similar. Both involve contacts between excitable tissues. Neuron to neuron at the neuronal synapse and neuron to skeletal muscle cell at the NMJ. Further, both presynaptic neurons release neurotransmitter at their terminal endings which diffuse across a narrow cleft to bind with receptor sites on the membrane of the postsynaptic cell, opening ion channels.

They differ in that each vertebrate skeletal muscle cell is innervated by a single neuron, whereas hundreds to thousands of neurons often converge upon a single postsynaptic neuron. Another difference lies in the fact that vertebrate neuromuscular junctions are excitatory only. There are no inhibitory junctions. Also, ACh is the only neurotransmitter to be identified with these junctions. The following descriptions refer to mammalian skeletal muscle unless otherwise indicated.

Skeletal muscle cells (muscle fibers) are typically innervated by large-diameter myelinated neurons. These neurons have single long axons which branch into filaments numbering from a very few to several thousand. Each filament ends by forming a neuromuscular junction with a skeletal muscle cell (Fig. 3-7). The neuronal filament terminates in a few flattened enlargements known as the *motor end plates*. These end plates are analogous to the presynaptic terminals in the neuronal synapse. Synaptic vesicles containing ACh are heavily concentrated in the end plates. The sarcolemmal membrane (muscle fiber membrane) beneath the end plate forms a many-folded depression. The folding of the membrane presents a greatly enlarged surface area equipped with receptor sites responsive to the ACh released by NMJ transmission.

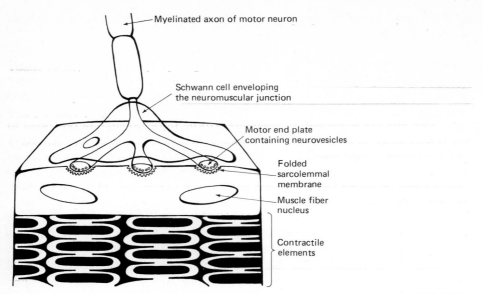

Figure 3-7 The neuromuscular junction. The bare terminal of a myelinated motor neuron makes a functional contact with the sarcolemma of a single skeletal muscle fiber. The terminal (motor end plate) forms a synaptic contact with a folded membrane depression in the sarcolemma. The neuromuscular junction is typically covered by one or more Schwann cells.

Activation of the Neuromuscular Junction

Neuromuscular junction transmission begins when an impulse reaches the motor end plate. The arrival of this impulse causes the release of ACh into the synaptic cleft, where it diffuses the short distance to the folded muscle fiber membrane. Here the ACh binds with receptor sites, causing the opening of both Na^+ and K^+ channels. Since the ionic distribution on either side of the sarcolemma is very similar to that which has already been observed for nerve cell membranes, Na^+ will diffuse inward while K^+ diffuses outward. Because the increase in Na^+ permeability is greater than for K^+ and because Na^+ is driven by both a chemical and electrical gradient, there is a net movement of positive charges into the cell, causing it to depolarize from its normal resting state of approximately −85 mV. Once the membrane starts to depolarize, it is no longer resting and its potential is now called an *end plate potential* (EPP).

Action potentials are not generated on the sarcolemmal membrane directly beneath the end plates but rather on that portion of the sarcolemma adjacent to the junction. Let's take a look at how this happens. Once the EPP is established, conditions exist for the development of an electrotonic current which spreads away from the junction through the sarcoplasm (muscle fiber cytoplasm) toward the still-polarized adjacent areas of the cell. As this current spreads away from the junction, it passes out through the adjacent sarcolemma, depolarizing it to the excitation threshold and producing an action potential.

This action potential then propagates as an impulse over the muscle cell, bringing about its contraction.

An important distinction between the neuronal synapse and the neuromuscular junction lies in the potency of a single synaptic discharge. A single synapse discharging once is almost never sufficient to produce an action potential in the second neuron of a neuronal synapse. We have previously described how a great many synapses firing simultaneously or a few firing repetitively at a very high rate are necessary to summate EPSPs to the excitation threshold of the postsynaptic neuron in order to produce an action potential. By contrast, a single neuromuscular junction firing once is almost always more than sufficient to produce an EPP capable of generating an action potential on the adjacent sarcolemma, bringing about impulse production and muscle fiber contraction. In fact the arrival of a single impulse at a single neuromuscular junction typically releases sufficient ACh to establish an EPP four times larger than necessary to generate the action potential. Thus we speak of a "safety factor" of 4 at the neuromuscular junction. This may seem like unnecessary waste of effort. However, if we consider that each muscle fiber receives only one neuronal input, the backup capability provided by this excess may not be out of line after all.

As is the case with the neuronal synapse, it is necessary to quickly remove the neurotransmitter after each discharge in order to keep the muscle cell from being continually stimulated, thereby eliminating the control the nerve fiber has over the contraction of the muscle cell it innervates. The great majority of ACh molecules are inactivated on the spot by the action of the enzyme acetylcholinesterase (AChE). The fraction of ACh not inactivated in this way diffuses out of the cleft or is reabsorbed by the end plate.

Drugs and Neuromuscular Junction Transmission

As with the neuronal synapse, a number of drugs are available which modify transmission at the neuromuscular junction. Curare is the classical competitive inhibitor at the junction. It competes with endogenously released ACh for the receptor sites. However, the curare–receptor site interaction does not cause depolarization and the establishment of an EPP. It thus blocks transmission of the signal from the nerve fiber to the muscle cell.

While curare is a naturally occurring drug, gallamine, benzoquinonium, and pancuronium are synthetic curarelike compounds which block neuromuscular transmission by similar mechanisms. Succinylcholine and decamethonium are also neuromuscular blocking agents but operate by a different mechanism. These compounds produce an initial depolarization of the sarcolemmal membrane which renders ACh incapable of producing a response in the already depolarized membrane. Several minutes later, as the membrane repolarizes, there is a secondary phase of decreased receptor sensitivity to ACh.

The neuromuscular blocking agents are primarily useful adjuncts to anesthesia for producing muscle relaxation. They are also useful for easing endotracheal intubation and for depressing spontaneous contraction of respiratory muscles under certain circumstances when artificial respirators are employed.

Neuromuscular transmission can be potentiated by the use of drugs which inhibit the action of the enzyme AChE. Neostigmine and physostigmine are reversible anticholinesterases. That is, they combine with AChE, for which they have a greater affinity than does ACh, and thus effectively tie up the enzyme so that it cannot degrade ACh. After a few hours, neostigmine and physostigmine uncouple from the enzyme for subsequent degradation elsewhere in the body, restoring normal function to the neuromuscular junction. Both drugs are potent anticurare agents as they allow ACh to build up in the synaptic cleft giving it a favorable competitive edge over curare for the available receptor sites. Diisopropylfluorophosphate is a potent compound which combines irreversibly with AChE, promoting long-term increases in neuromuscular transmission. It has had some therapeutic application but was primarily developed as a chemical warfare agent and is now principally of interest because of toxicological effects associated with its use as an insecticide. Its use produces a variety of signs and symptoms, including muscle fasciculations, sweating, abdominal cramps, respiratory distress, and even convulsions.

The therapeutic application of AChE inhibitors are limited by their lack of specificity since ACh levels are increased at ganglionic, postganglionic, and neuromuscular receptor sites. Neostigmine and physostigmine are primarily useful in the treatment of myasthenia gravis and glaucoma. Both are employed for the latter purpose, while neostigmine is commonly used for the treatment of myasthenia. In addition to its anticholinesterase effect, neostigmine has also been show to have a direct stimulating effect on skeletal muscle cell receptors.

THE NEUROEFFECTOR JUNCTION

The synapses made by autonomic nerve fibers with the cells of cardiac muscle, smooth muscle, and glands are more varied anatomically and chemically than are those at the neuronal synapse previously discussed and the neuromuscular junction. Nevertheless, these junctions are also characterized by the presynaptic release of neurotransmitters which diffuse to receptor sites on the effector cell membrane, producing changes in ion permeability and initiating physiological action such as muscle cell contraction or glandular activity.

Figure 3-8 illustrates a neuroeffector junction between a nonmyelinated postganglionic autonomic fiber and smooth muscle cells. Unlike the skeletal muscle junction, here we have several points at which transmitter is released to the muscle cell membrane. The nonmyelinated axon is shown to extend out of its groove at some places in an enveloping Schwann cell and to give rise there to enlargements which contain neurotransmitter-releasing vesicles. Recognize that these axons are not myelinated by the Schwann cell but are simply enveloped in grooves formed by infoldings of the cell. Impulse transmission along the axon causes release of neurotransmitter at these points with the subsequent excitation or inhibition of the muscle cells.

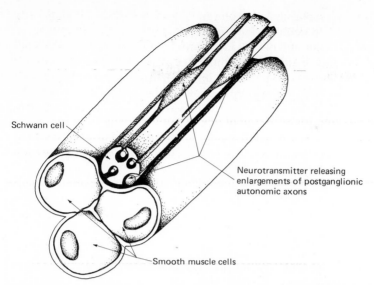

Schwann cell

Neurotransmitter releasing
enlargements of postganglionic
autonomic axons

Smooth muscle cells

Figure 3-8 Smooth muscle neuroeffector junction. Nonmyelinated postganglionic autonomic axons periodically extend out of their groves in Schwann cells to make functional contacts with neighboring smooth muscle cells. These extended enlargements contain transmitter-releasing neurovesicles. Recognize that these axons are not myelinated by the Schwann cells but are simply encased in groves formed by infoldings of the cells.

Like the neuronal synapse described earlier and unlike the neuromuscular junction, neuroeffector junctions can either excite or inhibit the effector cell. Postganglionic parasympathetic nerve fibers release ACh and give rise to either excitatory or inhibitory effects depending on the specific effector cell. These effects are summarized in Table 14-1 of Chap. 14, "The Autonomic Nervous System." Postganglionic sympathetic nerve fibers release either NE or ACh. The overwhelming majority of them, however, release NE. The effects of synaptically released NE are even more complex. Whether it is excitatory or inhibitory depends not only on the kind of effector cell innervated but also upon the type of receptor site located on the cell. These effects are summarized in Table 14-1.

Drugs and Neuroeffector Junction Transmission

A number of drugs active at neuroeffector junctions are covered in Chap. 14, "The Autonomic Nervous System." We will list a few here. Others will be examined later.

Acetylcholine, pilocarpine, and methacholine all directly stimulate cholinergic (ACh) receptors on autonomic effector organs. Physostigmine and neostigmine also potentiate activity at these receptors but act indirectly by their anticholinesterase activity. On the other hand, atropine is a potent antagonist at neuroeffector junctions by inhibiting the action of ACh on the receptor sites.

Norepinephrine, epinephrine, isoproterenol, and phenylephrine directly stimulate adrenergic (NE) receptors. Isoproterenol is specifically a beta receptor stimulant (agonist), while phenylephrine is an alpha receptor agonist. Conversely, phentolamine and phenoxybenzamine are effective alpha antagonists that block transmission at these junctions, while propranolol is a beta blocker. The concept of alpha and beta receptors is explored in Chap. 14.

REVIEW QUESTIONS

1 All of the following neurotransmitters have been identified in the peripheral nervous system, *except*
   a acetylcholine
   b serotonin
   c dopamine
   d norepinephrine
   e γ-aminobutyric acid

2 The following is (are) true at an excitatory neuronal synapse:
   a Transmitter interaction with receptor sites increases sodium conductance more than potassium conductance.
   b A single presynaptic terminal firing once is generally more than sufficient to establish an action potential in the postsynaptic neuron.
   c Released neurotransmitters establish an EPSP.
   d The neurotransmitter is always acetylcholine.

3 Neurotransmitters at an inhibitory neuronal synapse
   a interact with receptor sites and cause the postsynaptic membrane to depolarize
   b are never the same chemicals which operate at excitatory synapses
   c establish an IPSP
   d block the interaction of transmitters with excitatory receptor sites
   e all of the above

4 All of the following statements about the synaptic EPSP are true, *except:*
   a If the EPSP is subthreshold, a local response is seen.
   b The local response is nongraded but propagated.
   c The local response is an all-or-none response.
   d The magnitude of the EPSP increases with the number of presynaptic terminals which are firing.
   e Temporal summation is the establishment of a summated EPSP by the simultaneous firing of many synapses distributed over the dendrites and soma.

5 Indicate which of the following occur when the impulse reaches the presynaptic terminal:
   a Calcium ions enter the postsynaptic membrane.
   b Synaptic vesicles discharge their contents into the synaptic cleft.
   c The presynaptic membrane hyperpolarizes.
   d The presynaptic terminal swells.
   e All of the above.

6 A neuronal synapse is defined as
   a the contact between a neuron and a cardiac muscle cell
   b a neuromuscular junction
   c a neuroeffector junction

    d the contact between two neurons

    e none of the above

7 Neuronal synapses are characterized by

    a increased transmission in response to acidosis

    b the absence of fatigue

    c one-way transmission

    d synaptic delay

    e increased transmission in response to anticholinesterase drugs if the synapse is cholinergic

8 The simultaneous firing of many presynaptic terminals at an excitatory synapse causes

    a temporal summation

    b the establishment of a summated EPSP

    c no change in the membrane potential

    d hyperpolarization of the postsynaptic membrane

    e fatigue

9 A central excitatory state of 5 mV in the axon hillock of the alpha motor neuron to skeletal muscle fibers means:

    a The membrane potential is considered truly resting.

    b The neuron is firing repetitive action potentials.

    c The neuron is in a more excited state than if it were truly resting.

    d The hillock potential is 5 mV less polarized than if the membrane potential were in the resting state.

10 Indicate which of the following are true concerning the effects of drugs at the neuromuscular junction:

    a Transmission can be potentiated by neostigmine.

    b Curare blocks transmission.

    c Succinylcholine potentiates transmission.

    d Diisopropylfluorophosphate potentiates transmission.

    e All of the above.

Chapter 4

Muscle Tone and Spinal Reflexes

Muscles are always at least partially contracted. Even seemingly relaxed muscles possess a small degree of tension called *resting muscle tonus* or *tone*. This tone is ultimately controlled by impulses from the brain, though special receptors in the muscles themselves are also instrumental in its regulation. The brain relies on input from these receptors as well as those in tendons and joints to give it the information it needs to direct smooth and coordinated muscle movements. They constantly supply the brain with necessary information concerning the ever-changing tone in muscles as well as the present position of muscles at any time during a movement.

Many aspects of posture and movement depend on appropriately controlled and subsequently monitored tone in the large postural muscles. In this chapter we will examine how muscle tone is regulated both by the brain and spinal cord and how the brain is kept informed of the ever-changing status of this tone. A second objective will be to examine spinal reflexes. It is easy for the beginning student to treat reflexes lightly, associating them only with visible activities such as the knee jerk. In fact, the vast majority of reflex actions are unseen and unnoticed and yet are vitally important to normal function. Reflexes operating though the spinal cord are responsible for the smooth functioning of the gastrointestinal tract and bladder as well as all of the skilled movements of the trunk and limbs and the often-taken-for-granted activities of standing erect, walking, and running.

A PRELIMINARY OVERVIEW OF MUSCLE TONE

The muscle tone exhibited by otherwise relaxed muscles is necessary for these muscles to produce effective movements. If muscles relaxed completely (no resting tone), they would overlengthen, and too much time would be required to take up slack when a contraction was called for. On the other hand, too much tone would not allow for sufficient rest and recovery.

The principal regulator of muscle tone is the small stretch-sensitive intramuscular unit called the _muscle spindle._ Muscle spindles are encapsulated units within the belly of a muscle that lie parallel to the muscle fibers, stretching when the muscle is stretched and shortening when the muscle contracts. Thus they are uniquely situated to detect slight changes in muscle tone. When stretched, muscle spindles become activated, causing an increase in the impulse firing rate of afferent nerve fibers from the spindles to the spinal cord. Some of these _spindle afferents_ synapse on second-order neurons which conduct the stretch information up the spinal cord to the cerbellum and even the cerebral cortex. Since the firing rate of these neurons varies with the degree and velocity of stretch, the CNS is continually informed of the ever-changing status of muscle tone and movement.

Other spindle afferents directly excite large alpha motor neurons innervating skeletal muscle fibers. This reflex activation causes contraction (and shortening) of the muscle via the simple _myotatic_ or _stretch reflex_. This reflex functions as a servo-mechanism to maintain muscle tone at a preset level. If tone in a particular muscle decreases, allowing the muscle to lengthen, the spindles become stretched and trigger increased impulse firing in the spindle afferents, thereby increasing the firing rate of the alpha motor neurons to that same muscle and causing it to contract.

The stretch sensitivity of the spindles can be adjusted by action of the small gamma motor neurons in the anterior horn (lamina IX) of the spinal cord. This is an important capability, allowing the CNS to keep the spindles "in tune" with the muscles. These and other functions of the muscle spindles, as well as the tension-sensitive organs in tendons, will be discussed in this chapter.

THE MUSCLE SPINDLE

Anatomy

Muscle spindles are found in all skeletal muscles. They are more highly concentrated in muscle utilizing fine delicate control and less so in the large antigravity support muscles. The greatest percentage of spindles are located in

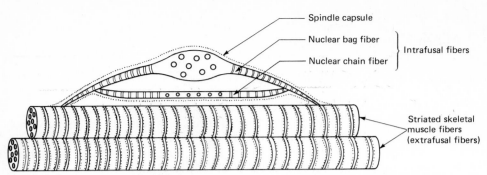

Figure 4-1 Schematic illustration of a muscle spindle, showing its relationship to two large striated skeletal muscle fibers. The encapsulated spindle is shown with one nuclear bag fiber and one nuclear chain fiber. The latter two are the intrafusal fibers of the muscle spindle. Notice that they are connected at their extremities to the large extrafusal skeletal muscle fiber. Notice also that the intrafusal and extrafusal fibers are parallel to each other.

the belly of the muscle. Spindles contain two types of *intrafusal fibers.* Both types are multinucleated contractile cells (Fig. 4-1).

   Nuclear bag fibers receive their name from the fact that their nuclei are clustered together in a baglike enlargement near the center of the fiber. *Nuclear chain fibers,* on the other hand, have no central enlargement, and their nuclei are spread out in a chainlike fashion in the equatorial region of the fiber. Both types are able to contract as contractile myofilaments are present in their striated peripheral portions. Nuclear bag fibers typically have greater diameters and are longer than chain fibers. A typical muscle spindle might contain up to eight chain and one or two bag fibers. The shorter chain fibers are often attached to the bag fibers, which in turn attach to the endomysium of the *extrafusal muscle fibers.* Extrafusal fibers are the large contractile fibers of the muscle, while the intrafusal fibers are the nuclear bag and chain fibers within the encapsulated muscle spindles.

Innervation of the Spindles

Before examining the role of the muscle spindle in regulating and responding to changes in muscle tone, let's first begin by looking at its neural connections (Fig. 4-2). Each nuclear bag fiber has both motor and sensory innervation. One or two gamma motor neurons form several distinct motor end plates, or *plate endings,* with the contractile portions of the fiber. Firing of the gamma fibers contracts and shortens the bag fibers, a feature which we will see is important in setting the sensitivity of the spindle. Stretch of the nuclear bag fibers is detected by specialized stretch-sensitive endings of both group Ia and group II nerve fibers. The Ia fibers form *primary endings* (annulospiral endings) by wrapping around the central region of the bag fibers. Group II fibers form *secondary endings* (flowerspray endings) over the striated portions of the bag fibers.

   The nuclear chain fibers also have both motor and sensory innervation. Very small gamma motor neurons form rather nondistinct *trail endings* on the

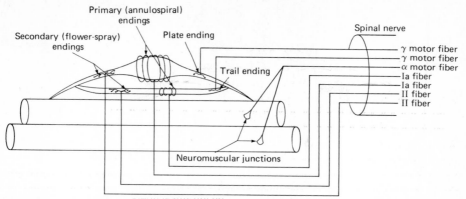

Primary (annulospiral)
endings

Secondary (flower-spray)
endings

Plate ending

Spinal nerve

Trail ending

γ motor fiber
γ motor fiber
α motor fiber
Ia fiber
Ia fiber
II fiber
II fiber

Neuromuscular junctions

Figure 4-2 Schematic illustration showing the afferent and efferent innervation of the muscle spindle. Also shown is the alpha motor neuron innervation of the extrafusal skeletal muscle fibers.

contractile portion of the chain fibers rather than the more distinct plate endings of bag fibers. Group Ia and II nerve fibers also form primary and secondary endings with the chain fibers.

The Myotatic (Stretch) Reflex

When a muscle is stretched, the spindles in that muscle are also stretched. Stretch of the nuclear bag and chain fibers in the spindles stimulates the primary and secondary endings of the Ia and II afferent fibers, causing them to send impulses into the cord. Many of these fibers (particularly the Ia fibers) synapse directly on alpha motor neurons supplying the same muscle which was initially stretched. This causes the muscle to contract and shorten, relieving the initial stretch. Such neurons are called *homonymous alpha motor neurons*. This "stretch-resulting-in-relieved-stretch" is known as the *myotatic* or *stretch reflex*. Once the muscle contracts and the stretch is relieved, the firing rate of the spindle afferents returns to the resting level (Fig. 4-3).

Skeletal muscles are attached to the skeleton in order to bring about movements of the body. It is usually necessary for muscles opposing a reflex movement (antagonists) to relax while those producing the movement (agonists) contract. This reciprocal action requires the incorporation of *inhibitory interneurons* in the spinal cord. Branches (collaterals), typically from the Ia spindle afferents, synapse in the posterior horn of the spinal cord gray matter. Here they stimulate inhibitory interneurons which depress activity in the alpha motor neurons to those muscles antagonistic to the desired movement. The *patellar tendon* or *knee jerk reflex* illustrates this point in Fig. 4-4.

When the tendon is tapped with a reflex hammer, the anterior thigh (quadriceps) muscles and many of its muscle spindles are stretched. Accordingly, volleys of impulses are sent into the spinal cord over the spindle afferents. Those fibers synapsing directly on homonymous alpha motor neurons bring about contraction of the quadriceps, causing the leg to kick in the classic

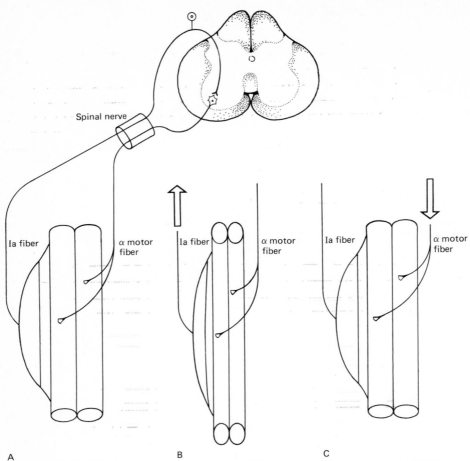

Spinal nerve

Ia fiber   α motor   Ia fiber   α motor   Ia fiber   α motor
                  fiber   fiber   fiber

A   B   C

Figure 4-3 The myotatic or stretch reflex. *A.* Muscle is relaxed. *B.* Extrafusal fibers are stretched, a condition which also stretches the muscle spindle, causing an increased firing rate along the spindle afferents (Ia fibers, in this case). *C.* Ia fibers monosynaptically stimulate the homonymous alpha motor neurons to the extrafusal fibers, causing them to contract, thus relieving the original stretch.

response. Of course the posterior thigh muscles (hamstrings) must relax in order to allow this to happen. This is accomplished by spindle afferent stimulation of inhibitory interneurons (Renshaw cells). Once activated, they depress firing in the alpha motor neurons to the antagonistic muscles. Renshaw cells release the inhibitory neurotransmitter GABA at their synapses. Notice that the same spindle afferents which increase the firing rate in the homonymous alpha motor neurons decrease activity in the antagonistic motor neurons. The latter is accomplished through *"feed-forward"* inhibition. Keep in mind that the spindle afferents are excitatory neurons releasing ACh at their synapses. The desired inhibition of the antagonistic alpha motor neurons is "fed forward" through the inhibitory interneuron, the Renshaw cell.

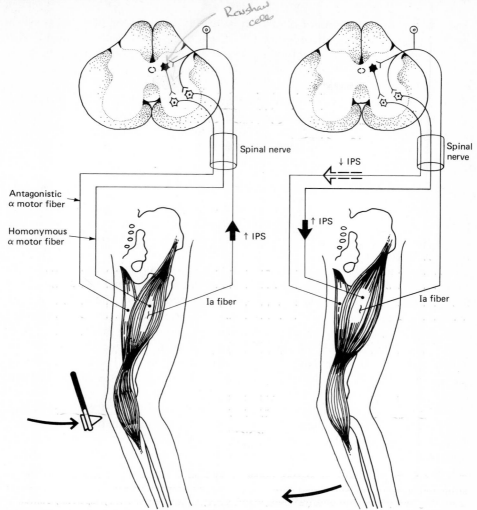

Figure 4-4   The knee jerk reflex is a visible example of the stretch reflex. Tapping the patellar tendon with a reflex hammer stretches the muscles of the anterior thigh and their muscle spindles. This increases the firing rate along the spindle afferents, monosynaptically stimulating homonymous alpha motor neurons and polysynaptically inhibiting (through inhibitory Renshaw cells) the antagonistic muscles of the posterior thigh. Consequently, the leg kicks out and the stretch is relieved.

The Gamma Efferents and Spindle Sensitivity

Up to this point we have only been concerned with the action of the muscle spindle afferents on alpha motor neurons. Now let's examine how the sensitivity of the spindles can be adjusted to maintain a preset level of muscle tone.

Recall that the spindle afferents are stimulated whenever the intrafusal fibers are stretched taut. Now if the intrafusal fibers are already partially contracted, only a slight amount of stretch is needed to pull them taut, increasing the firing rate of the spindle afferents. On the other hand, if the intrafusal fibers are relaxed and slack, a considerably greater stretch of the muscle is needed in order to pull them taut and fire the spindle afferents. In other words, *the muscle spindle is more sensitive to stretch when its intrafusal fibers are partially contracted then when they are not.* The degree of contraction of the intrafusal fibers and thus the sensitivity of the muscle spindle is controlled by the activity of the gamma motor neurons. The greater the firing rate of the gamma efferents, the greater the degree of intrafusal contraction, and the greater the sensitivity of the spindle.

Spindle Maintenance of a Preset Muscle Tone

Recognize that when muscles isotonically contract they shorten. Similarly, relaxation causes them to lengthen. Now let's assume that a given muscle is set to maintain a certain degree of contraction or tone. If the muscle relaxed too much it would lengthen and its spindles would stretch, initiating the stretch reflex. This would cause the muscle to contract, thereby relieving the stretch brought on by the initial relaxation. Similarly, if the muscle contracted too much, it would shorten and its spindles would become increasingly slack. This would decrease the stimulation of the spindle afferents, thereby decreasing the stimulation of the homonymous alpha motor neurons and causing the muscle to partially relax. As a result of this "servomechanical" nature of the muscle spindles, muscle tone remains very constant at any preset level. Increases in tension are reflexly countered by relaxation, while decreases in tension are countered by contraction.

It is important to recognize that tone is regulated by the stretch reflex and is not a characteristic of the muscle itself. This can be demonstrated by the immediate loss of muscle tone which occurs when the reflex arc is interrupted at any point. For example, sectioning either the anterior or posterior roots of spinal nerves results in the immediate loss of tone to all those muscles involved.

"Tuning" the Muscle Spindles

In order to remain sensitive to the slightest change in muscle tone it is important that the spindles not be allowed to go completely slack. Under normal conditions intrafusal spindle fibers are partially contracted. In this state, a slight relaxation or stretch of the muscle will be detected by the spindles as will a slight contraction or shortening. The firing rate of the spindle afferents will increase or decrease accordingly, and the spindles are said to be "in tune" with the muscle.

One of the important roles of muscle spindles is to keep the brain and particularly the cerebellum continually informed of even slight changes in muscle tone. This is accomplished via collaterals from the spindle afferents which synapse on neurons of the spinocerebellar tracts. The second-order neurons of these tracts conduct information concerning the state of muscle tone and movement to this important coordinating center of the brain (Fig. 4-7).

Now consider what would happen if the motor cortex of the brain directed a particular muscle to maintain a higher level of contraction (tension). Without a simultaneous contraction of the spindle intrafusal fibers in that muscle, the spindles would go slack and the firing rate of the spindle afferents would drop off to zero, producing a "silent period." Consequently, the spindles would no longer be able to detect slight increases or decreases in muscle tone and they would be "out of tune" with the muscle (Fig. 4-5). If, as neurophysiologists sus-

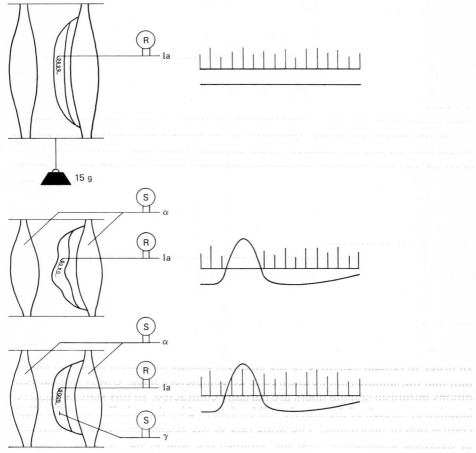

Figure 4-5 Muscle spindle "unloading" and "loading." In the upper record, a sustained tension of 15 g produces a steady discharge on the spindle afferent fibers recorded at R. In the middle record, stimulation of the alpha motor nerve fibers at S causes the extrafusal muscle fibers to contract allowing the spindle to go slack, thus "unloading" it and producing a "silent period" on the spindle afferent recording. In the bottom recording, both the alpha and gamma motor neurons are stimulated simultaneously, producing no "silent period" and keeping the spindle "tuned in" to the tone of the extrafusal muscle fibers. In each record the upper trace is the discharge on the spindle afferent fiber while the lower record is the recorded muscle tension. (*Drawn from Hunt and Kuffler, 1951.*)

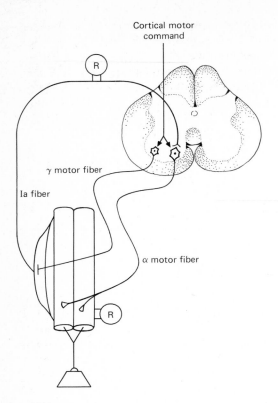

Cortical motor
command

R

γ motor fiber

Ia fiber

α motor fiber

R

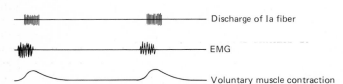

Discharge of Ia fiber

EMG

Voluntary muscle contraction

Figure 4-6 Alpha-gamma coactivation during the performance of a voluntary muscle contraction. Electromyographic recording just prior to discharge of spindle afferent fibers demonstrates that voluntary muscle contraction is not due to a "follow-up" length servomech-
anism controlled by the gamma efferents. The record instead demonstrates that the alpha
and gamma motor neurons are simultaneously stimulated during a voluntary contraction. In
this experiment, percutaneous recording needle electrodes were carefully placed into the peripheral nerves from the fingers of a human subject who was asked to voluntarily contract his
finger against a weight. Separate electrodes recorded the electromyogram. (*Drawn from
Eyzaguirre, 1975.*)

pect, detecting slight changes in muscle tone is an important feature of muscle spindles, these would no longer be contributing, and the cerebellum would be out of touch with tension changes in the muscle. Fortunately, activity in the gamma efferent nerve fibers prevent this from happening by increasing the degree of intrafusal fiber contraction at approximately the same time that the alpha motor neurons contract the extrafusal fibers. By this "coactivation" of alpha and gamma motor neurons, spindles are kept "in tune" with their muscles (Fig. 4-6).

The role of the gamma efferents in adjusting the sensitivity of the muscle spindles has already been discussed. The basal rate of firing of the gamma efferents and, through them, the contractile state and sensitivity of the spindles are regulated by the brain through pathways descending in the spinal cord. The principal route is the medial reticulospinal tract. This tract, which originates in the reticular formation of the brainstem, receives input from many areas of the brain, including the cerebral and cerebellar cortexes.

Cerebellar "Awareness" of Muscle Tone

The cerebellum is an important center for the central coordination of muscle activity. As such, it is necessary for the cerebellum to be continually informed of progressing body movements and changes in muscle tone. As previously mentioned, this is accomplished by collaterals from the spindle afferents which synapse in the nucleus dorsalis of the spinal cord. Some of the second-order nerve fibers from this nucleus ascend the cord in the *posterior spinocerebellar tract* (PSCT) to enter the cerebellum via the inferior cerebellar peduncle on the same (ipsilateral) side of the body as the entering spindle afferents. They terminate in the cerebellar cortex of the vermis (Fig. 4-7). Other second-order nerve fibers from the nucleus dorsalis cross over to the opposite (contralateral) side of the spinal cord and ascend to the brainstem in the *anterior spinocerebellar tract* (ASCT), where they cross back to enter the cerebellum via the superior cerebellar peduncle and terminate in the vermal cortex.

By "tapping off" the signals from the spindle afferents and conducting them cranially over these pathways, the cerebellum is continually kept informed of the ever-changing status of muscle tone. Electrophysiological studies indicate that group II fibers appear to be concerned with relaying information concerning changes in muscle length, while Ia fibers are concerned with changes both in length and contraction velocity.

In Chap. 13 we will closely examine the role of the cerebellum in muscle coordination. However, it is important to recognize here that the cerebellum functions as a coordinator examining the performance of a muscle during a given movement and comparing it with the intended movement directed by the cerebral cortex. If the intended performance and the actual performance don't match up exactly, the cerebellum can take corrective action to synchronize them through its own output to the motor system. Therefore it is important for

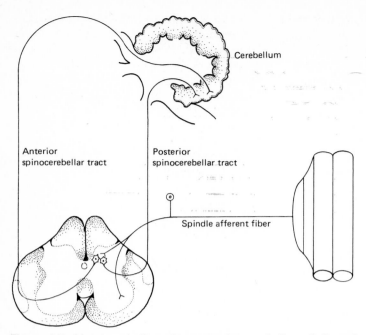

Figure 4-7 Muscle spindle pathways to the cerebellum. Collaterals from the spindle afferents synapse in the nucleus dorsalis of lamina VII. Second-order neurons then conduct the signals ipsilaterally up the cord to the cerebellum via the posterior spinocerebellar tract (PSCT). Other second-order neurons conduct the signals contralaterally to ascend the cord via the anterior spinocerebellar tract (ASCT). In either case, signals arising from spindles on the right side of the body enter the right side of the cerebellum to terminate in the vermal cortex. The same is true for the left side.

the cerebellum to continually receive input from the muscle spindles on the progression of any given movement. Input from Golgi tendon organs and joint receptors is also necessary for movement coordination.

THE GOLGI TENDON ORGAN

The tendons of skeletal muscle contain special receptors called *Golgi tendon organs*. These receptors are sensitive to the changes in tension generated by muscles as they contract. Little is known about their structure except that they are in intimate contact with the peripheral endings of group Ib afferent fibers. It is through impulses generated in these afferent fibers that changes in muscle tension detected by the tendon organs are relayed to the spinal cord and brain. As muscles contract and tension is applied to their tendons, the tendon organs are stimulated, which in turn propagate impulses over group Ib fibers into the cord, where they take several divergent routes (Fig. 4-8).

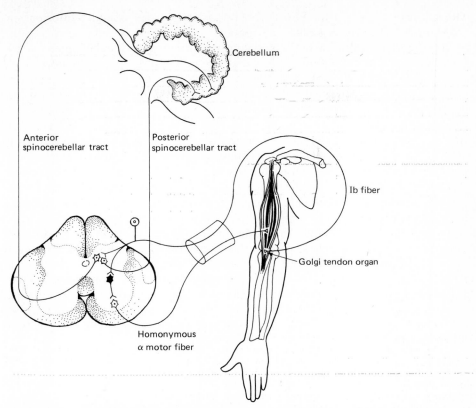

Figure 4-8 Neural pathways associated with the Golgi tendon organs. Signals from the Golgi tendon organs concerning the tension developed by a contracting muscle are relayed to the cerebellum via the posterior spinocerebellar tract (PSCT) and the anterior spinocere-bellar tract (ASCT). Ib fibers from the Golgi tendon organs synapse in the nucleus dorsalis of lamina VII. From here, second-order neurons of the PSCT and ASCT conduct signals to the cerebellum. If the tension developed by the contracting muscle is dangerously high, collater-alls from IB fibers stimulate inhibitory interneurons which reflexly inhibit homonymous alpha motor neurons, causing the muscle to relax. This is the lengthening reflex.

Function of the Golgi Tendon Organ

The sensitivity of the tendon organs is considerably less than that of the muscle spindles. As little as 1 or 2 g of tension is sufficient to increase the firing rate of the spindle afferents. On the other hand, the group Ib afferent fibers from the tendon organs don't register impulse conduction until the tension reaches as high as 100 g. When tension in the tendons begins to exceed this level, the ten-don organs become sufficiently stimulated to produce impulse firing in the group Ib fibers. Like the spindle afferents, the group Ib fibers send collaterals into the nucleus dorsalis of lamina VII of the spinal cord gray matter. Subsequently, both ASCT and PSCT second-order neurons conduct information from the tendon organs to the cerebellum.

If the tension developed in a strongly contracting muscle becomes excessive, it is not inconceivable that the tendon could pull free from the bone, certainly an undesirable situation. However, before this can happen the tendon organs become sufficiently stimulated to send large volleys of impulses into the cord to directly stimulate the alpha motor neurons to antagonistic muscles and inhibitory interneurons to homonymous alpha motor neurons. The resulting feed-forward inhibition to the strongly contracting muscle causes it to suddenly relax, relieving the strain on the tendon and preventing possible damage. This sudden relaxation of a muscle in the face of dangerously high tension is called the *lengthening reaction* or the *"clasp-knife" reflex* because of its similarity to the way a pocketknife suddenly snaps closed when the blade is moved to a certain critical position.

It was originally thought that little if any information from the tendon organs or the muscle spindles reached the conscious level in humans. The vast majority of the signals from these receptors which ascend the cord were thought to be directed exclusively to the cerebellum for subconscious evaluation. However, recent evidence now indicates that input from muscle spindles, tendon organs, and joint receptors is also relayed to the cerebral cortex and is probably responsible for the conscious sensation associated with the position and movement of limbs.

A PRELIMINARY OVERVIEW OF SPINAL REFLEXES

A reflex can be defined as a specific response to an adequate sensory stimulus. Strictly speaking, this response most often involves a muscular contraction or a glandular secretion. The spinal reflexes we will examine here all involve muscular contractions.

A *reflex arc* is the neural circuit over which the reflex operates (Fig. 4-9). In its simplest form it involves an afferent neuron conducting impulses from the point of stimulation into the spinal cord and an efferent neuron conducting impulses out to an efferent muscle or group of muscles. This is a *monosynaptic* or *simple reflex* because it utilizes only two neurons and one synapse. If one or more interneurons in the cord link the afferent and efferent fibers, the reflex is *polysynaptic*. If the afferent and efferent fibers occupy one or just a few cord segments the reflex is *segmental. Intersegmental reflexes* involve several cord segments. If centers in the brain are included in the reflex pathway, the reflex is *supraspinal*.

We noted earlier that it is easy to underestimate the importance of reflexes. For example, one tends to think of a simple act such as setting a dinner plate on the table as a purely voluntary act directed exclusively by the conscious motor cortex of the brain. In fact, however, the successful completion of this simple task requires the additional input of polysynaptic reflexes of the segmental, intersegmental, and supraspinal types. Most of the neural circuits making up such

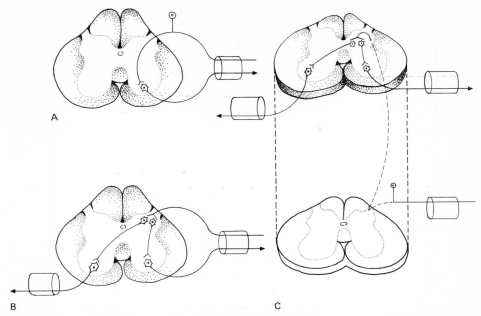

Figure 4-9 Schematic illustration of several reflex arcs. *A.* A simple monosynaptic reflex. Only two neurons and one synapse are involved. The stretch reflex may be the only monosynaptic reflex in man. *B.* Two polysynaptic reflexes. *C.* Two polysynaptic reflexes which are also intersegmental; that is, the efferent fibers of the reflex are at a different segmental cord level than the afferent fiber. By contrast, the monosynaptic and polysynaptic reflexes in *A* and *B* are segmental.

reflexes are very complex and poorly understood. Nevertheless, they undoubtedly involve special application of certain basic reflex types such as the stretch reflex and others. Let's look at an example of a somewhat complex spinal reflex which is at least partially understood.

The Flexor-Crossed-Extensor Reflex

A strong, painful, or potentially damaging stimulus delivered to cutaneous or joint receptors can reflexly cause a sudden bodily withdrawal away from the stimulus. Stepping on a tack is a good example of this reflex in action. The person will typically flex (withdraw) the stimulated foot and leg while extending the other leg in order to propel the body away from the tack. This is a polysynaptic, bilateral reflex incorporating both excitatory and inhibitory interneurons. Delivery of the stimulus to the receptors in a limb increases the firing rate of pain-carrying group III and IV afferents into the posterior horn, where they synapse with interneurons (Fig. 4-10). Excitatory interneurons ipsilaterally stimulate alpha motor neurons to the flexors in that limb while contralaterally stimulating extenders in the opposite limb—thus the term *flexor-crossed-*

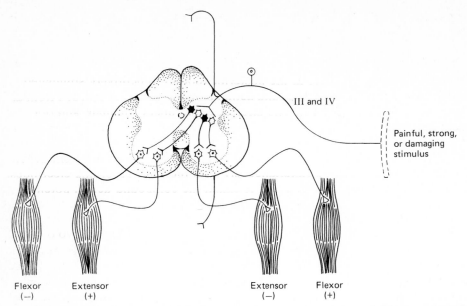

III and IV

Painful, strong, or damaging stimulus

Flexor (−)   Extensor (+)   Extensor (−)   Flexor (+)

Figure 4-10 The flexor-crossed-extensor reflex. When a strong, painful, or potentially damaging stimulus is delivered to cutaneous, muscle, or joint receptors of a limb, the limb is reflexly withdrawn away from the stimulus. The receptors associated with group III and IV afferents send impulses into the cord where they stimulate excitatory interneurons which ipsilaterally stimulate alpha motor neurons to limb flexors and contralaterally stimulate alpha motor neurons to limb extenders. Simultaneously, inhibitory interneurons ipsilaterally inhibit alpha motor neurons to limb extenders and contralaterally inhibit alpha motor neurons to limb flexors.

extensor reflex. At the same time, inhibitory interneurons ipsilaterally inhibit extenders of the stimulated limb while contralaterally inhibiting flexors of the opposite limb.

This reflex is often intersegmental. This should not be surprising when one considers that many muscles are involved in such movements. In the cat, for example, a painful stimulus delivered to one hind leg will not only reflexly withdraw that leg, but will extend to both hind legs and forelegs on the opposite side as well. This means that the group III and IV afferents not only stimulated interneurons at the same segmental level at which they entered the cord, but activated synapses at higher and lower cord levels as well. The ascending and descending collaterals travel in the *fasciculus proprius* (ground bundles) of the white matter. The fibers in these tracts carry intersegmental connections.

ELECTROPHYSIOLOGY OF SPINAL REFLEXES

Neuronal synaptic connections in the spinal cord are difficult to examine experimentally because of their great density and complexity. The peripheral fibers of a reflex are much easier to study. Consequently, some knowledge concerning synaptic activity in the cord can be obtained by electrically stimulating afferent fibers while recording from synaptically stimulated efferent fibers.

Monosynaptic and Polysynaptic Reflexes

When afferent nerve fibers in the posterior root are repetitively stimulated by an electronic stimulator, compound action potentials can be recorded from anterior root fibers (Fig. 4-11). The afferent nerve fibers stimulate anterior root neurons either directly or indirectly, which then conduct recordable impulses out their efferent fibers. A compound action potential is the sum of several individual action potentials. It is obtained when action potentials from several nerve fibers are recorded simultaneously with the same recording electrodes.

Notice that when the stimulus is small, the compound action potential is also small. With increases in stimulus strength, more posterior root neurons and hence more anterior root neurons are excited and the size of the action potential increases. With yet further increases in stimulus strength, two observations can be made. First, there is again an increase in the size of the compound action potential as more neurons are recruited, and secondly we see the appearance of slightly delayed potentials. These latter potentials are due to polysynaptic relays. Because of the delay caused by the additional synapses, the resultant impulses reach the recording electrodes later than the monosynaptic relays. These polysynaptic responses do not appear if the stimulus strength is too low because of the failure to sufficiently stimulate the interneurons. The more interneurons involved, the stronger the initial stimulus needs to be in order to maintain excitability through the multiple synapses. As the stimulus strength is still further increased, relays involving even greater numbers of synapses are recruited. Finally, when the posterior root neurons are maximally

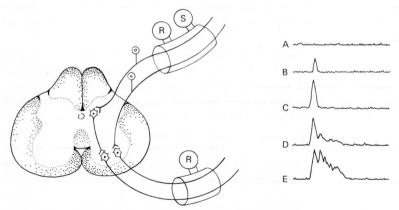

Figure 4-11 Monosynaptic and polysynaptic relays. When the strength of the stimulus delivered to the posterior root fibers is small, the size of the compound action potential recorded on the anterior root is also small. As the stimulus strength increases, more posterior root fibers are stimulated, and the action potential increases in size. With still further increases in stimulus strength, delayed action potentials caused by polysynaptic relays begin to appear. The stimulus strength increases in traces A through E. (*Drawn from Lloyd, 1943.*)

stimulated, the response will level off and further increases in stimulus strength will not change the magnitude of the response.

Determination of Synaptic Delay Time

When the stimulating electrodes are placed into the lateral region of the spinal cord itself, stimulation directly excites both afferent neurons and interneurons (Fig. 4-12).

By painstaking and careful placement of these stimulating electrodes, only one synapse separates the afferent neurons and interneurons from the efferent neurons of the anterior horn. As the stimulating current is increased, both afferent neurons and interneurons will be sufficiently stimulated to conduct impulses to their synapses and excite the alpha motor neurons so that compound action potentials are recorded in the anterior root. As the stimulus strength increases, more and more afferents and interneurons are stimulated and the size of the compound action potential is observed to increase also. With still further increases in stimulus strength, some of the anterior motor neurons are stimulated directly by the electrode current spread through the cord. Since no synapses are involved in this instance, an earlier compound action potential is also recorded. The difference in time delay between the appearance of these two action potentials represents the *synaptic delay*. Values of 0.5 ms are typi-

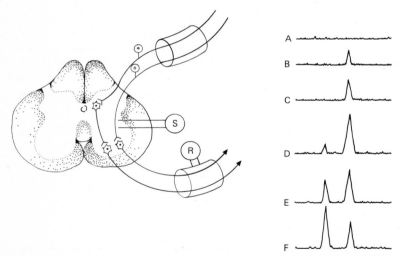

Figure 4-12 Determination of synaptic delay time. With the stimulating electrodes placed in the lateral region of the spinal cord, a small current will stimulate both afferent neurons and interneurons directly, causing a compound action potential to appear under the recording electrode on the anterior root. As the current strength is increased, more presynaptic fibers are fired and the size of the action potential increases still further. Additional increases in stimulus strength cause some of the anterior motor neurons to be directly stimulated, producing an earlier action potential than before because no synapses need be crossed. The difference in time between the appearance of the two potentials represents the synaptic delay time. Still further increases in the stimulus strength show an increase in the size of the first and a decrease in the second compound action potential due to the presynaptic neurons finding the anterior motor neurons in a refractory state. The stimulus strength increase in traces A through F. (*Drawn from Renshaw, 1940.*)

cal in this kind of experiment. The delay represents the time it takes for Ca^{2+} ions to enter the presynaptic terminal and bring about the subsequent release of neurotransmitter, followed by diffusion across the cleft and activation of receptor sites on the postsynaptic membrane. Still further increases in the stimulus strength produce an increase in the amplitude of the first potential and a decrease in the amplitude of the second potential because of the interneurons finding the motor neurons in a refractory state.

Facilitation and Occlusion in a Neuronal Pool

Nerve cell axons often branch into hundreds and even thousands of neuronal filaments before synapsing with other neurons. As many as 100 neurons are often supplied by a single axon in this manner. Some of these postsynaptic neurons receive many synaptic inputs from a single presynaptic neuron while others receive only a few. All of the nerve cells which receive synaptic input from a single presynaptic neuron make up the *neuronal pool* of that neuron. When a neuron supplying a neuronal pool is firing impulses repetitively, some of the neurons in the pool are sufficiently stimulated to establish EPSPs of threshold level, while others (those receiving few synaptic inputs from the neuron) are not. Those stimulated to threshold level are in the *liminal* or *discharge zone* of the pool, while the others are in the *subliminal* or *facilitation zone* (Fig. 4-13).

Neuron pools overlap. That is, some of the neurons in the neuronal pool of one input neuron are likely to be included in the neuronal pool of a second and even a third and fourth input neuron. While the neurons in the facilitation zone of one input neuron are not sufficiently stimulated to reach threshold by the action of that neuron alone, they may be raised to the excitation threshold and begin to fire impulses if they are also in the facilitation zone of a second simultaneously firing input neuron (Fig. 4-14). This phenomenon is called *facilitation*. Facilitation in this case means that the postsynaptic output from a neuronal pool evoked by the simultaneous firing of two input neurons is greater than the sum of each fired separately. When the discharge zones of two neuronal pools overlap, the opposite effect is observed. In this case the postsynaptic output from a neuronal pool evoked by the simultaneous firing of two input neurons is less than the sum of each fired separately (Fig. 4-15). This is called *occlusion*.

Convergence and Divergence

Convergence and divergence are important means by which the central nervous system channels and sorts different information. There are many examples of each throughout the nervous system. Synaptic input to the large alpha motor neuron in the spinal cord anterior horn is a good example of convergence (Fig. 4-16). We see that several nerve fibers converge on the motor neuron, each exerting some measure of influence over the central state of this cell. The primary sources are probably the corticospinal tract fibers from the brain. However, we also know that it receives input from the spindle afferents, group Ib fibers from Golgi tendon organs, Renshaw cells, and several other pathways descending in the spinal cord. Because of this funneling of input,

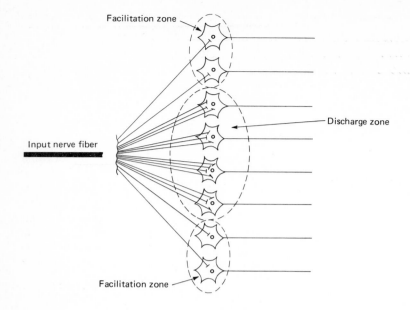

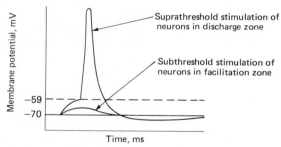

Figure 4-13 When the input neuron to a neuronal pool is firing impulses, some of the neurons in the pool will be sufficiently stimulated to reach their excitation thresholds and conduct impulses. Others receiving only a few synapses from the input neuron will not reach threshold and won't fire. Those stimulated to threshold are in the discharge of liminal zone, while those not reaching threshold are in the facilitation or subliminal zone.

Sherrington has called the motor neuron the *final common pathway* in motor output.

Remember that the firing rate of a neuron depends on the level of its central excitatory state (CES). The higher the CES in excess of the excitation threshold, the higher the firing rate. Of course if the CES is less than the excitation threshold, the motor neuron will not fire at all.

It is often important that information arising in one area of the body be transmitted to several different regions in the nervous system. This spread of information is accomplished by the process of *divergence*. Figure 4-16 illus-

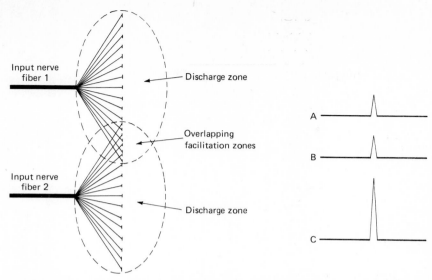

Figure 4-14   Neuronal pool facilitation caused by the overlap of facilitation zones. While the neurons in the subliminal zone of one presynaptic neuron are not sufficiently stimulated to reach threshold by the firing of that neuron alone, if they are also in the subliminal zone of a second presynaptic neuron discharging at the same time as the first, the central excitatory state of these sublimal zone neurons may be raised to the threshold of excitation. In A we see a compound action potential trace caused by the firing of input nerve fiber 1 only. In B we see the compound action potential recorded by firing input nerve fiber 2 only. In C we see neuronal pool facilitation as the postsynaptic discharge produced in the neuronal pool by the simultaneous firing of input nerve fibers 1 and 2 is greater than the sum of each firing separately.

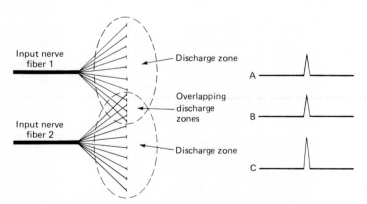

Figure 4-15   Neuronal pool occlusion caused by the overlap of discharge zones. In A we see a compound action potential trace caused by the firing of input nerve fiber 1 only. In B we see the compound action potential trace recorded by firing input nerve fiber 2 only. In C we see neuronal pool occlusion in that the postsynaptic discharge produced in the neuronal pool by the simultaneous firing of input nerve fibers 1 and 2 is less than the sum of each firing separately.

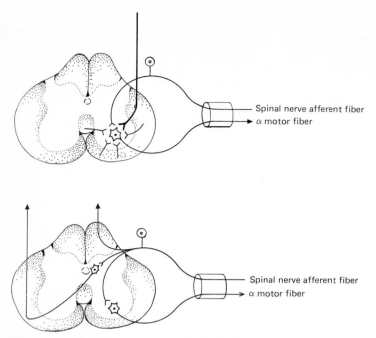

Spinal nerve afferent fiber
α motor fiber

Spinal nerve afferent fiber
α motor fiber

Figure 4-16 Convergence and divergence. In the upper drawing the presynaptic terminals of several different neurons converge on the anterior motor neuron in the spinal cord. Convergence (many neurons synaptically influencing a single neuron) occurs throughout the nervous system. The top drawing is but one example. The firing rate of the output neuron is determined by the type, number, and firing rate of the converging input neurons. In the lower drawing a spinal afferent fiber is shown to diverge in several directions. Again, this is but one example of divergence.

trates the divergence of signals entering the spinal cord via a spinal afferent fiber which diverges and takes three separate routes. Two of these are directed cranially via ascending pathways in the spinal cord, while the third is routed to a spinal reflex. In another respect, the transmission of impulses from a single input neuron to the various neurons in its neuronal pool is also divergence.

Parallel and Recurrent Circuits

It is easy to picture neurons lined up in single file with the first stimulating the second and so on. In nature, however, neural pathways are typically more complex. Two exceptions to the single-file concept are illustrated in Fig. 4-17. In a *parallel circuit,* an incoming neuron stimulates a second neuron both directly and indirectly (via one or more interneurons). Consider a neuron (A) which directly excites a neuron (B) through an excitatory synapse. In addition, neuron A stimulates an interneuron (C), which in turn excites neuron B. It should be apparent that if neuron A is stimulated, recording electrodes placed on neuron B will register two spikes. The first is caused by neuron A directly

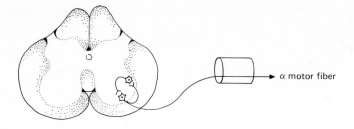

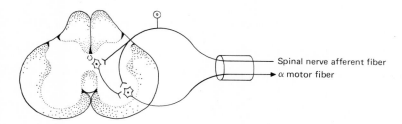

Figure 4-17 Recurrent and parallel circuits. A recurrent circuit is illustrated in the top drawing. In this case a collateral branch of the motor neuron loops back and stimulates an interneuron which returns to synapse with the motor neuron. Such circuits may be polysynaptic, involving several interneurons, some of which may be excitatory while others are inhibitory. A parallel circuit is illustrated in the lower drawing. In this case, a spinal nerve fiber stimulates a motor neuron both directly and indirectly via a parallel interneuron. Parallel and recurrent circuits occur in all parts of the nervous system, not just in the spinal cord as illustrated here.

stimulating neuron B, and the second is caused by the delay through the interneuron C synapse. The delay of this *afterdischarge* (second spike) is determined by the number of interneurons involved in the parallel circuit. The interneurons may be excitatory or inhibitory.

When a collateral branch of a neuron synapses with an interneuron which then returns to resynapse with itself, either directly or indirectly, a *recurrent circuit* is formed. Like parallel circuits, recurrent circuits may be either excitatory or inhibitory.

REVIEW QUESTIONS

1   Gamma efferent fibers are distributed to
    a   extrafusal muscle fibers
    b   intrafusal muscle fibers
    c   vascular smooth muscle
    d   tendons of skeletal muscles
    e   cutaneous touch receptors

2 The following is (are) true: If tone in a particular muscle decreases, allowing the muscle to lengthen, then
   a firing in spindle afferents decreases
   b homonymous alpha motor neurons are reflexly stimulated
   c muscle spindle intrafusal fibers are stretched
   d the myotatic reflex will cause the muscle to contract
   e all of the above
3 Muscle spindles are most highly concentrated in
   a muscles which are generally involved in fine delicate control
   b the bellies of muscles
   c large antigravity support muscles
   d tendons of skeletal muscles
4 The following is (are) true concerning neuronal contacts with intrafusal fibers:
   a Gamma motor fibers form plate endings and trail endings.
   b Group Ia fibers form annulospiral endings with the medial portions of the fibers.
   c Alpha motor neurons form flowerspray endings with the intrafusal fibers.
   d Secondary endings are associated with group II fibers.
   e All of the above.
5 Muscle spindle sensitivity is increased by
   a increased firing in the alpha motor neurons
   b increased firing in the gamma motor neurons
   c skeletal muscle stretch
   d intrafusal fiber stretch
   e none of the above
6 Golgi tendon organs
   a are considerably more sensitive than muscle spindles
   b are innervated by group Ib afferent fibers
   c are important structures in the stretch reflex
   d are involved in the clasp-knife reflex
7 The neurons in a neuronal pool
   a may be in the discharge zone or the facilitation zone
   b all receive input from the same presynaptic input neuron
   c are in the subliminal zone if they receive only enough input to establish a subthreshold EPSP
   d never overlap the neurons in an adjacent neuronal pool
8 The "final common pathway" concept of the alpha motor neuron is an example of
   a parallel circuits
   b convergence
   c recurrent circuits
   d divergence
   e synaptic delay
9 Relaxation of the antagonistic muscles in the knee jerk reflex is mediated through
   a a monosynaptic reflex
   b a polysynaptic reflex
   c Ia afferent fibers from the muscle spindles
   d homonymous alpha motor neurons
   e interneurons
   f none of the above

10 If the facilitation zones of two adjacent neuronal pools overlap, the postsynaptic output from one of the pools evoked by the simultaneous firing of input neurons to both pools is greater than the sum of each input neuron fired separately. This phenomenon is called
   a   occlusion
   b   discharge
   c   repetition
   d   excitation
   e   facilitation
   f   limination
   g   none of the above

Chapter 5

Skeletal Muscle Contraction
and the Motor Unit

Most of the important contributions to our current understanding of muscle contraction and coordination have been made since the turn of the century. Early observations utilizing the sartorius muscle of the frog helped to demonstrate the characteristics of the individual muscle twitch and also established that contracting muscles produce heat and are sensitive to the effects of temperature. Ultrastructural studies of individual muscle fibers (cells) were just beginning at this point, while the "sliding filament" theory describing muscle contraction is just over 30 years old.

Researchers have learned that muscle contraction cannot proceed in the absence of adenosine triphosphate (ATP) and Ca^{2+} ions. Most of our assumptions about the role of these two components during contraction is explained by the use of models. Current models are most often based on the classic work of A. F. Huxley, who in 1957 proposed a theory concerning the interaction of the filaments actin and myosin in the contraction process of skeletal muscle. In this chapter we will examine a current model of the contraction process.

We will also establish in this chapter that the functional units of skeletal muscle are not individual muscle fibers, but larger systems called *motor units*. The motor unit consists of a motor neuron and the group of skeletal muscle fibers which it innervates. An entire muscle may be composed of thousands of such units representing millions of individual muscle fibers.

SKELETAL MUSCLE CONTRACTION

A single skeletal muscle is composed of many thousands to millions of long, narrow contractile cells called *muscle fibers* (Fig. 5-1). These fibers are clustered together in parallel bundles called *fasciculi*. Each muscle fiber is 10 to 80 μm in diameter and is composed of hundreds to thousands of even smaller units called *myofibrils*. Myofibrils contain the proteins *actin* and *myosin*, which are the sliding *myofilaments* that are activated during muscle contraction.

Each individual muscle fiber is innervated by a single branch from a motor neuron. This branch (telodendron) forms a neuromuscular junction (NMJ) with the muscle cell membrane (sarcolemma). Impulses arriving on the nerve fiber are transmitted to the sarcolemma and ultimately cause the contraction of the muscle fiber. A muscle fiber is a multinucleated cell whose *sarcoplasm* (cytoplasm) contains mitochondria and stores of glycogen. The availability of glycogen, which is easily converted to glucose, ensures that the mitochondria will have sufficient amounts of this readily available nutrient as an energy source for the synthesis of ATP, a high-energy phosphate molecule needed to energize the contractile process. In times of low muscle activity, excess ATP is temporarily converted to *creatine phosphate*.

Most of the millions of individual muscle fibers within a single muscle run the entire length of the muscle. Because they run parallel to each other, the tensions developed by the individually contracting fibers summate to produce the overall tension developed by the muscle. In a sustained contraction, the individual muscle fibers alternate firing with each other so that some are contracting while others are relaxing. This process helps avoid fatigue yet maintains a smooth and prolonged muscle contraction.

Individual myofibrils present a striated appearance of alternating light and dark bands (Fig. 5-1). The wide dark bands (A bands) represent the region of relatively thick parallel-running myosin filaments. The white bands (I bands) represent the region of parallel-running actin filaments. The I band is bisected by a thin dark zone, the Z line. A narrow light region (H zone) bisects the A band. This distance between two Z lines is a *sarcomere*, typically 2 μm long in the resting muscle fiber.

During contraction, opposing actin filaments slide toward each other over the myosin, shortening the sarcomere and causing a narrowing of the I band. Because the bands and lines of each of the thousands of parallel myofibrils within a muscle fiber are adjacent to each other, the banded appearance is also characteristic of the entire muscle fiber.

Calcium Release by the Longitudinal Sarcoplasmic Reticulum (LSR)

Transmission at the neuromuscular junction was described in Chap. 3. Recall that the arrival of impulses at the end plate of the motor neuron causes the release of ACh into the synaptic cleft between the end plate and the folded muscle fiber membrane. This typically produces an end plate potential (EPP) in excess of the excitation threshold, generating impulses which travel over the

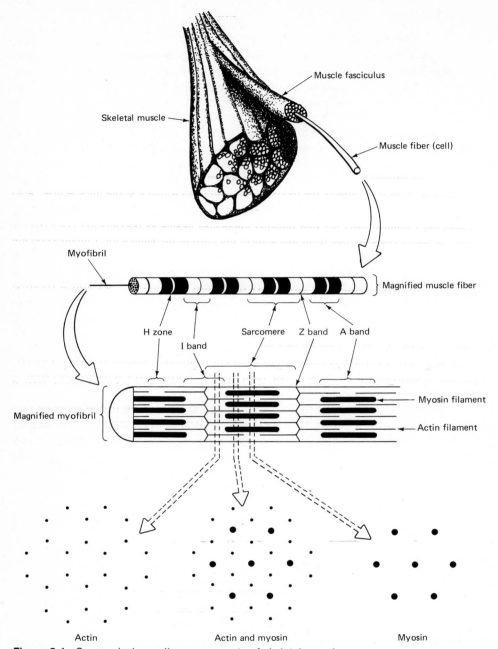

Figure 5-1 Successively smaller components of skeletal muscle.

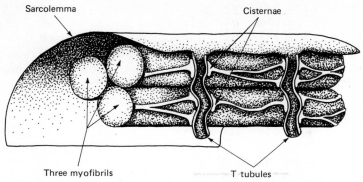

Sarcolemma

Cisternae

Three myofibrils

T tubules

Figure 5-2   A view of three of the thousands of myofibrils within a single muscle fiber. Also shown are two T tubules which pass through the muscle fiber. These channels are continuous with extracellular fluid surrounding the muscle fiber. Lying among the myofibrils, between the T tubules, are Ca^{2+}-rich reticular organelles known as *longitudinal sarcoplasmic reticula* (LSR). The cisternae (enlarged ends of the LSR) lie up against the T tubules and are particularly rich in Ca^{2+}.

muscle fiber membrane and ultimately deep into the muscle fiber and activating the contractile process. Extracellular fluid-filled channels called *T tubules* travel through the muscle fiber at right angles to the surface (Fig. 5-2). In humans these channels typically traverse that part of the muscle fiber where actin and myosin overlap. Among the myofibrils between the T tubules, are Ca^{2+}-rich organelles known as the *longitudinal sarcoplasmic reticula* (LSR). The cisternae (enlarged ends of the LSR near the T tubules) are particularly rich in Ca^{2+} ions (Fig. 5-2).

When impulses are generated on the sarcolemma, they travel over its surface and down the T tubule (Fig. 5-3). The arrival of the impulse in the vicinity of the cisternae causes the sudden (within microseconds) release of large quan-

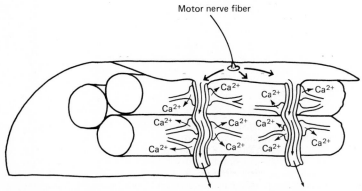

Motor nerve fiber

Figure 5-3   Impulse projection at the neuromuscular junction and the subsequent transmission of an impulse across the sarcolemma down the T tubules, causing the release of Ca^{2+} ions by the cisternae into the myofibrils.

tities of Ca²⁺ ions into the sarcoplasm where the actin and myosin overlap. These free Ca²⁺ ions then contribute toward activating armlike extensions of the myosin filaments, known as *cross-bridges,* which subsequently attach to the actin filaments and slide them inward toward the center of the sarcomere, causing the muscle fiber to shorten. As long as the Ca²⁺ remains in the sarcoplasm, the muscle fiber will remain contracted. Once impulses stop traveling across the sarcolemma, the Ca²⁺ is immediately and actively reabsorbed back into the cisternae and the muscle fiber relaxes.

Myosin Filaments

Each myosin filament is composed of approximately 200 myosin molecules, each of which has a molecular weight of 450,000. Each molecule has a light meromyosin shaft and a heavy meromyosin armlike extension, the cross-bridge (Fig. 5-4). The shaft is formed by two twisted strands of polypeptide which are more or less continuous with two twisted strands in the cross-bridge arm. At

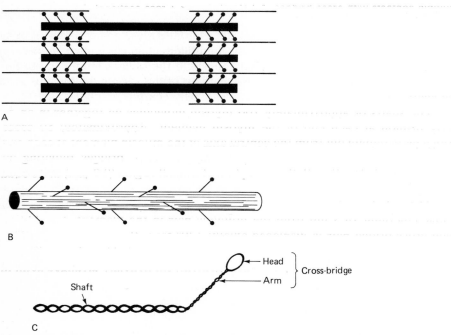

Figure 5-4 Three schematic views of myosin. *A.* Three myosin filaments showing cross-bridge pairs in close approximation to actin filaments on either end. *B.* A section of myosin filament showing cross-bridges radiating out in a regular and orderly fashion. Each cross-bridge pair is displaced axially 120 degrees from the previous pair, placing every third pair in the same spatial plane. *C.* A single myosin molecule. Approximately 200 myosin molecules make up a single myosin filament. Each molecule has a light meromyosin shaft and a heavy meromyosin armlike extension, the cross-bridge. The shaft is formed by two twisted strands of polypeptide which are more or less continuous with two twisted strands in the arm of the cross-bridge. At the top of the arm is a head composed of globular protein.

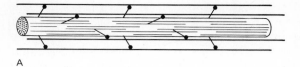

A

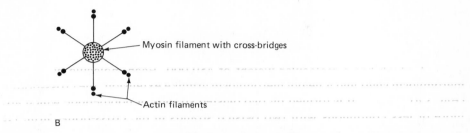

— Myosin filament with cross-bridges

— Actin filaments

B

Figure 5-5 A portion of a myosin filament and six helically arranged actin filaments making multiple contacts with cross-bridges. *A.* Lateral view. *B.* Cross-sectional view.

the tip of the arm is a head composed of globular protein. The heavy meromyosin of the arm and head form the cross-bridge. The cross-bridge is hinged to allow movement between the head and the arm and again between the arm and the shaft.

The shafts of approximately 100 myosin molecules lie together in an orderly fashion at each end of the myosin filament. Approximately 50 cross-bridge pairs radiate out from the central axis of the myosin filament at each end. The myosin filament is about 1.6 μm long with cross-bridges radiating out from most of its length with the exception of a small region (0.2 μm) at its equatorial point.

The radiation of cross-bridge pairs is regular and orderly with each cross-bridge emerging 14.3 nm from the previous pair in the filament. In addition, each cross-bridge pair is displaced axially 120° from the previous pair. Thus every third pair is in the same spatial plane and is separated by a linear distance of 42.9 nm. Because of this spatial arrangement, six helically arranged actin filaments can make multiple contacts with the cross-bridges at each end of the myosin filament (Fig. 5-5).

Actin Filaments

The actin filament is composed of two kinds of actin. These are G actin and F actin. G actin is composed of small protein molecules (molecular weight, 47,000) capped by a molecule of adenosine diphosphate (ADP). This unit complex, about 5.4 nm in length, is polymerized to form a long strand of F actin. An actin filament is formed when two F actin strands are helically twisted together around tropomyosin, which lies in the groove between the two. Troponin, associated with the tropomyosin, configurationally "covers"

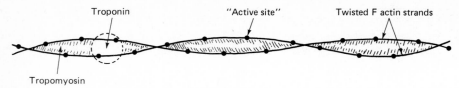

Figure 5-6 A portion of an actin filament. The filament is formed by two F actin strands helically twisted around tropomyosin, which lies between the two. Troponin, associated with the tropomyosin, configurationally "covers" the ADP "active sites" of the F actin strands when the muscle fiber is relaxed. When Ca^{2+} ions are present, the troponin (which has a high affinity for Ca^{2+}) binds with them and undergoes a change which causes the active sites to become uncovered. This allows the heads of the myosin cross-bridges to bind with them.

the ADP sites of the individual G actin molecules when the muscle fiber is relaxed (Fig. 5-6). The ADP sites occurring every 2.7 nm along the actin filament are the active sites to which the heads of the myosin cross-bridges attach. In the resting muscle no attachments are made as the troponin effectively prevents interaction of the two. However, when the muscle fiber is stimulated and Ca^{2+} ions are released by the cisternae, the troponin (which has a high affinity for Ca^{2+} ions) binds with them and is configurationally reoriented so as to

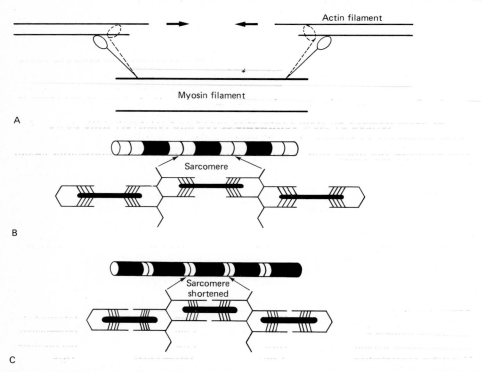

Figure 5-7 Schematic illustration of the contractile process in skeletal muscle. *A.* Two cross-bridges uncocking and sliding actin filaments forward. *B.* A muscle fiber in the relaxed state with sarcomere extended. *C.* A muscle fiber in the contracted state with a shortened sarcomere. Notice that the I band is also shortened when the muscle fiber contracts.

uncover the active ADP sites, allowing the heads of the myosin cross-bridges to bind.

The Contractile Mechanism

In the resting state, the actin and myosin are not in contact because of the interference of the troponin. Thus the sarcomere is at its relaxed 2-μm length. The heads of the cross-bridges are in a "cocked" state, storing potential energy. When the cocked heads bind with the ADP active sites (following Ca^{2+} release), some unknown trigger uncocks the heads, causing them to pivot at their hinges with the arms and sliding the actin filaments inward. The entire arm also pivots slightly (Fig. 5-7).

Sarcoplasmic ATP causes the heads of the cross-bridges to let go of the actin filaments and provides the energy for recocking them. The head of the cross-bridge itself probably provides the adenosine triphosphatase (ATPase) activity for this process. Subsequently the recocked heads bind with other active sites, uncocking them and sliding the actin filaments still further along, and so on. Consequently the sarcomere is shortened with a noticeable decrease in the width of the I band.

THE MOTOR UNIT

Recall that a *motor unit* consists of a motor neuron and the group of skeletal muscle fibers which it innervates. Three types of motor units are found in skeletal muscle. The largest of these are the *type A* motor units, which are characterized by high contractile speed and power. The term largely refers to the relative number of muscle fibers in the motor unit. *Type B* motor units are the smallest and are characterized by slow contractile speed and relatively little power, but a high resistance to fatigue. *Type C* motor units seem to represent a compromise between the other two. They are intermediate in size, contractile speed and power, and susceptibility to fatigue. These and other characteristics of the three types of motor units are listed in Table 5-1.

Table 5-1   Characteristics of Motor Unit Types

Characteristic	Type A	Type B	Type C
Size of motor unit	Large	Small	Intermediate
Size of muscle fiber	Large	Intermediate	Small
Type of muscle fiber	A	B	C
Contraction speed	Fast	Slow	Intermediate
Contraction tension	High	Low	Intermediate
Tetanization frequency	High	Low	Intermediate
Maximum tetanic tension	High	Low	Intermediate
Myoglobin concentration	Low	Intermediate	High
Glycogen concentration	High	Intermediate	Low
Mitochondrial ATPase	Low	Intermediate	High
Capillary supply	Low	Intermediate	High
Resistance to fatigue	Low	High	Intermediate

The specific contraction requirements of a particular muscle determine the type of motor units found in that muscle. Muscles which must produce great tension but are only called on periodically will likely incorporate a high percentage of type A motor units in their organization. Such muscles trade off resistance to fatigue in favor of contractile speed and power. On the other hand, muscles which must support the body against gravity in maintaining the upright posture must be continually active and demonstrate a high resistance to fatigue. Such muscles would be expected to incorporate a high percentage of type B units in their design. Still other muscles need to incorporate the best features of both and include a percentage of type C units along with the others.

A single muscle often contains all three types of motor units. Nevertheless, limb muscles often show a preponderance of type A or type B units and are thus often classified as "fast" (phasic) or "slow" (tonic) muscles, respectively. The gastrocnemius is an example of the former, while the soleus is an example of the latter. In order to appreciate the characteristics of each type of motor unit, let's compare the contractile characteristics of these two muscles.

Properties of the Soleus and Gastrocnemius Muscles of the Cat

The soleus and gastrocnemius muscles are well suited for comparison. While each has a different origin, they insert together into the common tendon of the calcaneus and serve to extend the foot. Nevertheless, their histology and contractile characteristics are quite different, reflecting the tonic role of the soleus in providing continual support of the body against gravity and the more transient role of the gastrocnemius in powering the phasic activities of walking, running, and jumping.

The soleus is a good example of a slow-twitch tonic muscle. Its fibers must be continually active while a person is standing in order to give support against gravity. It plays a similar role in the cat. Consequently it must be resistant to fatigue. Appropriately we find that its fibers contain a large amount of mitochondria, enabling it to easily produce the large amounts of ATP needed to power its continual contractions. Similarly its fibers are amply supplied with capillaries able to saturate the oxygen-carrying pigment myoglobin, which is abundantly found in its type B muscle fibers. This is a necessary feature for the aerobic production of ATP by its mitochondria. The red color of the soleus and other such muscles is due to the color of the myoglobin as well as the blood in the muscle's abundant capillary supply.

Pale muscles such as the gastrocnemius are often noted for periodic strong contractions rather than continual use. They are characterized by larger sarcoplasmic reticula than are found in red muscles such as the soleus. This enables them to release large amounts of Ca^{2+} quickly, producing rapid and strong contractions. Because such muscles lack large amounts of myoglobin, mitochondria, and extensive capillary supplies, their ability to aerobically produce ATP after a period of strong activity is considerably less than that of most red muscles. Hence they are also more susceptible to fatigue. The correlation between color and speed of contraction is not always perfect, however, and the reader should be cautious about thinking of red muscle as being synonymous with slow twitch and pale muscles with fast twitch.

Types of Muscle Fibers

Like motor units, muscle fibers are also classified by type. When muscles are specifically treated to assay them quantitatively for mitochondrial ATPase, three types of fibers can be identified. The largest of these contain relatively few mitochondria, are poorly supplied with capillaries, show little mitochondrial ATPase, contain relatively little myoglobin, and are pale in color. These are *type A muscle fibers*. They correspond to type A motor units. *Type C muscle fibers* represent the opposite extreme. They are the smallest fibers, contain the highest amount of myoglobin, are dark in color, are amply supplied with capillaries, contain many mitochondria, and show the highest ATPase activity. They correspond to type C motor units. *Type B muscle fibers* are intermediate in size, mitochondrial concentration, ATPase activity, capillary supply, and myoglobin concentration. They correspond to type B motor units.

The soleus is composed almost exclusively of type B fibers. The gastrocnemius, on the other hand, contains all three types; however, type A fibers constitute about 50 percent of the fiber population, and because of their relatively large size actually make up about 70 percent of the bulk of the muscle. The rest is composed of type B and type C fibers.

Size and Firing Rate of Motor Unit Neurons

Certain characteristics of motor units are determined by the properties inherent in the motor neuron itself. The motor units in the soleus muscle are innervated by small, slowly conducting alpha motor neurons. On the other hand, the neurons which innervate the large type A muscle fibers of the gastrocnemius muscle are larger and have greater conduction velocities.

The size of the neuron cell body is directly related to the diameter of the conducting fiber. Small-diameter nerve fibers have small cell bodies. Experimentation has shown that the smaller the cell body, the lower the excitation threshold for the production of an action potential. Therefore, the excitability of a neuron is an inverse function of its size, and less input stimulation is subsequently required to fire it. Therefore the participation of a motor unit in a graded muscle activity is dictated by the size of its motor neuron. Now recall that if the firing rate of a neuron depends on the degree to which its central excitatory state (CES) exceeds the excitation threshold (ET), it is not surprising to find that a CES of 30 mV would produce a higher firing rate in a small motor neuron with a low excitation threshold than it would in a larger neuron with a higher threshold (Fig. 5-8).

The number of muscle fibers in a motor unit is also directly related to the size of its motor neuron. Small motor nerve fibers form small motor units and large motor nerve fibers form large motor units. Since small motor neurons fire more frequently than larger neurons because of their relatively greater suscep-

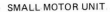

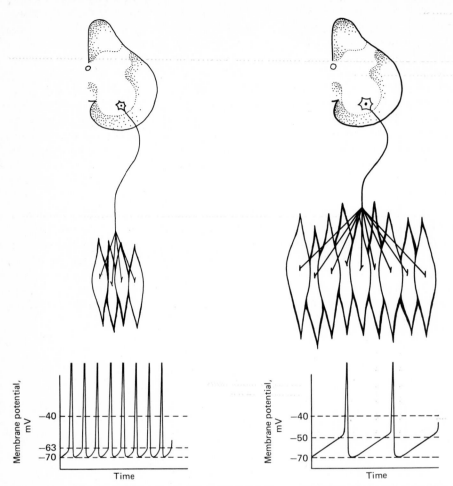

Figure 5-8   The excitability of a motor neuron, and hence the firing of its motor unit, is an in-verse function of its size. Assuming a steady central excitatory state (CES) on the motor neuron of 30 mV, the small motor unit will fire at a faster rate than the large motor unit because it has a lower excitation threshold (−63 mV) than the larger unit (−50 mV). The lower excitation threshold is due to the small size of the motor neuron.

tibility to discharge, it follows that the muscle fibers in these small motor units are more heavily "used" than those associated with larger units. Because of this high firing rate, small motor units must be relatively resistant to fatigue. Therefore it is not surprising to find their overwhelming incorporation into muscles which are often continually active and require high fatigue resistance such as the soleus.

Conversely the gastrocnemius, a phasic muscle, is subject to intermittent bursts of high activity. Its motor units have higher excitation thresholds because of the relatively larger motor neurons innervating its type A muscle fibers. These units will become active only when the input stimulation to the motor neuron pool in the spinal cord reaches a sufficiently high level. Nevertheless, the resting muscle tone found in the gastrocnemius and other such muscles is probably due to the activity in its type B and C motor units, which are more susceptible to firing and thus maintain a steady discharge frequency. Any long-term resistance to fatigue which these muscles possess is also probably due to the activity in its type B and C motor units. There is much evidence that world class long-distance runners have a higher than normal percentage of type B and C motor units in their phasic muscles, enabling them to cover many miles of continuous running without significant muscle fatigue.

Contractile Tension

Large motor units produce more tension than smaller motor units. This is possible because the large units incorporate more muscle fibers than small units. We also know that motor units obey the *all-or-none principle*, which means that if the motor unit fires at all, all of its muscle fibers contract together. Now because all the fibers in a muscle run parallel to each other, the tension produced by each is added to all the others, producing the combined tension of the motor unit. Examination of Fig. 5-9 will show that the contractile tension

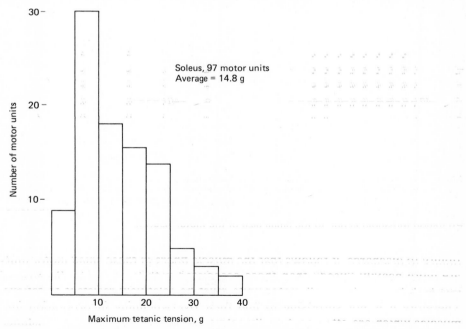

Figure 5-9 Maximal tetanic tensions of 97 soleus motor units, arranged in 5-g groups and plotted against the number of units in each group. (*Drawn from McPhedran, Wuerker, and Henneman, 1965.*)

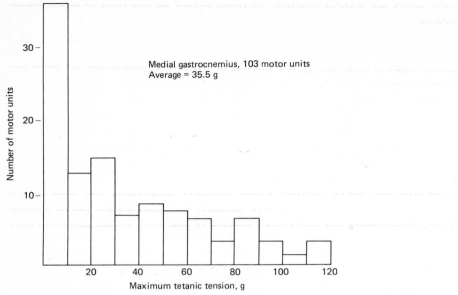

Figure 5-10   Maximal tetanic tensions of 103 medial gastrocnemius motor units, arranged in 10-g groups and plotted against the number of units in each group. (*Drawn from Wuerker, McPhedran and Henneman, 1965.*)

developed by the motor units within a single muscle are not identical. Instead they represent a wide range which gives the muscle a choice of variable tension which it would not otherwise possess.

The maximal tetanic tension of a representative sample of 97 motor units of the soleus muscle are plotted in 5-g groups against the number of units in each group. To obtain the records, a stimulating current was delivered to 97 individual motor nerve fibers in the ventral root of the VIIth lumbar and Ist sacral nerves of the cat. Muscle tension was measured by connecting the soleus muscle in series with a transducer.

Notice that the maximum tension developed by the largest motor units of the soleus was 40 g. The average tension was 14.8 g per unit. Compare this with the higher tension developed by 103 representative motor units from the gastrocnemius muscle when it was similarly examined (Fig. 5-10). In this case the motor units are plotted in 10-g groups against the number of units in each group. As might be expected from the relatively large motor units found in the gastrocnemius muscle, the average tension per unit is higher (35 g per unit) with its largest units producing up to 120 g.

Contractile Speed

Certain characteristics of the motor unit are functions of qualities inherent in the muscle fibers themselves. Nevertheless, the different qualities possessed by muscle fibers are also determined to some extent by the type of nerve fibers which innervate them. During fetal development, at the time of their first innervation, all the limb muscle fibers in mammals are similar in contractile behavior. However, following innervation, each motor unit develops a speed of contraction which is determined by its motor neuron. Fast-twitch muscle fibers are innervated by the large motor neurons, while slow-twitch muscle fibers are innervated by smaller motor neurons.

There seems to be little doubt that the neuron exerts a trophic influence on the development of the muscle fiber. In a telling experiment with 1-day-old kittens, J. C. Eccles showed that the type of motor innervation determines to some extent the speed of muscle contraction which develops. He separated the nerve to one fast-twitch and one slow-twitch muscle of the hind leg. He then reconnected the nerve portion which formerly innervated the slow-twitch muscle to the fast-twitch muscle. He similarly reconnected the nerve portion formerly innervating the fast-twitch muscle to the slow-twitch muscle. After reinnervation had been successfully completed and the kitten had recovered, he noted that the former fast-twitch muscle now contracted more slowly while the former slow-twitch muscle now contracted more quickly. Evidence now indicates that changes in twitch velocity following such reinnervation experiments probably results from alteration in the ATPase activity of the myosin and the rate of Ca^{2+} ion release by the cisternae of the LSR.

Examination of Fig. 5-11 will show that the soleus is a slow-twitch muscle. When the time to the peak of contraction of 81 randomly selected motor units is plotted against the number of units in each 10-ms group, we see that there is a wide range of contraction times within the muscle. The shortest time is 58 ms and the longest is 193 ms, with the greatest number falling between 80 and 90 ms.

The slow-twitch nature of the soleus muscle can be seen when it is compared to the gastrocnemius. When the contraction times of 83 randomly selected gastrocnemius motor units were plotted against the number of units in

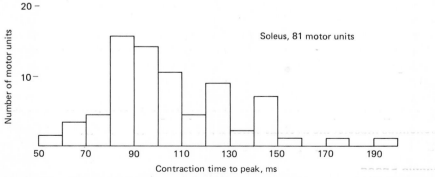

Figure 5-11 Contraction times of 81 soleus motor units arranged in 10-ms groups and plotted against the number of units in each group. (*Drawn from McPhedran, Wuerker and Henneman, 1965.*)

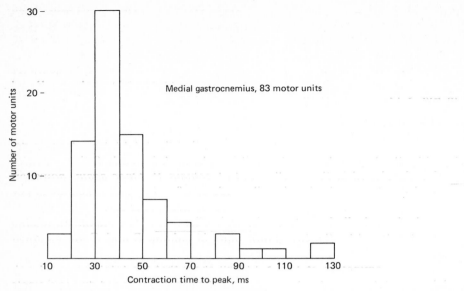

Figure 5-12 Contraction times of 83 medial gastrocnemius motor units arranged in 10-ms groups and plotted against the number of units in each group. (*Drawn from Wuerker, McPhedran, and Henneman, 1965.*)

each 10-ms group, it was observed that they fall into two groups: a large one from 18 to 70 ms and a smaller one from 84 to 129 ms (Fig. 5-12).

There is a relationship between the contraction velocity and the tension developed by a motor unit. As a group, large motor units (those producing the most tension and innervating the greatest number of muscle fibers) contract quickly, while smaller motor units produce less tension and contract more slowly.

Stimulating Frequency Required for Tetanization

If a contracting muscle is stimulated again before it has had a chance to fully relax, a second contraction will fuse with the first, producing tetanus. The minium stimulating frequency necessary to do this depends on the duration of the previous twitch (single contraction in response to a single stimulus). Motor units with brief contraction times (larger units) require a higher stimulating frequency to produce tetanus than do smaller slow-twitch units. In Fig. 5-13 a large and small motor unit from the gastrocnemius of the cat were stimulated repeatedly at 5, 10, 20, 50, and 100 stimuli per second. Notice that the large unit in column A showed little tetanus until the frequency reached 20 per second and didn't develop maximum tension until the frequency reached 100 per second. By comparison, the small motor unit in column B began to tetanize at the relatively low frequency of 10 per second and was nearly maximal at 20 per second. Column C shows the response of a soleus motor unit similar in size to the small gastrocnemius motor unit in column B. Remember that most of the motor units in the gastrocnemius muscle have shorter contraction times than most of the soleus units. It is not surprising to find that the average frequency required for tetanization of the gastrocnemius motor units is greater than we find in the soleus motor units. Nevertheless, the gastrocnemius does contain some small motor units with contraction speeds and tetanization frequencies similar to small units in the soleus. These two are compared in columns B and C in Fig. 5-13.

Maximum Tetanic Tension

A second examination of Fig. 5-13 will show that the total tetanic tension developed by the large soleus motor unit in column A is nearly 8 times greater than that developed in the smaller unit of column B. Once again, however, because the gastrocnemius is primarily made up of motor units which are larger than those found in the soleus, the maximum tentatic tension developed by its motor units is typically larger (not shown in Fig. 5-13). The maximum tetanic tensions developed by the two motor units in column B and C are identical because the size of the motor units is identical.

Further examination of Fig. 5-13 will show that the total tension developed during a tetanic contraction is greater than that developed during a single twitch. The reason for this is not known, but may be due to a less-than-maximum amount of Ca^{2+} release by the LSR during a single twitch. It may require

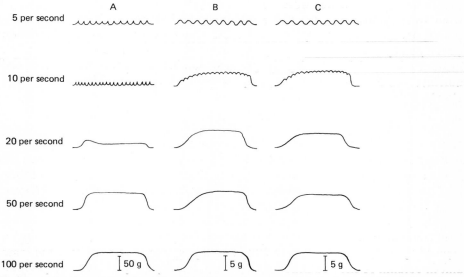

Figure 5-13 Tetanic tensions developed by a large motor unit from the medial gastrocnemius (column A), a small motor unit from the gastrocnemius (column B), and a motor unit from the soleus of approximately the same size as the small gastrocnemius unit (column C). Notice that the large motor unit in column A requires a higher frequency of stimulation in order to tetanize it and it develops a higher maximal tetanic tension than the other units. (*Drawn from Wuerker, McPhedran, and Henneman, 1965.*)

several consecutive twitches to release enough Ca^{2+} to activate all of the cross-bridges and produce maximum tension. The ratio between the twitch tension and the maximum tetanic tension is between 0.2 and 0.25 for both slow- and fast-twitch muscles.

Resistance to Fatigue

An ideal muscle would be able to develop great tension when needed, doing it quickly and smoothly. In addition, it would be able to maintain a high level of activity for prolonged periods of time without fatiguing. Actual muscles exhibit some of these characteristics, but not all of them. Therefore a good-compromise all-purpose muscle is one which contains different types of motor units, each capable of producing one or more of the desired characteristics. As previously noted, muscles which of necessity are used intensely for prolonged periods of time are generally composed of small motor units innervating small muscle fibers rich in myoglobin, mitochondrial ATPase, and capillary supply. They contract slowly and produce minimum tension but can operate for extended periods of time without fatiguing because of their ability to produce large amounts of ATP. Recall also that motor units of such muscles are heavily "used" because of their low excitation thresholds, which produce high firing rates in their motor neurons. Such muscles have clearly had to compromise between contractile speed and power and the need to resist fatigue, choosing the latter as the more important feature for their particular role. The soleus is such a muscle.

Since not all muscles of the body are exclusively involved in tonic or phasic activity, it is not surprising to find that most muscles are a heterogeneous mixture of all three types of motor units, varying the ratio between the types of units in order to achieve the best possible compromise of contractile characteristics suited for their particular range of activities.

Innervation Ratio and Fine Control

A single motor nerve fiber can innervate any number of muscle fibers from one up to several thousand. The innervation ratio represents the number of muscle fibers innervated by a single motor nerve fiber. A small motor unit might have an innervation ratio as low as 10:1. Some of the large motor units of the gastrocnemius have been estimated to be as high as 2000:1. The innervation ratio of its motor units confers certain qualities to a muscle, as we have already seen.

An additional quality not previously examined is the smoothness with which fine increases in tension can be added to a contracting muscle. Muscles primarily composed of small motor units are capable of finer, more gradual changes in contractile tension and thus are capable of finer movements than muscles composed primarily of larger motor units. For example, certain muscles of the fingers have innervation ratios as low as 10:1. This means that if a slight increase in tension is called for in order to perform a certain delicate task, the recruitment of one more motor unit will add the tension of only 10 more muscle fibers. This allows for very fine and controlled increments in tension. This is a very important feature in muscles which are often called upon to perform fine delicate and controlled movements. The trade-off which these muscles make in gaining fine control is the lack of contractile speed and power, features which aren't that important in such muscles anyway.

Compare this with the gastrocnemius muscle of the calf whose largest motor units have innervation ratios as high as 2000:1. Obviously, firing one more motor unit in this muscle adds the combined tension produced by 2000 additional muscle fibers. This obviously increases the overall tension of the muscle but certainly by a less finely controlled increment than in finger muscles. Of course the ability to add large amounts of tension quickly is obviously more important in the gastrocnemius than are finely graded increments of low tension.

Order of Motor Unit Recruitment during a Progressing Muscle Contraction

As a motor act proceeds from little to maximum strength, motor units with precise characteristics are progressively recruited in a logical order. First are the smallest tonic motor units, followed by larger tonic units, and finally by the largest tonic units. Now if the motor act requires fine control only and not a great deal of tension, the recruitment of motor units might stop here. However, if strength is also required, the higher-threshold phasic units are recruited next. Depending on how much strength is required for the particular motor act, appropriate numbers and types of additional phasic motor units will be recruited. Again, the order will be the smallest phasic units (those with the lowest thresholds) followed by larger and finally the largest phasic units.

Recognize that tonic motor units, because of their low tetanization frequencies, can alternate firing to give finely controlled yet long-lasting and smooth contractions at low tension. Thus because of their relatively long twitch durations, some tonic units can begin to relax while others begin to contract while continuing a smoothly maintained level of muscle tension. Phasic units, on the other hand, lack fine control in sustaining smooth contractions because of their short twitch durations, which make tetanus, and hence a smooth alteration of motor unit firings, less likely.

Factors Determining the Final Strength of Contraction

The final strength of any muscle contraction is determined by two factors. The first is the firing rate of the motor units involved, while the second relates to the number and types of units incorporated in the contraction. We have already seen that increasing the firing rate of an individual motor unit will increase the final strength of contraction. Recall that the maximum tetanic tension of a motor unit is considerably greater than the tension produced by a single twitch (Fig. 5-13). It is important to recognize that tetanus in this case is a normal and certainly desirable physiological event adding progressively to the tension developed by the motor unit. We should also recognize that the recruitment of additional motor units adds to the final strength of contraction. Also, because phasic motor units develop higher tension than tonic units, the final strength is partially a function of which type is employed.

REVIEW QUESTIONS

1 A motor neuron and the group of skeletal muscle fibers which it innervates is called a
   a motor unit
   b motor pool
   c neuronal pool
   d discharge group
   e none of the above
2 A single muscle cell is a
   a myofibril
   b fasciculus
   c muscle fiber
   d myofilament
3 The following is (are) true during the contraction of a skeletal muscle:
   a Z lines shorten.
   b Sarcomeres shorten.
   c A bands shorten.
   d I bands shorten.
   e All of the above.
4 Muscle contraction is slightly preceded by
   a calcium ion interaction with light meromyosin
   b calcium ion release by the cisternae of the sarcoplasmic reticula
   c uptake of calcium ions by the sarcoplasmic reticula
   d the release of norepinephrine at the neuromuscular junction
5 The largest motor units
   a have relatively little capillary supply
   b are type B motor units
   c have low myoglobin concentrations
   d have low resistance to fatigue
   e have large muscle fibers
6 The soleus muscle is a good example of
   a a muscle with high fatigue resistance
   b a fast-twitch muscle
   c a tonic muscle
   d a muscle with a low tetanization frequency
   e an antigravity muscle
   f all of the above
7 The smallest muscle fibers
   a are type C muscle fibers
   b contain the least amount of myoglobin
   c are poorly supplied with capillaries
   d have the least ATPase activity
   e correspond to type C motor units

8 If a motor act required skillful manipulation but only a mild degree of contractile tension, it would probably
   a incorporate primarily small tonic units
   b incorporate large phasic units
   c incorporate motor units with a high innervation ratio
   d incorporate primarily low-threshold motor units

9 Motor units with very short contraction times
   a are easily tetanized
   b produce relatively high tetanic tension
   c typically have low resistance to fatigue
   d comprise most of the units in the soleus muscle
   e none of the above

10 All of the following are factors which determine the final strength of a muscle's contraction, *except*
   a the firing rate of the motor units involved
   b the maximum tetanic tension of the motor units involved
   c the number of motor units recruited
   d the type of motor units recruited
   e the number of muscle fibers in the muscle

Chapter 6

Neurophysiology of Movement and Descending Motor Pathways

Sherrington called the motor neuron the final common pathway. All the subtle signals converging from several descending tracts as well as afferent input from the periphery are somehow integrated on the motor neuron, which subsequently conducts the appropriate signal out to the muscle. Because so many different pathways converge on the motor neuron, the contribution of any single tract to the final motor act is extremely difficult to determine.

Several descending pathways have been shown to effect changes in the activity of motor neurons. The anatomical courses of these pathways have been extensively studied from their origins in various areas of the brain to their synaptic contacts with the motor neurons. The precise physiological roles of these pathways have been studied but the information is limited because of several factors. Principal among them is the fact that most of the work has concerned the motor neurons innervating hind limbs of the cat. Studies on primates have been continuing, but a big problem is the somewhat suspect attempt to wed the neurophysiology of the cat's movement performance to the neuroanatomy of the human's.

Another problem lies in the fact that a common tool for studying the function of nerve pathways is electrical stimulation. While there seems to be little alternative to this procedure, the meaningfulness of artificially induced volleys of impulses is questionable when one considers that the natural influences on motor neurons are spatially and temporally varied and probably achieve their effects by virtue of a pattern of impulses rather than a repetitive volley. Recent attempts have been made to study the neurophysiology of movement by recording neuromuscular potentials accompanying spontaneous movement. This is certainly a desirable approach but is also limited by the fact that even simple body movements are neurally very complex. Thus attempts to relate the anatomical and physiological events associated with these movements are difficult and hard to interpret.

Nevertheless, much has been learned concerning the role of the nervous system in such activities as walking, running, and the regulation of postural movements. It now appears that there are "pattern generators" or "prewired" groups of neurons within the central nervous system producing a wide variety of basic motor programs. "Command" neurons activate these pattern generators when a particular movement is called for. In this chapter we will examine some of these pattern generators as well as the role of the brain and its descending pathways in initiating and regulating movement.

UPPER AND LOWER MOTOR NEURONS

Electrophysiological studies have shown that the motor cortex resembles a map showing a distorted image of the body turned upside down and reversed left to right. This organization will be examined in Chap. 16. For the present discussion it is sufficient to know that some motor pathways to the skeletal musculature of the body arise directly from cells within the cerebral motor cortex, while others arise from subcortical areas of the brain and brainstem.

Neurons that originate in the cerebral motor cortex, the cerebellum, or various brainstem nuclei that send axons into the brainstem and spinal cord to activate cranial or spinal motor neurons are called *upper motor neurons*. Those cranial and spinal motor neurons which actually innervate muscles are the *lower motor neurons*. The latter include the alpha and gamma motor neurons of spinal nerves. Upper motor neurons are found entirely within the CNS, while the fibers of lower motor neurons are part of the PNS.

Upper motor neurons are clustered together to form descending tracts in the brain and spinal cord. Such tracts are commonly named according to their site of origin and the region of their distribution. An example is the corticospinal tract, which originates in the cerebral cortex and is distributed to the spinal cord. Another is the rubrospinal tract, which originates in the red nucleus (nucleus ruber) of the midbrain and is distributed to the spinal cord. The lower motor neurons of spinal nerves are somatotopically organized in the anterior horn of the spinal cord gray matter. In general, those innervating the distal limb musculature are located in the lateral aspects of the anterior horn, while those innervating proximal limb muscles are found in the intermediate region. The most medial group of motor neurons innervates the musculature of the appendicular and pelvic girdles.

PATTERN GENERATORS AND THE CENTRAL PROGRAM
FOR MOVEMENT

Upper motor neurons don't simply stimulate lower motor neurons and produce movement. The highly skilled and coordinated movements of which humans are capable would seem to require a more complex and involved system. While little is known of the highly involved and integrated activity which occurs in the brain's neural circuits during even a simple body movement, it now appears that highly coordinated and very complex systems of interneurons regulate the precise timing and sequencing of muscle activity which is observed in such movements. There is also increasing evidence that groups of interneurons cause specific patterns of impulses to fire in the lower motor neurons associated with a given coordinated movement. The central theory is that these interneurons form *pattern generators* within the CNS which produce the basic motor program. At the spinal cord level the pattern generator is composed of a set of local control centers located in the gray matter. There are neurons within these centers which coordinate muscular synergies and generate timing signals. *Command neurons* activate these pattern generators when a particular coordinated movement is required. The result of such activation is that the lower motor neurons fire in a properly sequenced and timed pattern to produce a coordinated movement.

Identification of specific command neurons for a particular human movement is a difficult process and a speculative one at best. It may be that upper motor neurons from the brain and brainstem function in this respect for voluntary movements and reflex postural adjustments. In some invertebrates, however, the activation of a single interneuron is sufficient to excite an entire coordinated muscle behavior. For example, stimulation of the giant axon of the crayfish produces a coordinated tail flip which propels it away from the stimulus. Similarly, stimulation of the Maunther cells of teleost fishes produces a tail flip propelling the fish away from the stimulus. These cells are part of the reticulospinal tract neurons in the fish and apparently serve as command neurons that activate the pattern generator which carries the motor program for tail flip.

It is presumptuous to assume that all movements proceed in accordance with pattern generators and prewired motor programs. Nevertheless, it may be that certain basic coordinated movements of the limbs and trunk may proceed in a very general way under the influence of such programs, while the initiation and fine tuning of the movement requires input from descending and sensory pathways. The upper motor neurons of some descending motor pathways no doubt serve as command neurons for certain movement patterns. Variations in the discharge patterns of these neurons determines the variability of the programmed response. There is evidence that a change in the firing frequency of certain command neurons leads to a change in the intensity of the response. If the coordinated movement involves a postural system, altering the firing rate alters the magnitude of postural adjustment. If a locomotor system is involved, the frequency of the movement cycle will vary with changes in the frequency of command neuron firing. Other command neurons produce the same motor pattern regardless of their firing rates. Their role seems to be simply turning the program on and off. Still others may regulate the magnitude of the programmed response. Most of the vertebrate work involving motor programs has dealt with locomotor activity in the cat. Perhaps we can get a feel for the intricate features of such programs by an examination of this work.

Locomotion in the Mesencephalic Cat

Removal of the telencephalon (cerebral hemispheres) and the rostral portion of the thalamus in an acute cat preparation remarkably leaves the animal with practically normal locomotion. It can walk spontaneously on its own and it can be forced to run by electrical stimulation of a region in the subthalamus called the *subthalamic locomotor region* (SLR). However, spontaneous walking movements cease in acute preparations where the brainstem is sectioned caudal to the subthalamus but just rostral to the midbrain. This is a *mesencephalic preparation*, meaning the highest intact brain component is the midbrain or mesencephalon. There are several advantages to the study of locomotion in such a preparation. Perhaps most important is that relatively normal locomotor movements can be initiated by the electrical stimulation of an area in the tectum of the midbrain called the *mesencephalic locomotor region* (MLR). Such a cat preparation can also be placed on a treadmill to facilitate natural movements while its head is fixed in a stereotaxic apparatus enabling the experimenter to conveniently stimulate various brainstem areas and observe the results (Fig. 6-1).

Walking and running movements in a mesencephalic cat are similar to those observed normally. A single *step cycle* is accomplished when a limb touches down, lifts off and moves forward, and then touches down again. The step cycle is composed of a stance phase (limb in contact with the ground) and a

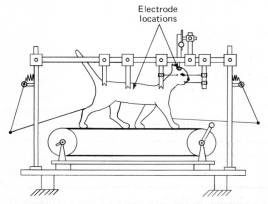

Electrode
locations

Figure 6-1   Experimental setup for evaluating locomotion in the mesencephalic or subthalamic cat. The cat is fixed in a stereotaxic device with its limbs on a treadmill. Electrodes are inserted into the brainstem and spinal cord for stimulating and recording. Limb movements are recorded by a potentiometric transducer. (*Drawn from Shik, Severin, and Orlovsky, 1966.*)

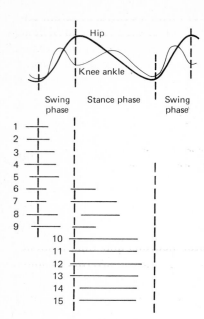

Figure 6-2 Illustration showing the joint movements and muscular activity of the mesencephalic cat during locomotion produced by mesencephalic locomotor region (MLR) stimulation. Curves deflect upward when joints are flexing. Muscles illustrated are: (1) rectus femoris; (2) tensor fasciaelatae; (3) tibialis anterior; (4) extensor digitorum longus; (5) iliopsoas; (6) biceps pars posterior; (7) gracilis; (8) sartorius; (9) semitendinosus; (10) soleus; (11) gastrocnemius, plantaris; (12) vastus; (13) adductor, semimembranosus; (14) biceps pars anterior; (15) gluteus. (*Drawn from Gambaryan, Orlovsky, Protopopova, Severin, and Shik, 1971.*)

swing phase (limb lifted off and moving forward). Muscle group activity during the step cycle proceeds in a logical order. At the end of the stance phase, when the limb is at its most caudal position, the flexors become active, lifting the leg and initiating the swing phase. During the swing phase, the relaxation of the flexors combined with onset of extensor activity and inertia all propel the limb forward. Because the extensors begin to contract prior to the stance phase, the limb is able to support the weight of the body as the limb touches down. Extensor activity continues throughout the stance phase until just at the end, when it begins to diminish and is replaced by increasing flexor activity preceding another step cycle (Fig. 6-2).

Increasing the stimulation of the MLR causes an increase in the stepping frequency of the mesencephalic cat. However, this increased frequency is apparently due to an increased muscular force moving the treadmill faster with the rate of stepping increasing indirectly to keep up with it. The increased force is apparently due to the increased recruitment of more alpha motor neurons and motor units rather than to any increase in the firing rates of the currently active units. Thus MLR stimulation directly increases the level of muscular force and indirectly the stepping frequency. If the level of MLR stimulation is held constant and the treadmill is either speeded up or slowed down by the experimenter, the stepping frequency of the mesencephalic cat will speed up or slow down accordingly.

It is very interesting to note that while stepping is a complex process involving a repetitive sequence of muscular contractions and relaxations with very precise timing, all that is necessary to get it started is to stimulate the MLR in the mesencephalic cat or the SLR in the subthalamic cat. Thus it seems likely that stepping is an automatic process with a central program controlled by a pattern generator in the CNS. Stimulation of the MLR and SLR activates this program and can in fact vary its intensity. The pattern generator for stepping with the hind limbs of the cat appears to reside in the spinal cord. In chronic cat preparations where the lower thoracic spinal cord was completely sectioned shortly after birth, the animals are capable of a full variety of stepping gaits in accordance with the speed of the treadmill. Thus it seems likely that the pattern generator resides in the spinal cord, at least for hind limb movements. Transection of the spinal cord at a high enough level to include the forelimbs (high cervical) does not ordinarily allow for satisfactory locomotor movements, and thus has not been adequately evaluated in this regard.

Input to the Pattern Generator

Signals arrive at the pattern generator in the spinal cord both from the periphery and from supraspinal levels. The Ia afferents from muscle spindles monosynaptically stimulate homonymous alpha motor neurons and thus influence the activity of an ongoing motor program. Similarly, signals arriving at spinal cord interneurons from supraspinal levels via upper motor neurons also exert an influence over the performance of a motor program.

It is important to note that the stretch reflex is not always productively useful at all times during the step cycle. Thus it is not surprising to find that the sensitivity of the reflex is varied cyclically with the step. It is "tuned in" when the reflex is useful and "tuned out" when activation of the reflex would be counterproductive to a particular phase of the step cycle. Muscle spindle sensitivity can be controlled by the pattern generator since it can apparently direct the timing of both alpha and gamma motor neuron firing. Thus during the phase of the stepping cycle when a muscle is passively stretched (i.e., the gastrocnemius at the end of the stance phase) the sensitivity of its muscle spindles is decreased. This prevents the stretch reflex from activating muscle contraction during the "wrong" phase. Thus the spindles are "tuned out" when the muscle is passively stretched and "tuned in" again when the muscle becomes active during the step cycle. Let's now examine the descending motor pathways which influence motor activity.

DESCENDING MOTOR PATHWAYS

Descending motor pathways are defined as those which initiate or modify performance and which originate in the brain. While several tracts have been anatomically identified and physiologically studied, it is still speculative to assume that we fully understand what contribution any given tract makes to a spontaneous movement. To electrically stimulate a descending tract, observe a movement response, and then assume that the observed response represents the function of the tract is surely dangerous. The tract may have other, perhaps more important, functions to perform which are not observed in the movement. Or possibly the participation of the tract in a spontaneous movement of the same kind may be of considerably different magnitude. Nevertheless, stimulation of descending motor pathways does produce activity in groups of flexor and extensor muscles. Examination of these effects may give us valuable clues as to the role of these pathways in normal spontaneous movement.

The Corticospinal Tracts

The corticospinal tracts are often called the *pyramidal tracts* because they form pyramid-shaped enlargements on the anterior surface of the medulla. They are primarily concerned with controlling skilled movements of the distal extremities and, in particular, facilitation of those alpha and gamma motor neurons which innervate the distal flexor muscles (Fig. 6-3). There is also evidence that they inhibit distal extensor muscles. The upper motor neurons of these tracts originate in the precentral gyrus of the cerebral cortex. From here their fibers pass without synapsing all the way to their terminal destinations in the spinal cord gray matter. After leaving the cortex, the fibers descend through the posterior limb of the internal capsule (Fig. 16-4), through the middle portion of the cerebral peduncles to the basilar portion of the pons, and on into the medulla oblongata where they form the medullary pyramids. Most of the fibers (85 percent) cross over (decussate) to the opposite side in the pyramidal decussation, where they continue to descend in the lateral funiculus of the spinal cord as the *lateral corticospinal tract* (LCST). The tract descends all the way to sacral levels with fibers continually leaving it in order to synapse on interneurons in laminae IV, V, VI, VII, and VIII. Some even synapse directly on alpha and gamma motor neurons in lamina IX (Fig. 6-3). Those corticospinal fibers which do not decussate in the medulla continue descending on the same (ipsilateral) side of the cord and become the *anterior corticospinal tract* (ACST). This tract does not extend below the midthoracic level. Fibers leave the tract at various levels to cross over in the anterior white commissure to synapse on interneurons in lamina VIII.

Corticospinal Stimulation of Motor Neurons   Electrical stimulation of the cortical areas from which the corticospinal tracts arise excites many more motor neurons to distal forelimb muscles in the baboon than it does motor neurons to proximal muscles. In fact, proximal limb muscles are frequently not activated at all by cortical stimulation. The more dextrous the distal muscles are, the greater effect the corticospinal tracts seem to have on their activity. Following cortical stimulation, larger EPSPs are seen in the motor neurons to skilled distal flexors than are observed in proximal muscle motor neurons.

Destruction of the Corticospinal Tracts   Studies have shown that following complete bilateral pyramidal tract section in monkeys, they are still able to perform a wide range of activities using the body and limbs and are able to walk and climb in a normal manner. Their principal and most dramatic shortcoming is in their ability to perform skillful manipulative tasks with the fingers and hands. In similar tests of manipulative skills in monkeys with unilateral

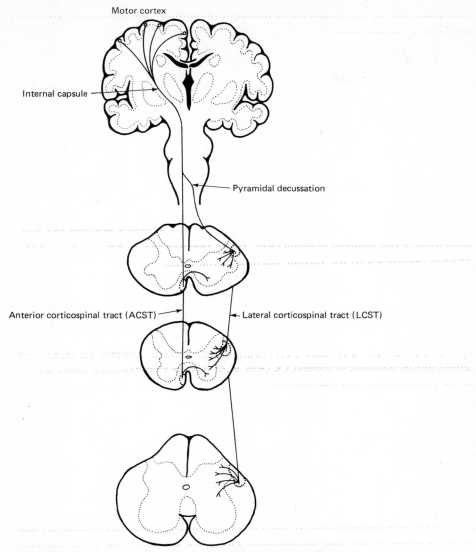

Figure 6-3 Diagram showing the course of the corticospinal (pyramidal) tracts. Lateral corticospinal tract fibers are distributed to all levels of the spinal cord synapsing primarily on interneurons in laminae IV to VIII. Some even synapse directly on alpha and gamma motor neurons in lamina IX. Fibers of the anterior corticospinal tract cross to the opposite side in the anterior white commissure to synapse on interneurons in lamina VIII.

pyramidal tract sections, it was found that skilled movements in the affected hand were dramatically reduced relative to the normal hand. However, the animals were still able to move the whole limb around the joints of the pectoral and pelvic girdles with no trouble and they showed no difficulty in performing

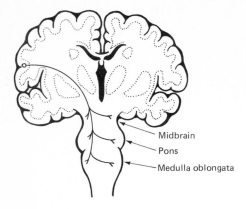

Midbrain

Pons

Medulla oblongata

Figure 6-4 The distribution of cortico-bulbar tract fibers. Fibers originate in the precentral gyrus of the lower quarter of the motor cortex. They descend through the internal capsule with fibers of the corticospinal tract to terminate in the motor nuclei of cranial nerves III and IV in the midbrain; V, VI, and VII in the pons; and IX, X, XI, and XII in the medulla oblongata. The fibers of this tract project bilaterally.

combined movements of the limbs and the body. Thus it seems probable that the corticospinal system is directed effectively to facilitating movements requiring skill and dexterity of the distal musculature.

The Corticobulbar Tract

This tract is composed of fibers originating in the precentral gyrus of the lower quarter of the motor cortex. The descending fibers leave the motor cortex and pass through the posterior limb of the internal capsule just anterior and medial to the corticospinal tract fibers. From here they continue on through the cerebral peduncles just medial to the corticospinal tract fibers to terminate in the motor nuclei of cranial nerves III and IV in the midbrain; V, VI, and VII in the pons; and IX, X, XI, and XII in the medulla. The corticobulbar fibers from one side of the brain project to the motor nuclei on both sides of the brainstem (Fig. 6-4).

The Rubrospinal Tract

The fibers of this tract originate in the red nucleus (nucleus ruber) of the midbrain. They cross over near their point of origin and descend contralaterally in the lateral funiculus of the cord adjacent to the lateral corticospinal tract (Fig. 6-5). Before leaving the brainstem, some fibers of the tract enter the reticular formation. As the tract descends through the spinal cord, fibers leave it and synapse on interneurons in laminae V, VI, and VII. Cells in the posterior portion of the red nucleus give rise to axons influencing motor neurons of the neck and upper limbs, while fibers from the anterior portion descend to lumbar levels where they influence lower limb muscles.

Ablation studies in which the tracts are experimentally cut have shown that the corticospinal and rubrospinal tracts have somewhat similar effects on the motor neurons. When the rubrospinal tracts of monkeys were damaged on top of earlier pyramidal tract sections, the loss of skilled control of the distal musculature became even more severe and yet there was little or no loss of control in the proximal muscles. Lawrence and Kuypers concluded that a later-

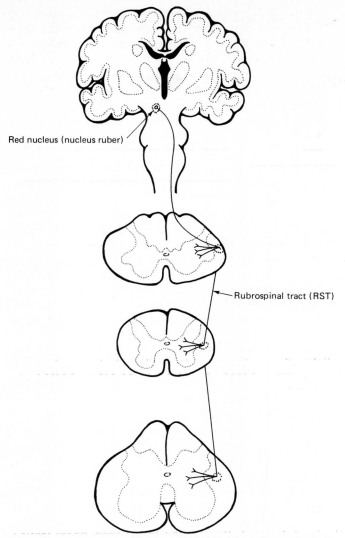

Red nucleus (nucleus ruber)

Rubrospinal tract (RST)

Figure 6-5 The course of rubrospinal tract fibers. The fibers of this tract originate in the red nucleus (nucleus ruber) of the midbrain. They cross over near their point of origin and descend contralaterally in the lateral funiculus to synapse upon interneurons in laminae V, VI, and VII at all cord levels.

ally placed group of descending fibers, which they called the lateral system (corticospinal, rubrospinal, and possibly other tracts), is primarily concerned with delivering cortical control to the distal limb musculature. Independent electrical stimulation of the intact rubrospinal tract facilitates flexor and inhibits extensor alpha and gamma motor neurons to the distal muscles.

Considering that the red nucleus receives input from the same area of the cerebral cortex as the corticospinal tracts, the similarity of their actions may not be too surprising. The red nucleus also receives input from the deep cerebellar nuclei and possibly the basal nuclei as well. Nevertheless, as previously pointed out, the reader should bear in mind that ablation and electrical stimulation studies give us an incomplete picture of the function of a descending, or for that matter any, tract in the central nervous system. Further, whatever information is obtained relates to the unnatural experimental situation and not necessarily to normal function in the intact spontaneous animal.

The Reticulospinal Tracts

The reticular formation is an indistinct group of cell bodies clustered in the core of the brainstem. They don't form distinct nuclear groups like those found elsewhere in the CNS. The reticulospinal tracts represent groups of fibers which originate in the reticular formation and descend into the spinal cord (Fig. 6-6). Those fibers which originate in the medullary reticular formation show both a crossed and an uncrossed component which descend in the lateral funiculus of the spinal cord as the *lateral reticulospinal tract* (LRST). The descending fibers in this tract periodically leave and synapse principally on interneurons in lamina VII. Those fibers arising chiefly in the pontine reticular formation represent the *medial reticulospinal tract* (MRST). Fibers in this tract descend ipsilaterally in the anterior funiculus to all levels of the cord, periodically leaving to synapse in laminae VII and VIII.

The reticulospinal tracts exert both somatic and autonomic control. The somatic control involves both facilitation and inhibition of alpha and gamma motor neurons at all cord levels. Some cells in the medulla and medullary reticular formation (the inhibitory center of Magoun and Rhines) exert a strong inhibitory effect through the reticulospinal tracts on all types of alpha and gamma motor neurons. On the other hand, cells in the upper medullary and pontine reticular formation exert a strong facilitatory effect on alpha and gamma motor neurons. Accordingly, the idea of an "inhibitory" and "excitatory" center in the brainstem has been postulated. It may be that many of the modulating effects of the cerebral cortex and the cerebellum are mediated through these "centers" since both feed into the reticular formation.

The reticulospinal tracts influence autonomic effects through their influence on preganglionic neurons in the intermediolateral horn of the spinal cord gray matter. Most of these fibers are derived from the lateral reticulospinal tract with a smaller number coming from the medial reticulospinal tract. It is undoubtedly simplistic to assume that the reticulospinal tracts are the only descending tracts regulating autonomic control. Some fibers of the corticospinal and vestibulospinal tracts have also been implicated.

The Vestibulospinal Tracts

The vestibulospinal tracts originate in the vestibular nuclei of the brainstem. Those fibers originating in the lateral vestibular (Deiter's) nucleus descend ipsilaterally in the anterior funiculus and form the *lateral vestibulospinal tract*

Deiter's Nucleus

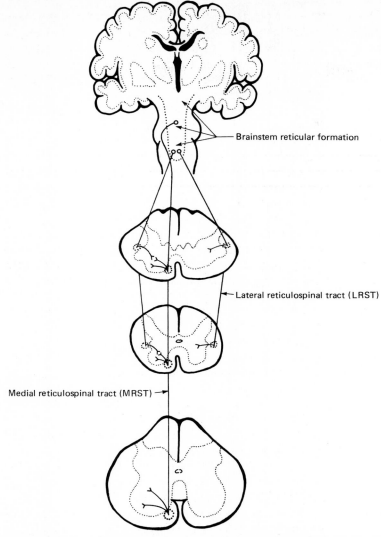

Brainstem reticular formation

Lateral reticulospinal tract (LRST)

Medial reticulospinal tract (MRST)

Figure 6-6   The distribution of reticulospinal tract fibers. The lateral reticulospinal tracts originate in the medullary reticular formation and descend bilaterally in the lateral funiculi to synapse in laminae VII. The medial reticulospinal tracts arise chiefly in the pontine reticular formation and descend in the anterior funiculi to synapse in laminae VII and VIII.

(LVST) (Fig. 6-7). The fibers of this tract terminate in laminae VII, VIII, and IX at all levels of the cord. The vestibulospinal tracts facilitate extensor and inhibit flexor alpha and gamma motor neurons. Input from the vestibular apparatus to the vestibular nuclei via cranial nerve VIII presupposes an antigravity or postural role for the lateral vestibulospinal tract. Activity in this tract is also influenced by input to the vestibular nuclei from the cerebellum. Arising from

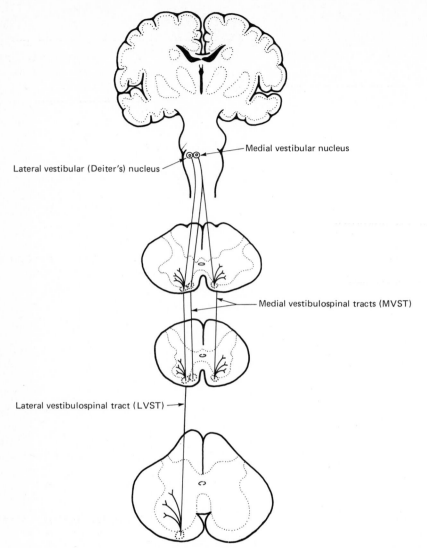

Lateral vestibular (Deiter's) nucleus

Medial vestibular nucleus

Medial vestibulospinal tracts (MVST)

Lateral vestibulospinal tract (LVST)

Figure 6-7 The course of vestibulospinal tract fibers. Both crossed and uncrossed fibers descend from the medial vestibular nucleus as the medial vestibulospinal tracts. They descend in the anterior funiculi and their fibers synapse in laminae VII, VIII, and IX. The lateral vestibulospinal tract is composed of uncrossed fibers which descend from the lateral vestibular (Deiter's) nucleus to synapse in laminae VII, VIII, and IX.

the medial vestibular nucleus are the fibers of the *medial vestibulospinal tract* (MVST). While there is a small crossed component, most of its fibers descend ipsilaterally only as far as the midthoracic cord, where they too synapse in laminae VII, VIII, and IX. The function of this tract may be similar to that of the lateral vestibulospinal tract, but its precise role is largely unknown.

Interstitiospinal Tract

The descending fibers of this tract arise in the interstitial nucleus of Cajal (an accessory nucleus of III) in the tegmentum of the midbrain. They descend ipsilaterally only to the cervical level of the cord, where they synapse in laminae VI, VII, and VIII. The tract may play a role in reflex movements of the head and neck in response to visual stimuli, but its function is largely unknown and probably more complex.

Tectospinal Tract

The descending fibers of this tract arise chiefly in the tectum of the superior colliculus. Some of them decussate and others don't. In either case they only descend to cervical levels where they synapse in laminae VI, VII, and VIII. The tract has been implicated in mediating visual reflexes but, again, its function is largely unknown.

REVIEW QUESTIONS

1 Corticospinal tract neurons can be classified as
   a   upper motor neurons
   b   sensory fibers
   c   motor fibers
   d   pyramidal tract fibers
2 The highest intact brain region in a mesencephalic preparation is
   a   the midbrain
   b   the thalamus
   c   the medulla oblongata
   d   the pons
3 According to a current theory concerning basic motor programs such as walking, their timing and sequencing are coordinated by
   a   stretch reflexes
   b   behavior patterns
   c   step cycles
   d   descending motor pathways
   e   pattern generators
4 A complete bilateral pyramidal tract section in monkeys
   a   renders the animals unable to walk and climb
   b   renders them unable to perform skillful manipulative tasks with the fingers and hands
   c   renders them unable to move the whole limb around the joints of the pectoral and pelvic girdles
   d   causes total paralysis of the skeletal muscles
   e   produces no noticeable motor deficiencies
5 Rubrospinal tract fibers
   a   from the posterior portion of the nucleus ruber influence lower limb muscles
   b   primarily originate in the contralateral red nucleus

    c   when sectioned, produce responses similar to corticospinal (pyramidal) tract section

    d   are included in what Lawerence and Kuypers call the *lateral system*

    e   when electrically stimulated, facilitate extensor and inhibit flexor alpha and gamma motor neurons to the distal muscles

6   Reticulospinal tract fibers

    a   exert both somatic and autonomic control

    b   originating in the medullary reticular formation form the ipsilateral anterior reticulospinal tract

    c   originating in the medulla and medullary reticular formation exert a strong inhibitory effect on alpha and gamma motor neurons

    d   originating in the upper medullary and pontine reticular formation exert a strong facilitatory effect on alpha and gamma motor neurons

7   Lateral vestibulospinal tract fibers

    a   facilitate extensor and inhibit flexor alpha and gamma motor neurons

    b   originate in the medial vestibular nucleus

    c   arise primarily from a contralateral vestibular nucleus

    d   descend only to the midthoracic level

    e   all of the above

8   Each of the following motor tracts descend to all cord levels, *except*

    a   the lateral corticospinal tract

    b   the anterior corticospinal tract

    c   the corticobulbar tract

    d   the anterior reticulospinal tract

    e   the interstitiospinal tract

9   In acute cat preparations, the animal loses all spontaneous walking movements when

    a   the motor cortex is destroyed

    b   the telencephalon (cerebral hemispheres) is removed

    c   the brainstem is sectioned caudal to the subthalamus but rostral to the midbrain

    d   the telencephalon and rostral portion of the thalamus are removed

10   Lower motor neurons

    a   are found entirely within the CNS

    b   include the alpha and gamma motor neurons of the spinal nerves

    c   have their cell bodies located in the brainstem and spinal cord

    d   originate in the cerebellum

    e   are part of the peripheral nervous system

    f   none of the above

Receptors

The central nervous system is kept continually informed of the ever-changing external and internal environment of the body by way of centrally directed signals which arise in its many and varied receptors. These receptors report on a wide variety of sensory modalities including changes in temperature, pressure, touch, sound, light, taste, smell, body and limb movements, and even blood pressure and chemistry. Scientists have recognized for almost 100 years that certain afferent nerve fibers of the peripheral nervous system are in contact with specialized nonneural receptive structures which detect and transmit sensory information from the periphery to the CNS. The nonneural receptive structure together with its afferent nerve fiber is often called a *receptor*.

Nature has evolved a variety of morphological structures which function as receptors. The earliest studies of sensation led to the idea that each morphological receptor type was responsible for the transduction of a particular modality of sensation. This early hypothesis has been modified in light of evidence that receptors respond to more than one type of stimuli.

CLASSIFICATION OF RECEPTORS BY ADEQUATE STIMULI

An *adequate stimulus* is that form of stimulation to which a receptor has the lowest threshold. For example, a certain type of receptor will respond to a slight mechanical displacement by increasing the impulse firing rate in its afferent nerve fiber. The same receptor may also respond when subjected to extreme temperature changes. However, if it has a lower threshold for mechanical than for thermal changes, it is classified as a mechanoreceptor and not a thermoreceptor. Accordingly, receptors are often classified as follows:

Receptor type	Adequate stimulus
Mechanoreceptors	Mechanical displacement
Thermoreceptors	Temperature change
Nociceptors	Pain
Chemoreceptors	Chemicals
Photoreceptors	Light

Recognize that this classification does not mean that the adequate stimulus is the only stimulus to which a particular receptor will respond. It simply says that the receptor has the lowest threshold for (is most easily simulated by) the adequate stimulus.

Mechanoreceptors, thermoreceptors, and nociceptors in cutaneous, subcutaneous, and deep connective tissue are collectively called *somatosensory receptors*. While the morphological endings of many of these are unknown, the remainder are classified as either free endings, endings with expanded tips, or encapsulated endings (Fig. 7-1).

Free nerve endings represent receptors with no nonneural element. Instead, the afferent fibers simply end in bare terminals which are directly suscep-

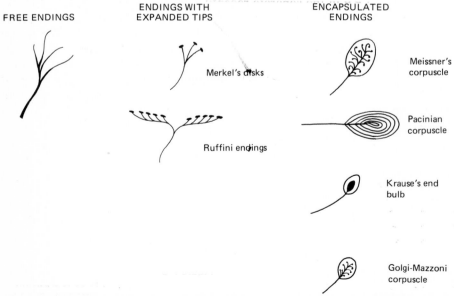

Figure 7-1 The basic types of nerve endings found in cutaneous, subcutaneous, and deep connective tissue.

tible to stimulation. Similarly, endings with expanded tips such as Merkel's disks and Ruffini endings are all neural structures which respond directly to adequate stimulation. However, receptors with encapsulated endings are characterized by a nonneural element surrounding the afferent endings of the nerve fibers. In receptors of this type the adequate stimulus must first be transduced through the nonneural capsule to the endings of the afferent nerve fiber.

THE NATURE OF THE RECEPTOR POTENTIAL

When a stimulus is applied to a receptor, it may or may not be strong enough to elicit impulse production in the afferent nerve fiber. The application of the stimulus causes the membrane of the receptor cell to depolarize, producing a *receptor potential* (RP). If the receptor potential reaches the excitation threshold of the nerve fiber membrane, the fiber will generate impulses. Further, as long as the receptor potential is maintained above the excitation threshold, impulses will continue to travel down the fiber away from the receptive element. A distinction can be made between receptors in which the receptive element is a specialized ending of the nerve fiber sharing a continuous membrane and receptors in which the receptive element is a separate structure not continuous with the membrane of the nerve fiber. In the former (*one-element*) receptor, the RP established in the receptive element produces impulses in the adjacent membrane by depolarizing this membrane with electrotonic currents. In the latter (*two-element*) receptor the RP is generated in the separate receptive element, which in turn stimulates and produces impulses in the afferent nerve fiber. The mechanism by which a RP in the separate receptive element does this is not well understood. It may be that the close proximity of the two allows for a current spread between them or, as is suspected in some cases, a chemical transmitter may be released from the receptive element to the afferent nerve fiber.

When not being stimulated, the membrane potential of the receptor is resting and polarized. However, when a stimulus is applied and its strength is steadily increased, the receptor membrane begins to depolarize and a RP is established (Fig. 7-2).

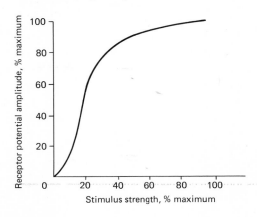

Figure 7-2 The relationship between the strength of stimulus applied to a pacinian corpuscle in the cat mesentery and the receptor potential developed. (*Drawn from Loewenstein, 1961.*)

It is thought that the receptor potential is produced by changes in the ionic current across the membrane of the receptive element. The depolarization phase of the receptor potential is very likely caused by the inward diffusion of Na^+ ions. Repolarization is less well understood but is probably caused by ionic changes also. The receptor potential increases as a function of the stimulus strength and is therefore graded. However, it must be understood that Fig. 7-2, which shows the relationship between the two, is based on a pacinian corpuscle from the cat mesentery and does not represent all types of receptors. Mathematical attempts have been made to predict the receptor potential from the strength of the stimulus but have thus far been inaccurate when applied to different types of receptors.

Receptor Potentials and Impulse Generation

It is important to understand that in an afferent neuron which conducts impulses following stimulation of its receptive element, the impulses are not generated in the receptive element itself. Instead, they are initiated at some point central to the receptor. Only the receptor potential is initiated in the receptive element. In one-element receptors like the pacinian corpuscle illustrated in Fig. 7-3, the trigger for the production of impulses is the spread of an electrotonic current from the receptive element to the "active zone" of the nerve fiber just central to the receptor.

When a slight mechanical displacement is applied to the corpuscle of the receptor, changes in ionic conduction occur in the membrane of the afferent fiber within it, depolarizing its membrane and producing a small receptor potential. The RP generates a small electrotonic current which spreads a short distance down the fiber central to the point of stimulation. No impulses are recorded in the afferent fiber, however, as the electrotonic current is too small to reach and subsequently depolarize the "active zone" (first node of Ranvier). However, as the strength of the applied stimulus is systematically increased, the size of the RP and thus the electrotonic current increases also. When the current is sufficiently strong to not only reach but also depolarize the membrane of the first node to the excitation threshold, an action potential is generated at the node which propagates by ordinary saltatory conduction down the length of the fiber. Further, the first node continues to produce action potentials and generate impulses as long as the membrane of the first node remains above the excitation threshold. Notice that impulses are not generated in the same region of the receptor that produces the receptor potential. Thus it is commonly said that the receptor potential is a graded but nonpropagated event, while the action potential is nongraded but propagated. Nerve fibers continue to conduct impulses as long as the stimulus is applied and the excitation threshold of the active zone is exceeded. The firing rate depends on the magnitude of the receptor potential (Fig. 7-4), which itself depends on the strength of the applied stimulus.

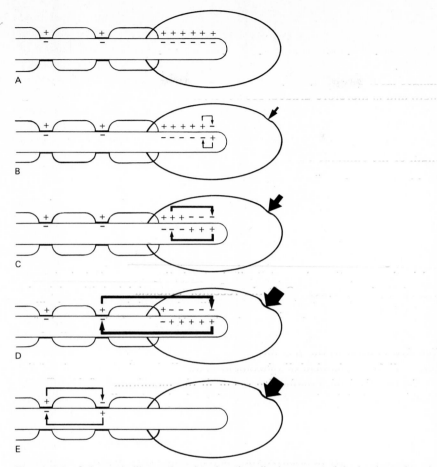

Figure 7-3 Schematic illustration showing that displacement of the laminated pacinian corpuscle ultimately produces impulses in the myelinated afferent nerve fiber. No impulses are
generated until the receptor potential is large enough to produce an electrotonic current
which reaches (and subsequently depolarizes) the first node of Ranvier to the excitation
threshold. *A.* No displacement, no receptor potential, no electronic current, no impulse conduction. *B.* Slight displacement, small receptor potential, weak electronic current, no impulse
conduction. *C.* Greater displacement, larger receptor potential, stronger electronic current,
no impulse conduction. *D.* Still greater displacement, larger receptor potential, stronger electronic current, first node begins to depolarize, no impulse conduction. *E.* Action potential
produced at first node, impulse conduction.

Adaptation by Receptors

When a receptor is strongly stimulated a high initial firing rate is established in
the nerve fiber which decreases somewhat with time. Even when the stimulus is
continually applied with the same intensity, the firing rate decreases within a
few seconds. This decrease in the firing rate in spite of constant stimulation is
called *adaptation.*

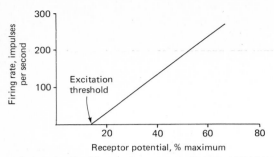

Figure 7-4 Graphic illustration of the relationship between the receptor potential and the firing rate in the afferent nerve fiber. Notice that if the receptor potential is too small, the excitation threshold is not exceeded and impulse firing does not occur. However, beyond this threshold, the firing rate increases as a function of the magnitude of the receptor potential. (*Drawn from Katz, 1950.*)

All receptors adapt to some extent with the possible exception of pain receptors. Certain receptors (i.e., hair receptors and pacinian corpuscles) adapt very quickly and are referred to as *rapidly adapting receptors*. As you can see in Fig. 7-5, their firing rates drop to zero within a second or two even in the face of constant stimulation. In other words their receptor potentials decreased below the excitation threshold and impulse conduction stopped. Other receptors (i.e., muscle spindles) adapt much more slowly and even then only to a limited degree. Their firing rates usually level off to a steady, although lower, rate than initially recorded. These are *slowly adapting receptors*. The receptor potential also decreases here, but generally not below the excitation threshold for impulse firing. It is apparent that rapidly adapting receptors are particularly

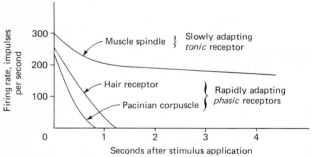

Figure 7-5 The difference in firing patterns between tonic and phasic receptors as they adapt to a continuous stimulation. Phasic receptors such as hair and pacinian corpuscle receptors adapt rapidly to the cutaneous stimulus because their firing rates drop to zero within seconds as their receptor potentials rapidly fall below the excitation threshold necessary for impulse production. On the other hand, a tonic receptor such as the muscle spindle adapts much more slowly as its receptor potential remains above the excitation threshold and it continues to signal the presence of the stimulus. (*Drawn from Guyton, 1976.*)

adept at signaling the presence of a stimulus only at the outset of stimulation. Consequently they are classed as *phasic receptors*. On the other hand, slowly adapting receptors continually signal the presence of a stimulus and are often referred to as *tonic receptors*.

MECHANORECEPTORS: A CLOSER EXAMINATION

Mechanoreceptors by definition respond to mechanical displacement. Pushing the skin on the back of one hand with the finger of the other hand, for instance, displaces a great number of cutaneous mechanoreceptors. Similarly, joint receptors respond to mechanical displacement during movement of a limb. While the body has many individual examples of mechanoreceptors, they can be conveniently grouped into three broad categories (Fig. 7-6). *Position and velocity mechanoreceptors* respond by firing impulses when the stimulating source is stationary as well as when it is moving. *Velocity mechanoreceptors*, on the other hand, fire only when the stimulating source is moving and stop or become "silent" once the mechanoreceptor has been displaced to a new fixed position. The third group, *transient mechanoreceptors*, fire only at the onset of a displacement.

While some mechanoreceptors fall in only one of the three groups, it is important to recognize that others show characteristics of two or even all three of the groups. There appear to be no receptors which respond strictly to position. Nevertheless, it is likely that all position receptors show some degree of velocity response.

When a mechanoreceptor is stimulated, its firing rate increases. As the degree of displacement increases so does the firing rate. At a certain level of displacement the firing rate stops increasing even in the face of continual dis-

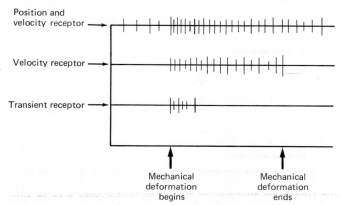

Figure 7-6 Position and velocity mechanoreceptors respond by firing when the stimulating source is stationary and when it is moving. Velocity receptors fire only when the stimulating source is moving and stop or become "silent" once the mechanoreceptor has been displaced to a new position. Transient mechanoreceptors fire only at the beginning of a displacement.

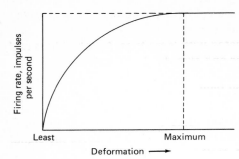

Figure 7-7 Graphic illustration of the dynamic range of a mechanoreceptor. When a mechanoreceptor is stimulated, its firing rate increases. As the degree of displacement increases, so does the firing rate. At a maximum degree of deformation, the firing rate will stop increasing even in the face of further displacement. The firing rate at the maximum degree of deformation minus the firing rate at the least deformation is the dynamic range of the receptor.

placement (Fig. 7-7). The firing rate at the greatest displacement minus the firing rate at the least displacement represents the *dynamic range* of the receptor.

Mechanoreceptors in Hairy Skin

All three types of mechanoreceptors are found in hairy skin. While these three types are also found in glabrous (hairless) skin, there are significant differences between individual receptors.

Position and Velocity Receptors   Two types of position and velocity receptors are found in hairy skin. *Type I* receptors are the peripheral ends of type A beta fibers associated with Merkel's disks. They are stimulated by indentation of the skin and respond with an irregular discharge. They show a good velocity response but a smaller position response. *Type II* receptors are the peripheral ends of type A beta fibers which terminate in Ruffini corpuscles. They are stimulated by deformation of the skin and respond with a regular discharge. Unlike type I receptors, they have a good position response but a smaller velocity response. Both type I and type II receptors are slowly adapting and are thus able to give rise to conscious sensation associated with both instantaneous and prolonged skin displacement.

Velocity Receptors   Four types of velocity receptors are found in hairy skin. *G_2 hair receptors* are the peripheral ends of type A beta fibers terminating around the base of guard hairs in the base of hair follicles. They respond to both slow and rapid movement of hairs and deflection of the skin. *Field receptors* are associated with type A beta fibers and their terminal morphology is unknown. They respond to indentation of the skin. *D hair receptors* are the terminal endings of type A delta fibers terminating around the base of both guard and down (fine) hair. They respond to both slow and rapid movements of these hairs as well as to skin deflection. *C mechanoreceptors* are rare, typically being associated with nonmyelinated type C fibers. Their terminal morphology is unknown and they respond only to slow displacement of the skin.

Transient Receptors   Two types of transient receptors are found in hairy skin. *Pacinian corpuscle receptors* are associated with the peripheral ends of certain type A alpha and beta fibers. They respond to mechanical "taps" and vibrations in the 50- to 500-Hz range. G_1 *hair receptors* are specialized processes at the base of hair follicles associated with large type A alpha fibers and they respond to high-velocity guard hair and skin displacement.

Mechanoreceptors in Glabrous (Hairless) Skin

Like hairy skin, glabrous skin also contains position and velocity, velocity, and transient receptors. Nevertheless, there are some morphological differences between them such as the type of afferent nerve fiber which carries the signal and the nature of the receptive element itself.

Position and Velocity Receptors The position and velocity receptors in glabrous skin are classified as slowly adapting (SA) receptors. It is likely that there is more than one type present. Nevertheless, *SA receptors* are associated with type A beta fibers and terminate in Ruffini-type corpuscles and possibly Merkel's disks. They respond to indentation of the skin.

Velocity Receptors Velocity receptors in glabrous skin are classified as rapidly adapting (RA) receptors. *RA receptors* are associated with type A alpha fibers and possibly terminate in Meissner's corpuscles. Like SA receptors they respond to skin indentation.

Transient Receptors The transient receptors in glabrous skin are also *pacinian corpuscles*. They have the same morphological and stimulating characteristics as those in glabrous skin.

Mechanoreceptors in Muscles and Tendons

Strict velocity receptors do not appear to be present in this group. However, transient receptors and several kinds of position and velocity receptors have been identified.

Position and Velocity Receptors The position and velocity receptors in this group include the muscle spindles, Golgi tendon organs, and pressure receptors. *Muscle spindles* are associated with both group Ia and group II nerve fibers and respond both to change and rate of change in muscle length. *Golgi tendon organs* are the terminal endings of group Ib fibers and they respond to the tension developed in fascia and contracting or stretched muscle insofar as it applies tension to tendons. *Pressure receptors* respond to pressure on the belly of the muscle primarily, and to any distortion of the fascia surrounding the muscle. They are associated with certain group III fibers and their terminal morphology is unknown.

Transient Receptors Transient receptors are again of the pacinian corpuscle type. They are associated with group II fibers and respond to both "taps" and vibrations in the 50- to 500-Hz range.

Mechanoreceptors in Joints

All three types of mechanoreceptors are represented in joints. However, their distribution is not uniform.

Position and Velocity Receptors   Position and velocity receptors are the most abundant type of mechanoreceptors found in joints. They fall into two categories. *SA type 1 receptors* are associated with myelinated fibers greater than 10 μm in diameter which terminate in Golgi-type organs. They are located in the joint ligaments and respond both to joint position and movement. *SA type 2 receptors* terminate in Ruffini-type endings and are associated with type A beta fibers. They respond to joint bending and discharge in the absence of movement to give position sense and during movement to give velocity sense.

Velocity Receptors   The velocity receptors signal phasic stimuli. Their terminal morphology is unknown but they are associated with type A alpha fibers and respond to joint movement, particularly of a bending and twisting nature.

Transient Receptors   This group represents the least common joint receptor responding to mechanical transients in joint movement. They signal "tap" stimuli and are associated with type A alpha fibers which terminate in pacinian-type corpuscles. They discharge whenever the joint is moved regardless of the direction, and their response is brief.

Mechanoreceptors in Special Sense Organs

The ear and the vestibular system make interesting use of mechanoreceptors. *Organ of Corti hair cells* respond to sound-induced movements of the basilar membrane of the inner ear. Special somatic afferent (SSA) fibers of cranial nerve VIII are stimulated when the hairs are bent. *Vestibular system hair cells,* located in the crista ampullaris and macula acustica of the vestibular apparatus, respond to angular movements, linear acceleration, and the position of the head in space. SSA fibers of cranial nerve VIII located at the base of the hair cells respond when the hairs are bent, pushed, or pulled.

Mechanoreceptors in the Viscera

A number of mechanoreceptors operate in the visceral organs and blood vessels. *Carotid sinus and aortic baroreceptors,* located in the walls of the carotid sinus and the aorta, respectively, respond to changes in blood pressure. Their terminal morphology is unknown, but general visceral afferent (GVA) fibers of cranial nerves IX (glossopharyngeal) and X (vagus), respectively, connect the receptive elements with the brainstem. *Alveolar stretch receptors* located in the walls of the pulmonary alveoli are the peripheral endings of GVA fibers of the vagus nerve. They respond to inflation and deflation of the lungs and their terminal morphology is unknown.

Gastrointestinal (GI) stretch receptors are located throughout the walls of

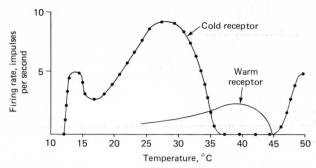

Figure 7-8 Diagram showing the relative response range of cutaneous thermoreceptors. (*Drawn from Zotterman, with permission, from Ann. Rev. Physiol. vol. 15. © 1953, by Annual Reviews Inc.*)

the GI tube from the pharynx to the rectum. They respond to stretch of the tube and subsequently conduct impulses to the CNS over GVA fibers of cranial nerves V (trigeminal), IX, and X as well as certain afferent fibers of the pelvic nerves. *Urinary bladder stretch receptors* are located in the walls of the detrusor muscle of the bladder. Their terminal receptive elements are associated with the GVA fibers of the pelvic nerve and they respond to filling of the bladder.

THERMORECEPTORS

Thermoreceptors respond to changes in temperature. Little is know about visceral temperature receptors and consequently most of our knowledge is limited to cutaneous thermoreceptors. Strict thermoreceptors (those with a lower threshold to thermal changes than to mechanical or noxious stimuli) are classified as warm or cold receptors. *Warm receptors* respond to temperature increases of greater than 0.1°C in the range from 30 to 43°C. *Cold receptors* respond to temperature decreases of greater than 0.1°C in the range from 35 to 15°C (Fig. 7-8). It is likely that the brain has learned to interpret the relative ratio of warm and cold receptor firing as indicative of a particular temperature in the region where the response of the two receptors overlap.

NOCICEPTORS

Receptors which respond primarily to injurious or painful stimulation are called nociceptors. Within this general category are four subgroups: mechanonociceptors, mechano-heat nociceptors, mechano-cold nociceptors, and polymodal nociceptors. Nociceptors are found in skin, muscles, joints, and the viscera.

Nociceptors in the Skin

Each of the four subgroups of nociceptors is represented in cutaneous tissue. While their terminal morphology is unknown, they are distinguished by their response patterns. Cutaneous *mechanonociceptors* are associated with type A delta fibers and respond to high shearing force. Cutaneous *mechano-heat nociceptors* respond to noxious levels of mechanical stimulation and heat in excess of 43°C. They are associated with certain myelinated type A delta fibers. On the other hand, cutaneous *mechano-cold nociceptors* are the terminal endings of certain nonmyelinated type C fibers. They are particularly adept at responding to noxious levels of mechanical stimulation and temperatures below 10°. *Polymodal nociceptors* respond to noxious levels of mechanical, heat, and chemical stimulation and represent the terminal endings of certain nonmyelinated type C fibers.

Nociceptors in Muscles, Joints, and Viscera

Two types of muscle nociceptors have been identified. *Pressure nociceptors* respond to strong pressure and excessive muscle stretch. Their terminal morphology is unknown and they are associated with myelinated group III fibers. *Group IV nociceptors* respond to strong pressure, temperature extremes, and anoxia. Their receptive elements are associated with nonmyelinated group IV fibers.

Little is known about joint and visceral nociceptors. Joint nociceptors are the peripheral ends of certain type A delta fibers. They respond to joint overextension and their terminal structures are unidentified. Pain receptors in the viscera are probably not located in the parenchyma of the internal organs themselves, but are found instead in the peritoneal surfaces, pleural membranes, dura mater, and the walls of blood vessels.

CHEMORECEPTORS

Chemoreceptors are defined as those receptors which respond most easily to chemical stimulation. *External chemoreceptors* include taste cells and olfactory cells, which give rise to the conscious sensations of taste and smell. *Internal chemoreceptors* respond to changes in circulating P_{CO_2}, P_{O_2}, and pH. They do not give rise to conscious sensation. Included in this category are the carotid body and aortic chemoreceptors and those chemoreceptors in the respiratory and vasomotor centers of the brainstem.

External Chemoreceptors

Taste Cells   The *taste cell* is the chemically sensitive element for the sense of taste. Taste cells cluster together in small units called *taste buds* (Fig. 7-9). The average taste bud contains 20 or so taste cells. Children have the greatest number of functional taste buds, and the number decreases with age so that the adult has about 10,000 functional buds. Each taste cell is typically columnar in shape and is characterized by numerous microvilli which project to a narrow opening at the top of the bud called a *taste pore*. The base of the taste cells are in close contact with the special visceral afferent (SVA) fibers of cranial nerves VII and IX.

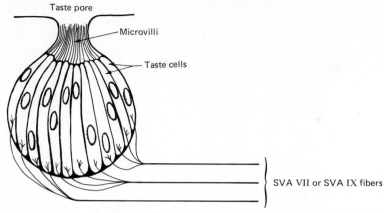

Figure 7-9 A taste bud. Each taste bud is a collection of several taste cells. The taste cells are columnar in shape and are characterized by numerous microvilli which project into a narrow opening at the top of the bud, called a taste pore. The base of the taste cells are in close contact with the SVA fibers of cranial nerves VII and IX.

Papillae Location Taste buds are chiefly located in raised areas of the tongue known as *papillae*. In addition, taste buds are located on the epiglottis, the tonsilar pillars, and other areas of the fauces (passage from mouth to pharynx). Numerous small *fungiform papillae* are located over the anterior surface of the tongue. These papillae contain a moderate number of buds, perhaps as many as 100 per papilla. Much larger *circumvallate papillae* form a V on the back of the tongue and contain up to 250 taste buds each. *Foliate papillae*, located behind the circumvallate papillae, contain fewer buds.

Afferent Innervation of the Tongue and Fauces Figure 7-10 illustrates that several afferent fibers conduct information from the tongue. Touch (not taste)

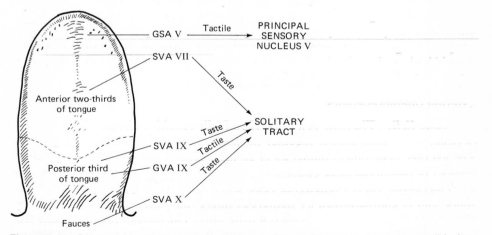

Figure 7-10 Diagram illustrating the cranial nerve afferent fibers which are responsible for carrying information from the tongue to the brainstem.

sensation from the anterior two-thirds of the tongue is transmitted over GVA fibers of cranial nerve V to the principal sensory nucleus of V in the pons, while tactile sensation from the posterior one-third of the tongue is conducted over GVA fibers of cranial nerve IX to the solitary tract of the medulla oblongata.

Taste sensation from the anterior two-thirds of the tongue is transmitted over SVA fibers of cranial nerve VII, while SVA IX fibers relay taste information from the posterior one-third. SVA X fibers conduct taste information from taste cells in the fauces. All of these afferent taste-conducting pathways terminate in the solitary tract.

Four Basic Taste Modalities   Four basic taste modalities are generally recognized. These are sweet, salty, sour, and bitter. Evidence suggests that all taste buds respond to some degree to all four stimuli. Nevertheless, buds on the tip of the tongue respond most strongly to sweet and salty stimuli, while chemicals giving rise to a sour sensation most effectively stimulate buds along the edge. Chemicals associated with the bitter sensation most effectively stimulate the base of the tongue.

The adequate chemical stimuli for the four basic taste modalities fall into characteristic chemical groups. For instance, the chemicals which give rise to the sour sensation are usually acids. The lower the pH, the more the taste cells are stimulated. Sweet stimuli are usually organic molecules such as sugars, glycols, aldehydes, and others. Alkaloids like quinine, caffeine, and nicotine give rise to the bitter sensation, while ionizable salts give rise to the sensation we describe as salty.

In order to stimulate the taste cells within a taste bud, the stimulating chemicals must dissolve in the saliva and then enter the taste pore. Here they stimulate the taste cells, which in turn stimulate the SVA endings of cranial nerves VII, IX, and X.

Adaptation of Taste Cell Chemoreceptors   When a taste stimulus is first applied to the tongue, the sensation is strong and then becomes weaker with time. The sourness becomes less sour, the sweetness becomes less sweet, etc. In other words, the taste cells adapt to the stimulus. This subjective awareness of decreasing sensation is paralleled by a decrease in the firing rate of the SVA neurons (Fig. 7-11).

Taste Discrimination   While taste buds respond to the four basic taste stimuli, they do so with different intensities. A particular taste bud may respond with a high-frequency discharge to a sweet stimulus but produce a low-frequency discharge to salty, bitter, and sour stimuli. As stated previously, those responding primarily to bitter stimuli are concentrated at the base of the tongue, while those responding with the greatest discharge frequency to sweet and salty stimuli are concentrated at the tip. Sour receptors are located along the edge. Figure 7-12 illustrates the different sensitivities of two taste buds.

Taste bud A is a "sweet" bud. That is, when a sweet stimulus is applied, a

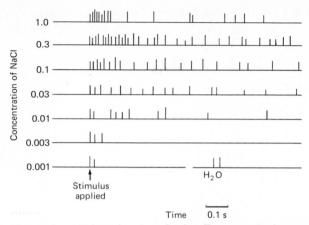

Figure 7-11 The response of a single nerve fiber to the application of different concentrations of salt to the tongue of the rat. (*Drawn from Pffafmann, 1955.*)

much higher firing rate is initiated in the SVA fibers from its taste cells than when a bitter, salty, or sour stimulus is applied. Taste bud B, on the other hand, is a "bitter" bud because it responds with the greatest discharge to bitter stimuli. The brain probably interprets a given taste by analysis of the discharge ratios of the different kinds of taste buds stimulated. For example, if the firing rate from bud A is 10 times greater than from bud B when a chemical stimulus is applied, the stimulus was probably quite sweet. On the other hand, if the relative firing rates were reversed with bud B responding with a firing rate 10 times greater than bud A, the applied stimulus was probably quite bitter. Since the only message a neuron can carry is an impulse, all of which are quite similar, it follows that the only variable is the pattern of firing (i.e., the rate, grouping patterns, etc.). Consequently a possible partial explanation of how the conscious cortex evaluates a given taste stimulus is by analysis of the relative discharge patterns of the four basic kinds of taste buds from each part of the tongue and

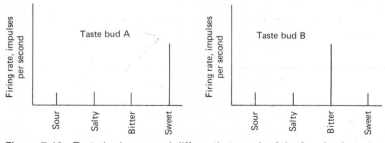

Figure 7-12 Taste buds respond differently to each of the four basic taste modalities. Taste bud A is nevertheless classified as a "sweet" taste bud because it responds with a much higher firing rate to the application of sweet stimulus than to the application of a bitter, salty, or sour stimulus. Similarly, taste bud B is a "bitter" taste bud because of its greater response to a bitter stimulus than to the other three.

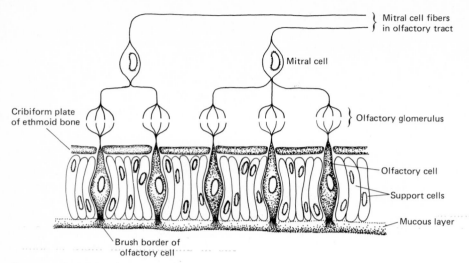

Figure 7-13 The relationship of the chemically sensitive olfactory cells to the olfactory epithelium and mitral cells of the olfactory tract.

fauces. Such an integrated discharge pattern could supply the necessary information to the brain to enable it to accurately sense even the most subtle differences in taste.

Olfactory Cells   The chemically receptive element for the sense of smell is the *olfactory cell.* These cells, located in the olfactory mucosa of the nasal cavity, project their peripheral processes into a mucous layer which is exposed to the air in the nasal cavity. Their central processes penetrate the cribiform plate of the ethmoid bone to synapse with mitral cells in tufted olfactory glomeruli (Fig. 7-13).

In addition to olfactory cells, the olfactory mucosa is also made up of support cells and mucus-secreting cells. The entire surface of the olfactory mucosa occupies a little more than 5 cm².

Conscious and Reflex Olfactory Pathways   The axons of mitral cells pass from the olfactory bulb centrally toward the brain as the *olfactory tract.* The tract then divides to form separate medial and lateral olfactory tracts. The *lateral olfactory tract* ultimately terminates in the periamygdaloid cortex of the temporal lobe. This pathway probably represents the conscious smell pathway. The *medial olfactory tract* may terminate in the septal nuclei, the contralateral amygdala, or the anterior continuation of the hippocampus.

The body reflexly responds to both pleasant and unpleasant odors. The reflex responses are classified as viscerosomatic or viscerovisceral, depending on the nature of the response. Viscerosomatic reflexes include the reflex movements of the eyes, facial muscles, neck and the rest of the body in response to both pleasant and unpleasant odors. Viscerovisceral reflexes include salivary and gastric secretions in response to certain pleasant odors and vomiting in response to very obnoxious odors. Both the medial and lateral olfactory tracts contribute to the reflex pathways.

Odorants Unlike taste, no subjective classification of basic olfactory modalities has been agreed upon. However, for any odorant to be an effective stimuli it must be volatile. Water and lipid solubility are also desirable qualities. Volatility is necessary to allow the chemical to be adequately drawn into the nasal cavities, while water solubility is necessary since the odorant must penetrate the olfactory mucosa in order to reach the brush borders of the olfactory cells. There is even some evidence that the odorant must penetrate the brush border membrane in order to effectively stimulate the olfactory cell, in which case lipid solubility would be a desirable feature. In any event, the odorant establishes a receptor potential in the olfactory cell, which then gives rise to impulse production in the mitral cells of the olfactory bulb. The mechanism of olfactory cell stimulation of the mitral cells in unknown, but there is some evidence that a chemical transmitter may be involved.

Olfactory Discrimination When an odorant of threshold concentration is presented to the olfactory epithelium, the subject is barely aware of its presence. If the concentration is increased, the sensation increases as well. Finally, the sensation reaches a maximum, and further increases in odorant concentration elicit no further increases in sensation.

Allowing for individual differences, maximum sensation is usually reached with an odorant concentration 10 to 50 times greater than threshold. This does not allow much dynamic range. It is considerably less, for instance, than the range for vision (about 500,000 to 1). It would appear that the olfactory system is better designed for odor detection than for odor quantification. Further support for the idea that odor detection is perhaps the principal role of the olfactory system is the adaptation which occurs in the face of a sustained stimulus. The firing rate of olfactory tract neurons might decrease by as much as 50 percent within the first second or two following odorant application. This rapid decrease declines after the first second or two, but the signal is very weak after a minute or so.

Electroolfactogram When an odorant is presented to the olfactory epithelium a monophasic action potential called the *electroolfactogram* (EOG) can be recorded. The amplitude of the EOG is a function of the odorant concentration, and in all probability represents the combined receptor potentials of many olfactory cells. Receptor potential recordings from individual olfactory cells has not yet been satisfactorily achieved.

Internal Chemoreceptors

Internal chemoreceptors include the carotid body and aortic chemoreceptors and the chemically sensitive cells in the respiratory and vasomotor centers of

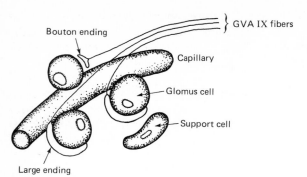

Bouton ending

GVA IX fibers

Capillary

Glomus cell

Support cell

Large ending

Figure 7-14   The chemoreceptive elements of the carotid body. The carotid bodies are particularly sensitive to changes in the arterial oxygen concentration. When the arterial P_{O_2} drops below 95 mmHg, the GVA IX fibers respond by an increase in their firing rates. It is not presently known whether the GVA endings themselves are directly stimulated by the oxygen drop or whether the glomus cells are the sensitive elements which in turn stimulate the bouton and large endings of the nerve fibers. (*Adapted from Eyzaguirre, Fed. Proc. 31:1385–1393, 1972.*)

the brainstem. The carotid body chemoreceptors have been subjected to more study than the others partly because of their relative accessibility. Recall that the internal chemoreceptors respond to changes in circulating P_{CO_2}, P_{O_2}, and pH but do not give rise to conscious sensation.

Functional Arrangement of the Carotid Body Chemoreceptors   The carotid bodies contain large glomus cells which make contact with the endings of the GVA fibers of the glossopharyngeal nerve. Two kinds of contacts are observed: small discrete *bouton endings* to single glomus cells and *large endings* in contact with several glomus cells (Fig. 7-14).

Carotid Bodies Respond to Changes in P_{CO_2}, P_{O_2}, and pH   The carotid bodies are particularly suitable for blood chemistry testing as about 20 ml per gram of carotid body tissue per minute is the flow rate of blood through the carotid bodies in the cat. This is among the highest tissue blood flow values found anywhere in the body. The carotid bodies are particularly sensitive to changes in the arterial oxygen concentration. When the P_{O_2} drops below the normal level of about 95 mmHg, the GVA fibers from the carotid bodies respond with an increase in their firing rates. It is not presently known whether the GVA endings themselves are directly stimulated by the oxygen drop or whether the glomus cells are the chemosensitive elements which then stimulate the bouton and large endings of the nerve fibers.

To a lesser extent, the carotid bodies are also sensitive to changes in blood P_{CO_2} and pH. Increasing the P_{CO_2} above the normal value of 40 mmHg or decreasing the arterial pH below the normal value of 7.4 produces increased firing in the GVA IX fibers. Because of the close relationship between P_{CO_2} and pH it is difficult to tell which event is the actual stimulus. Again, it is not known whether the glomus cells of the endings of the afferent fibers themselves are initially stimulated. There is some evidence that chemical transmission is involved, however, and this would point to the likelihood that the glomus cells themselves are the actual receptive elements subsequently stimulating the afferent endings of the GVA fibers by chemical transmission.

Evidence for Cholinergic Transmission   If a chemical transmitter operates in the carotid body chemoreceptor system, it is probably acetylcholine. ACh is present in carotid body tissue. So are the enzymes necessary for its synthesis (cholineacetyltransferase) and degradation (acetylcholinesterase). In addition, carotid bodies in vitro are sensitive to extremely small amounts of ACh, and this sensitivity is enhanced by physostigmine (an anticholinesterase). In vitro studies also show that the response of the carotid bodies to natural stimulation is decreased by the administration of curare and atropine.

A technique pioneered by Otto Loewi has been used to illustrate the cholinergic nature of the carotid bodies. In Fig. 7-15 two carotid bodies, each

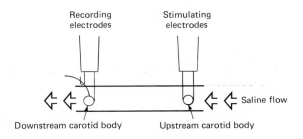

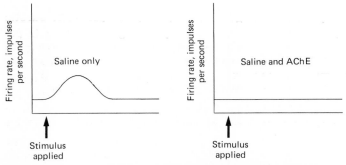

Figure 7-15   Experimental setup illustrating evidence for cholinergic transmission in the carotid body chemoreceptor. When a saline solution is washed over two excised carotid bodies with the upstream body stimulated and the nerve from the downstream carotid body fitted with recording electrodes, a subsequent response is noted in the downstream body after an appropriate delay. The implication is that a chemical was released into the saline stream from the upstream preparation which diffused downstream and subsequently stimulated the downstream preparation. Evidence that the chemical may be acetylcholine is supported by the fact that the addition of acetylcholinesterase (AChE) to the saline flow abolishes the response. (*Drawn from Eyzaguirre, 1968.*)

with its nervous innervation intact, are placed in a saline trough so that physiological saline can flow freely over both of them in a single direction. Stimulating electrodes are placed on the upstream preparation and recording electrodes are placed on the downstream preparation. When the two bodies are relatively close to each other (9 mm), stimulation of the upstream preparation produces, after an appropriate delay, increased firing in the nerve of the downstream preparation. The implication is that a chemical was released into the saline stream from the upstream preparation which diffused downstream, subsequently stimulating the downstream carotid body. Modification of this experiment indicates the chemical may be ACh. If the same procedure is run again with acetylcholinesterase (AChE) added to the saline flow, no response is observed.

CLASSIFICATION OF RECEPTOR BY AFFERENT NERVE FIBER TYPE

The receptors of the peripheral nervous system will be classified (Table 7-1) according to the type of afferent nerve fiber which conducts its signals to the cen-

Table 7-1   Classification of Receptor by Afferent Nerve Fiber Type

I   *General somatic receptors.* Respond to adequate stimulation of cutaneous receptors and the receptors in muscles, tendons, and joints
   A   *Mechanoreceptors*
      1   *Skin.* Type I and type II receptors, G_2 hair receptors, field receptors, D hair receptors, C mechanoreceptors, pacinian corpuscle (PC) receptors, G_1 hair receptors, SA receptors, RA receptors
      2   *Muscle and tendon.* Muscle spindles, Golgi tendon organs, pressure receptors, PC receptors
      3   *Joint.* SA type 1 receptors, SA type 2 receptors, "phasic" receptors, "tap" receptors
   B   **4**   *Thermoreceptors.* Warm and cold receptors
   C   **5**   *Nociceptors.* Pain receptors
II   *Special somatic receptors.* Respond to adequate stimulation of the organ of Corti of the inner ear, the retina of the eye, and the crista ampullaris and macula of the vestibular system
   A   *Mechanoreceptors.* Organ of Corti hair cells and vestibular system hair cells (type I and type II)
   B   *Photoreceptors.* Rods and cones of the retina
III   *General visceral receptors.* Respond to adquate stimulation of the viscera and blood vessels
   A   *Mechanoreceptors.* Carotid sinus and aortic baroceptors, alveolar stretch receptors, GI stretch receptors, urinary bladder stretch receptors
   B   *Thermoreceptors.* Warm and cold receptors
   C   *Nociceptors.* Pain receptors
   D   *Chemoreceptors.* Carotid body and aortic chemoreceptors
IV   *Special visceral receptors.* Respond to adequate stimulation of taste cells and the olfactory epithelium
   A   *Chemoreceptors.* Taste cells and olfactory cells

tral nervous system. Receptors located within the brain (i.e., chemoreceptors of the hypothalamus and those in the respiratory and vasomotor centers of the brainstem) are not included in this classification system because they are not associated with peripheral terminations of spinal and cranial afferent nerve fibers.

REVIEW QUESTIONS

1 That form of stimulation to which a receptor has the lowest threshold is called the
   a   least stimulus
   b   principal stimulus
   c   adequate stimulus
   d   liminal stimulus
   e   subliminal stimulus
2 All of the following are rapidly adapting phasic receptors, *except*
   a   muscle spindles
   b   hair receptors
   c   pacinian receptors
3 The firing rate of a mechanoreceptor at the greatest displacement minus the rate at the least displacement is the
   a   adequate range
   b   static range
   c   significant range
   d   dynamic range
   e   response range
4 All of the following are special somatic mechanoreceptors, *except*
   a   carotid sinus baroreceptors
   b   vestibular system hair cells
   c   organ of Corti hair cells
   d   alveolar stretch receptors
5 All of the following are mechanoreceptors, *except*
   a   pacinian corpuscles
   b   D hair receptors
   c   olfactory cells
   d   field receptors
   e   Golgi tendon organs
6 All of the following are general visceral receptors, *except*
   a   alveolar stretch receptors
   b   aortic baroreceptors
   c   aortic chemoreceptors
   d   urinary bladder stretch receptors
   e   muscle spindles
7 The carotid body chemoreceptors are most sensitive to changes in
   a   circulating P_{O_2}
   b   circulating P_{CO_2}
   c   blood pH
   d   blood phosphate levels

8 All of the following are true concerning carotid body chemoreceptors, *except:*

 a They are classified as external chemoreceptors.

 b They don't give rise to conscious sensation.

 c They are classified as two-element receptors.

 d They are innervated by GVA fibers of cranial nerve IX.

9 All of the following are true concerning Golgi tendon organs, *except:*

 a They are associated with group Ib fibers.

 b They are position and velocity receptors.

 c They are an integral part of the myotatic reflex.

 d They are general visceral mechanoreceptors.

10 All of the following are true concerning the receptor potential which is developed by displacement of the pacinian corpuscle, *except:*

 a It is graded and nonpropagated.

 b Its magnitude determines the firing rate of the receptor.

 c Its magnitude is determined by the degree of displacement.

 d It displays no adaptation.

Sensory Pathways

Strictly speaking, sensory pathways include only those routes which conduct information to the conscious cortex of the brain. However, in this chapter we will use the term in its more loosely and commonly applied context to include input from all receptors, whether their signals reach the conscious level or not.

GENERAL SOMATIC AFFERENT (GSA) PATHWAYS FROM THE BODY

Pain and Temperature

Pain and temperature information from general somatic receptors is conducted over small-diameter (type A delta and type C) GSA fibers of the spinal nerves into the posterior horn of the spinal cord gray matter (Fig. 8-1). These are monopolar neurons with cell bodies in the posterior root ganglia. After entering the cord, the fibers pass up or down in the *dorsolateral tract,* located between the tip of the posterior horn and the surface of the spinal cord near the posterior root, before finally synapsing in laminae III and IV.

Second-order neurons from these synapses cross over to the opposite side of the cord in the anterior white commissure, where they turn upward as the *lateral spinothalamic tract* (LSTT). At higher pontine levels this tract comes to

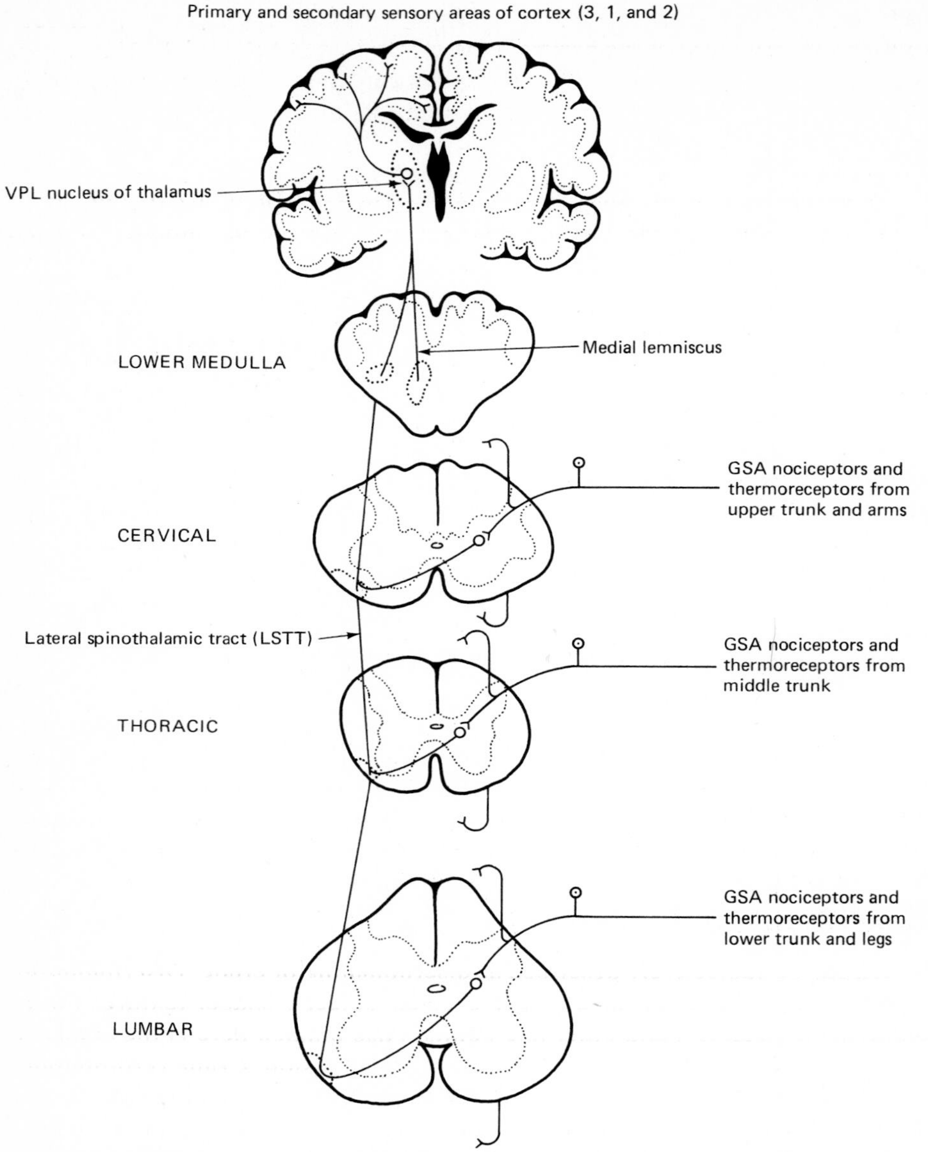

Primary and secondary sensory areas of cortex (3, 1, and 2)

VPL nucleus of thalamus

LOWER MEDULLA — Medial lemniscus

CERVICAL — GSA nociceptors and thermoreceptors from upper trunk and arms

Lateral spinothalamic tract (LSTT) — GSA nociceptors and thermoreceptors from middle trunk

THORACIC

GSA nociceptors and thermoreceptors from lower trunk and legs

LUMBAR

Figure 8-1 Schematic illustration showing the general somatic afferent (GSA) pathways for pain and temperature from the body.

lie close to the medial lemniscus, with which it travels to the *ventral posterior lateral nucleus* (VPL) of the thalamus. Some fibers of this tract don't enter the thalamus but end instead in the brainstem reticular formation. After synapsing in the thalamus, third-order neurons enter the posterior third of the internal capsule, pass through the corona radiata, and terminate in the primary and secondary sensory areas of the parietal lobe cortex (areas 3, 1, and 2). Notice that regardless of the level of entry into the spinal cord, pain and temperature stimulation delivered to one side of the body registers in the cerebral cortex of the opposite side.

Fast and Slow Pain   Pain sensation is often confusingly labeled "fast" or "slow" depending on the type of fiber which conducts the impulse and the speed with which the signal consciously registers. *Fast pain,* often called sharp or pricking pain, is usually conducted to the CNS over type A delta fibers. These ultimately excite lateral spinothalamic tract fibers which go directly to the VPL of the thalamus on the contralateral side. From here third-order fibers project to the cerebral cortex where they are somatotopically organized and sharply localized. Somatotopic organization means that each minute area of the sensory cortex receives input from a distinct peripheral area. A person can sharply localize a pain if he is able to tell exactly where it is originating. *Slow pain,* often called burning pain, is conducted to the CNS over smaller-diameter type C fibers. After entering the cord these fibers stimulate lateral spinothalamic tract neurons which send collaterals into the brainstem reticular formation. Fibers from the reticular formation diffusely project to the thalamus, hypothalamus, and possibly other areas as well, perhaps giving rise to the emotional component of pain. Pain signals following this route are poorly localized.

Dermatomes   A dermatome is the area of skin supplied by the afferent fibers in the posterior root of a single spinal nerve. Dermatomes tend to overlap each other so that stimulation of a specific point on the skin typically sends afferent signals into the cord over more than one posterior root. This is functionally important since destruction of a single posterior root does not totally eliminate sensation from the afflicted dermatome.

Touch and Pressure

Touch can be subjectively described as discriminating or crude. *Discriminating (epicritic) touch* implies an awareness of an object's shape, texture, three-dimensional qualities, and other fine points. Also implied here is the ability to recognize familiar objects simply by tactile manipulation. *Crude (protopathic) touch,* on the other hand, lacks the fine discrimination described above and doesn't generally give enough information to the brain to enable it to recognize a familiar object by touch alone. The tactile information implied here is of a much cruder nature than described for epicritic touch. The pathways to the brain for these two kinds of touch appear to be distinct.

Crude (Protopathic) Touch and Pressure   General somatic mechanoreceptors sensitive to crude touch and pressure conduct information into the cord over GSA nerve fibers (Fig. 8-2). The fibers pass up or down a few cord segments (neuromeres) in the dorsolateral (Lissauer) tract before synapsing

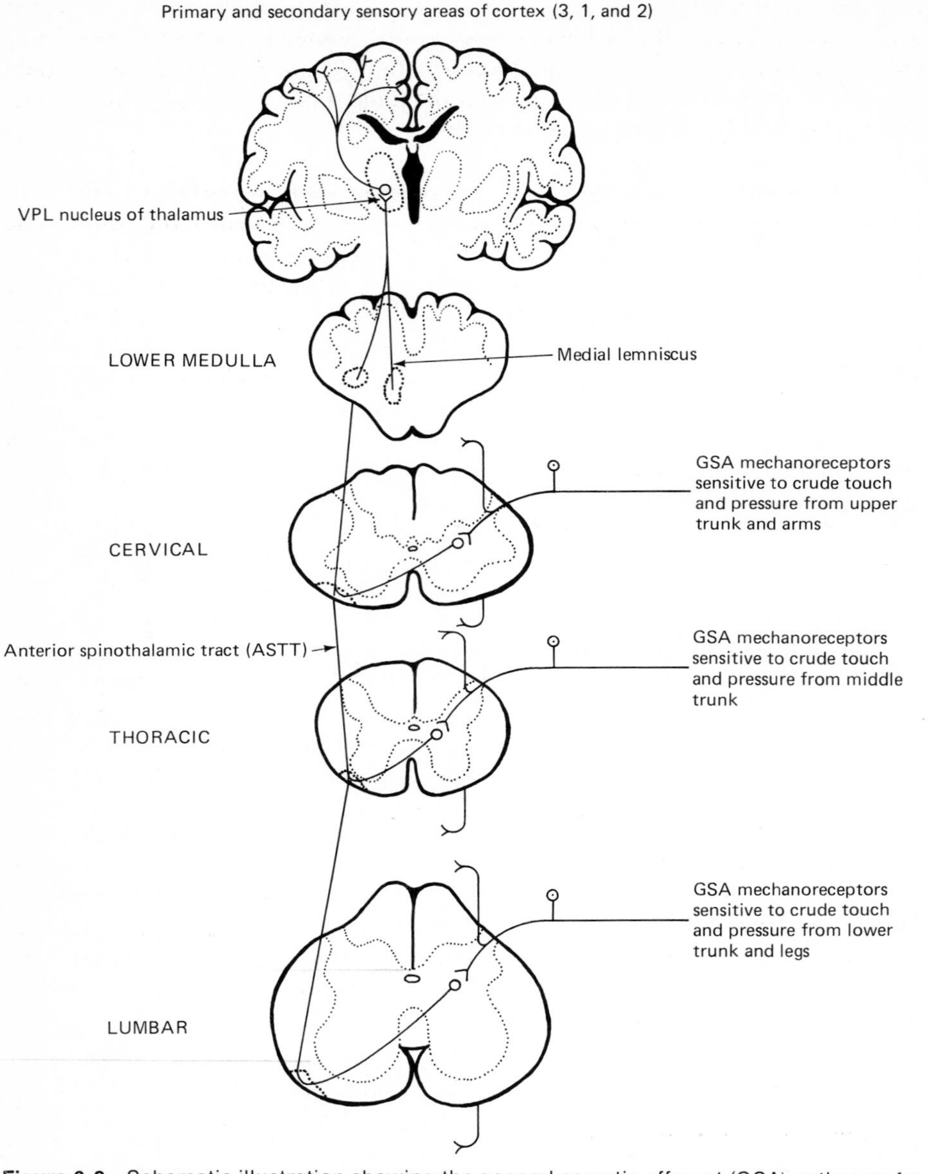

Primary and secondary sensory areas of cortex (3, 1, and 2)

Figure 8-2 Schematic illustration showing the general somatic afferent (GSA) pathways for crude (protopathic) touch and pressure from the body.

chiefly in laminae **VI, VII,** and **VIII.** Second-order neurons cross over to the opposite side in the anterior white commissure to the anterior funiculus, where they turn upward in the *anterior spinothalamic tract* (ASTT) to the VPL of the thalamus. At higher pontine levels the tract also comes to lie close to the medial lemniscus as it ascends to the thalamus. Third-order neurons project from the VPL to areas 3, 1, and 2 of the cerebral cortex. Some of the ASTT fibers send collaterals into the brainstem reticular formation. While some of these no doubt ultimately reach the thalamus by reticulothalamic projections, the principal fate and function of these collaterals is largely unknown.

Discriminating (Epicritic) Touch, Pressure, and Kinesthesia The conscious awareness of body position and movement is called the *kinesthetic sense.* It's important to recognize that there are many receptors throughout the body which continually conduct information to the brain concerning the body's position and movement and even the level of muscle tone. Such receptors are collectively called *proprioceptors.* However, not all of these signals reach the conscious level as a large portion are conducted instead to the brainstem and cerebellum for subconscious evaluation and integration. Only those proprioceptive signals reaching the conscious level contribute to the kinesthetic sense. The kinesthetic sense and discriminating touch and pressure pathways share a common route to the brain (Fig. 8-3).

General somatic mechanoreceptors sensitive to discriminating touch and pressure and body position and movement conduct signals into the cord over GSA fibers. They pass directly into the ipsilateral posterior funiculus, where they turn upward in the dorsal columns to terminate in the dorsal column nuclei of the medulla. Those fibers entering the cord below the midthoracic level (i.e., from the lower trunk and legs) ascend through the medial dorsal column as the *fasciculus gracilis* and terminate in the *nucleus gracilis.* Fibers entering the cord above the midthoracic level (i.e., from the upper trunk and arms) enter the more lateral dorsal column and ascend as the *fasciculus cuneatus* to terminate in the more lateral dorsal column nuclei, the *nucleus cuneatus.* As might be expected, the dorsal columns include the fasciculus gracilis and fasciculus cuneatus while the dorsal column nuclei include the nucleus gracilis and nucleus cuneatus. Second-order neurons from these nuclei cross over to the other side of the brainstem in the lower medulla as the *internal arcuate fibers,* which then turn upward in the medial lemniscus to the VPL of the thalamus. Third-order neurons then project through the posterior limb of the internal capsule to areas 3, 1, and 2 of the cerebral cortex.

Much of the proprioceptive information which reaches the conscious level giving rise to the kinesthetic sense originates in joint receptors. However, recent evidence indicates that signals from muscle spindles may also represent a significant contribution to kinesthetic sensation. On the other hand, the subconscious proprioceptive information which is shunted to the brainstem and cerebellum for evaluation and integration arises chiefly in muscle spindles and Golgi tendon organs.

Subconscious Proprioception

Most of the subconscious proprioceptive input is shunted to the cerebellum. Further, signals arising in proprioceptors on the left side of the body register on the left side of the cerebellum. By contrast, sensory signals arising in the left side of the body register on the right side of the cerebral cortex. After entering the cord, proprioceptive afferents (GSA fibers) terminate in laminae V, VI, and VII (Clarke's column) of the posterior horn. Second-order neurons (primarily conducting information from Golgi tendon organs) cross over to the opposite

Primary and secondary sensory areas of cortex (3, 1, and 2)

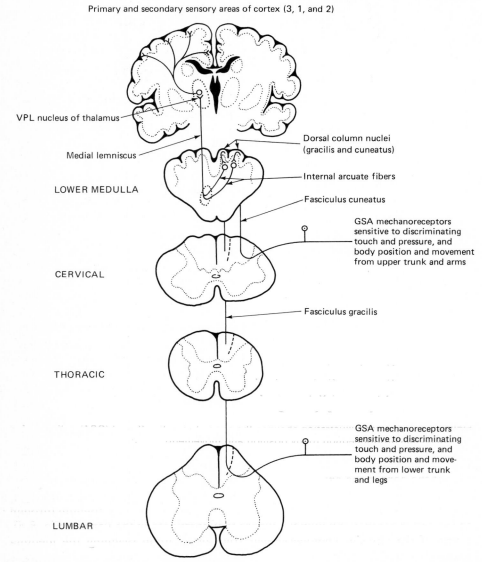

VPL nucleus of thalamus

Medial lemniscus

LOWER MEDULLA

Dorsal column nuclei (gracilis and cuneatus)

Internal arcuate fibers

Fasciculus cuneatus

GSA mechanoreceptors sensitive to discriminating touch and pressure, and body position and movement from upper trunk and arms

CERVICAL

Fasciculus gracilis

THORACIC

GSA mechanoreceptors sensitive to discriminating touch and pressure, and body position and movement from lower trunk and legs

LUMBAR

Figure 8-3   Schematic illustration showing the general somatic afferent (GSA) pathways for discriminating (epicritic) touch and pressure, and kinesthesia (awareness of body position and movement) from the body.

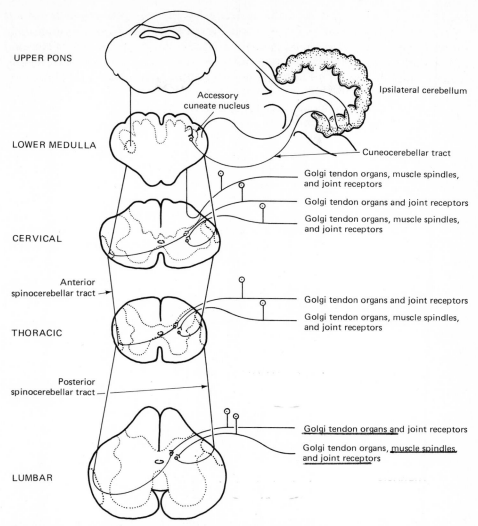

UPPER PONS

Ipsilateral cerebellum

Accessory
cuneate nucleus

LOWER MEDULLA

Cuneocerebellar tract

Golgi tendon organs, muscle spindles,
and joint receptors

Golgi tendon organs and joint receptors

Golgi tendon organs, muscle spindles,
and joint receptors

CERVICAL

Anterior
spinocerebellar tract

Golgi tendon organs and joint receptors

Golgi tendon organs, muscle spindles,
and joint receptors

THORACIC

Posterior
spinocerebellar tract

Golgi tendon organs and joint receptors

Golgi tendon organs, muscle spindles,
and joint receptors

LUMBAR

Figure 8-4   Schematic illustration showing the general somatic afferent (GSA) pathways for subconscious proprioception (body position and movement).

side of the cord in the anterior white commissure to the lateral funiculus, where they turn upward in the *anterior spinocerebellar tract* (ASCT). After reaching upper pontine levels the fibers cross back over and enter the cerebellum through the superior cerebellar peduncle, where they terminate in the vermis (Fig. 8-4). Some of the anterior spinocerebellar tract fibers upon reaching the medulla remain uncrossed and enter the cerebellum via the inferior cerebellar peduncle and terminate in the contralateral vermis. Other second-order neurons (those receiving information primarily from muscle spindles and tendon organs) leave

Clarke's column to ascend in the ipsilateral *posterior spinocerebellar tract* (PSCT) to the cerebellum. After reaching the medulla, the fibers enter the cerebellum via the inferior cerebellar peduncle to terminate in the ipsilateral cortex.

Some of the subconscious proprioceptive input from the cervical region follows an alternate route to the cerebellum. Some of the fibers travel a short distance in the dorsal funiculus, terminating in the accessary cuneate nucleus of the medulla. Second-order neurons project from here as the *cuneocerebellar tract* to enter the cerebellum via the inferior cerebellar peduncle.

Posterior Funiculus Injury   Certain clinical signs are associated with injury to the dorsal columns. As might be expected, these are generally caused by impairment to the kinesthetic sense and discriminating touch and pressure pathways. They include (1) the inability to recognize limb position, (2) astereognosis, (3) loss of two-point discrimination, (4) loss of vibratory sense, and (5) a positive Romberg sign. Astereognosis is the inability to recognize familiar objects by touch alone. When asked to stand erect with feet together and eyes closed, a person with dorsal column damage may sway and fall. This is a positive Romberg sign.

GENERAL SOMATIC AFFERENT (GSA) PATHWAYS FROM THE FACE

Pain, Temperature, and Crude Touch and Pressure

General somatic nociceptors, thermoreceptors, and mechanoreceptors sensitive to crude touch and pressure from the face conduct signals to the brainstem over GSA fibers of cranial nerves V, VII, IX, and X. The afferent fibers involved are processes of monopolar neurons with cell bodies in the similunar, geniculate, petrosal, and nodose ganglia, respectively. The central processes of these neurons enter the spinal tract of V, where they descend through the brainstem for a short distance before terminating in the spinal nucleus of V. Second-order neurons then cross over the opposite side of the brainstem at various levels to enter the *ventral trigeminothalamic tract*, where they ascend to the VPM of the thalamus. Finally, third-order neurons project to the "face" area of the cerebral cortex in areas 3, 1, and 2 (Fig. 8-5).

Discriminating Touch and Pressure

The pathway for discriminating touch from the face is illustrated in Fig. 8-6. Signals are conducted from general somatic mechanoreceptors over GSA fibers of the trigeminal nerve into the principal sensory nucleus of V, located in the middle pons. Second-order neurons then conduct the signals to the opposite side of the brainstem, where they ascend in the medial lemniscus to the VPM of the thalamus. Thalamic neurons then project to the "face" region of areas 3, 1, and 2 of the cerebral cortex.

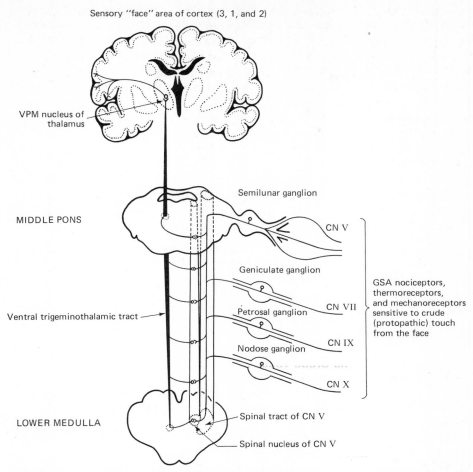

Sensory "face" area of cortex (3, 1, and 2)

VPM nucleus of thalamus

MIDDLE PONS

Semilunar ganglion

CN V

Geniculate ganglion

Ventral trigeminothalamic tract

CN VII

Petrosal ganglion

CN IX

Nodose ganglion

CN X

GSA nociceptors, thermoreceptors, and mechanoreceptors sensitive to crude (protopathic) touch from the face

LOWER MEDULLA

Spinal tract of CN V

Spinal nucleus of CN V

Figure 8-5 Schematic illustration showing the general somatic afferent (GSA) pathways for pain, temperature, and crude (protopathic) touch from the face. CN, cranial nerve.

Kinesthesia and Subconscious Proprioception

Proprioceptive input from the face is primarily conducted over GSA fibers of the trigeminal nerve. Curiously, however, the cell bodies of these monopolar neurons are located in the mesencephalic nucleus of V in the midbrain rather than the semilunar ganglia, where the cell bodies of other afferent neurons of the trigeminal nerve are located. The peripheral endings of these neurons are the general somatic mechanoreceptors sensitive to both conscious (kinesthetic) and subconscious proprioceptive input. Their central processes extend from the mesencephalic nucleus to the principal sensory nucleus of V in the pons (Fig. 8-7).

The subconscious component is conducted to the cerebellum, while the

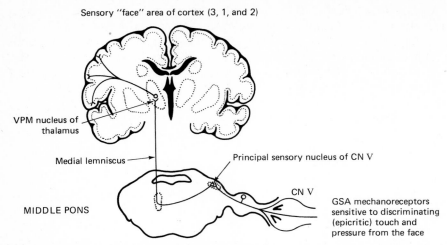

Sensory "face" area of cortex (3, 1, and 2)

VPM nucleus of thalamus

Medial lemniscus

Principal sensory nucleus of CN V

MIDDLE PONS

CN V

GSA mechanoreceptors sensitive to discriminating (epicritic) touch and pressure from the face

Figure 8-6 Schematic illustration showing the general somatic afferent (GSA) pathways for discriminating (epicritic) touch and pressure from the face.

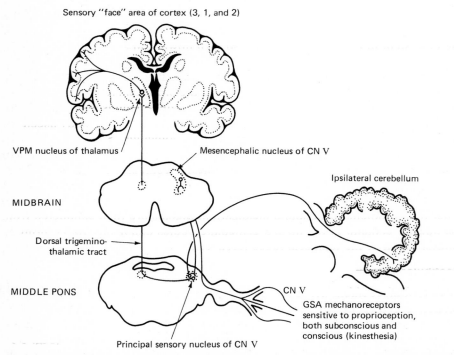

Sensory "face" area of cortex (3, 1, and 2)

VPM nucleus of thalamus

Mesencephalic nucleus of CN V

Ipsilateral cerebellum

MIDBRAIN

Dorsal trigemino-thalamic tract

MIDDLE PONS

CN V

GSA mechanoreceptors sensitive to proprioception, both subconscious and conscious (kinesthesia)

Principal sensory nucleus of CN V

Figure 8-7 Schematic illustration showing the general somatic afferent (GSA) pathways for both conscious proprioception (kinesthesia) and subconscious proprioception from the face.

conscious component travels to the cerebral cortex. Certain second-order neurons from the principal sensory nucleus relay proprioceptive information concerning subconscious evaluation and integration into the ipsilateral cerebellum. Other second-order neurons project to the opposite side of the pons and ascend to the VPM of the thalamus as the *dorsal trigeminothalamic tract*. Thalamic projections terminate in the face area of the cerebral cortex.

SPECIAL SOMATIC AFFERENT (SSA) PATHWAYS

Hearing

The organ of Corti with its sound-sensitive hair cells and basilar membrane are important parts of the sound transducing system for hearing. Mechanical vibrations of the basilar membrane generate membrane potentials in the hair cells which produce impulse patterns in the cochlear portion of the vestibulocochlear nerve (VIII). The principles of this system will be examined in Chap. 10. For now we will examine only the central pathways from the receptors to their terminations in the brain (Fig. 8-8).

Special somatic nerve fibers of cranial nerve VIII relay impulses from the sound receptors (hair cells) in the cochlear nuclei of the brainstem. These are bipolar neurons with cell bodies located in the spiral ganglia of the cochlea. Their central processes terminate in the dorsal and ventral cochlear nuclei on the ipsilateral side of the brainstem at the pontomedullary border. Most of the second-order neurons arising in the cochlear nuclei cross to the opposite side of the brainstem in the trapezoid body and turn upward in the *lateral lemniscus,* terminating in the inferior colliculus of the midbrain. Collaterals of the lateral lemniscus terminate in the nucleus of the trapezoid body, superior olivary nucleus, nucleus of the lateral lemniscus, and the brainstem reticular formation. Fibers arising in these nuclei also ascend in the lateral lemniscus. Those fibers from the cochlear nuclei which don't cross over in the trapezoid body ascend in the ipsilateral lateral lemniscus to the inferior colliculus. Sound signals also pass from one side to the other via contralateral projections from one lemniscal nucleus to the other as well as from one inferior colliculus to the other. Thus each lateral lemniscus conducts information from both sides, which helps to explain why damage to a lateral lemniscus produces no appreciable hearing loss other than problems with sound localization. Signals are then conducted from the inferior colliculi to the medial geniculate bodies and finally to the primary auditory area of the temporal lobes (area 41).

Vestibular System

The vestibulocochlear nerve serves two quite different functions. The cochlear portion, previously described, conducts sound information to the brain, while the vestibular portion conducts proprioceptive information. It is the central neural pathways of the latter function which we will examine now (Fig. 8-9). The mechanics and physiology of the system will be explained later in Chap. 11.

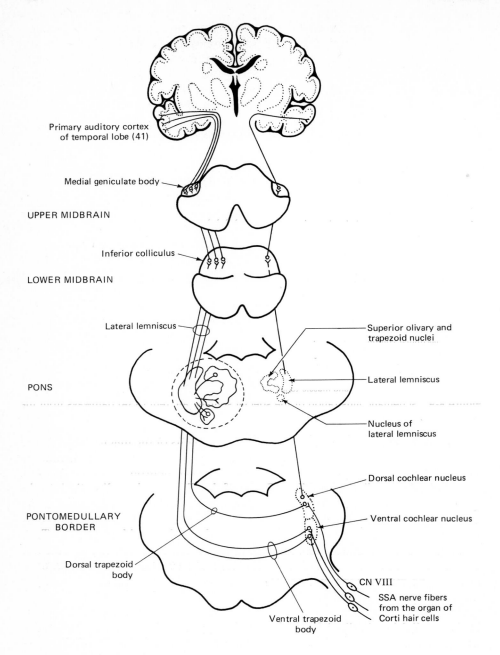

Primary auditory cortex
of temporal lobe (41)

Medial geniculate body

UPPER MIDBRAIN

Inferior colliculus

LOWER MIDBRAIN

Lateral lemniscus

Superior olivary and
trapezoid nuclei

Lateral lemniscus

PONS

Nucleus of
lateral lemniscus

Dorsal cochlear nucleus

PONTOMEDULLARY
BORDER

Ventral cochlear nucleus

Dorsal trapezoid
body

CN VIII

SSA nerve fibers
from the organ of
Corti hair cells

Ventral trapezoid
body

Figure 8-8 Schematic illustration showing the special somatic afferent (SSA) pathway for hearing. In addition to those fibers which cross in the trapezoid body, some fibers cross the midline in between the nuclei of the lateral lemnisci and between the two inferior colliculi (not pictured). Still others remain uncrossed and ascend in the ipsilateral lateral lemniscus.

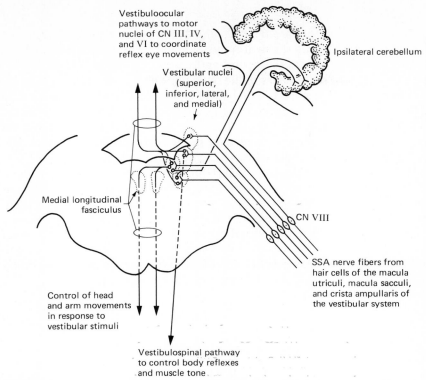

Vestibuloocular
pathways to motor
nuclei of CN III, IV,
and VI to coordinate
reflex eye movements

Ipsilateral cerebellum

Vestibular nuclei
(superior,
inferior, lateral,
and medial)

Medial longitudinal
fasciculus

CN VIII

SSA nerve fibers from
hair cells of the macula
utriculi, macula sacculi,
and crista ampullaris of
the vestibular system

Control of head
and arm movements
in response to
vestibular stimuli

Vestibulospinal pathway
to control body reflexes
and muscle tone

Figure 8-9   Schematic illustration of the special somatic afferent (SSA) pathways from the vestibular system.

Special somatic afferent fibers from the hair cells of the macula utriculi and macula sacculi conduct information into the vestibular nuclei on the ipsilateral side of the pons and medulla. These are bipolar neurons with cell bodies located in the vestibular ganglion. Some of the fibers project directly into the ipsilateral cerebellum to terminate in the uvula, flocculus, and nodulus, but most enter the cochlear nuclei and synapse there.

As might be expected, neuronal output from the cochlear nuclei effects bodily and eye movements in response to movements of the head as detected by the vestibular apparatus. The *vestibulospinal* path fibers which affect body reflexes and muscle tone in response to vestibular input originate primarily in the lateral vestibular nucleus. The medial vestibular nucleus is the principal origin of both crossed and uncrossed fibers which descend through the brainstem in the medial longitudinal fasciculus to the upper cord causing various reflex head and arm movements in response to vestibular stimuli. Finally, all four vestibular nuclei (medial, lateral, superior, and inferior) project both crossed and uncrossed fibers to the motor nuclei of cranial nerves III, IV, and VI in order to control and coordinate reflex eye movements. These *vestibuloocular* paths also travel in the medial longitudinal fasciculus.

Vision

The visual system receptors are the rods and cones of the retina. In Chap. 12 we will deal specifically with the neurophysiology of vision and visual reflexes. For now we will look only at the neural pathways.

Special somatic afferent fibers of the optic nerve (II) conduct visual signals into the brain. Examination of Fig. 8-10 will show that fibers from the lateral (temporal) retina of either eye terminate in the lateral geniculate body on the same side of the brain as that eye. On the other hand, SSA II fibers from the medial (nasal) retina of each eye cross over in the optic chiasm to terminate in the contralateral lateral geniculate body. The optic nerve is composed of fibers from the retina to the optic chiasm. Even though no synapses occur in the optic chiasm, the continuation of the visual pathway from the optic chiasm to the lateral geniculate body is called the *optic tract* rather than the optic nerve. After a synapse in the lateral geniculate body, the signal continues in the *optic radiation* to area 17 of the conscious visual cortex. Area 17 is the *primary visual area*, which receives initial visual signals. Neurons from this area project into the adjacent occipital cortex (areas 18 and 19) which is known as the *secondary visual area*. It is here that the visual signal is fully evaluated.

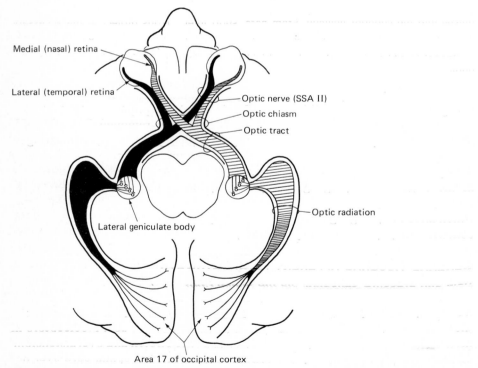

Figure 8-10 Schematic illustration of the special somatic afferent (SSA) pathways for vision. Signals projected to area 17 are referred to areas 18 and 19 for full visual interpretation.

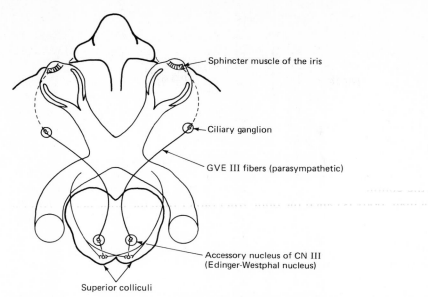

Sphincter muscle of the iris

Ciliary ganglion

GVE III fibers (parasympathetic)

Accessory nucleus of CN III
(Edinger-Westphal nucleus)

Superior colliculi

Figure 8-11   Schematic illustration of the visual reflex pathway involved in producing the pupillary light reflex. In response to a light shined into the eyes, SSA II fibers conduct impulses into the superior colliculi. From here, short interneurons project to the accessary nucleus of cranial nerve III (Edinger-Westphal nucleus) which is the origin of the GVE parasympathetic fibers of the oculomotor nerve (III). After entering the ciliary ganglion, postganglionic fibers innervate and constrict the sphincter muscle of the iris, constricting the pupil.

The visual reflex pathway involving the pupillary light reflex is illustrated in Fig. 8-11. This is the well-known reflex in which the pupils constrict when a light is shined into the eyes and dilate when the light is removed. Some SSA II fibers leave the optic tract before reaching the lateral geniculates, terminating in the superior colliculi instead. From here, short neurons project to the Edinger-Westphal nucleus (an accessory nucleus of III) in the midbrain, which serves as the origin of the preganglionic parasympathetic fibers of the oculomotor nerve (GVE III). The GVE III fibers in turn project to the ciliary ganglia, from which arise the postganglionic fibers to the sphincter muscles of the iris, which constrict the pupils when they contract.

GENERAL VISCERAL AFFERENT (GVA) PATHWAYS

Pain and Pressure Sensation via the Spinal Cord

Visceral pain receptors are located in peritoneal surfaces, pleural membranes, the dura mater, walls of arteries, and the walls of the GI tube. Nociceptors in the walls of the GI tube are particularly sensitive to stretch and overdistension.

General visceral nociceptors conduct signals into the spinal cord over the monopolar neurons of the posterior root ganglia. They terminate in laminae III and IV of the posterior horn as do the pain and temperature pathways of the

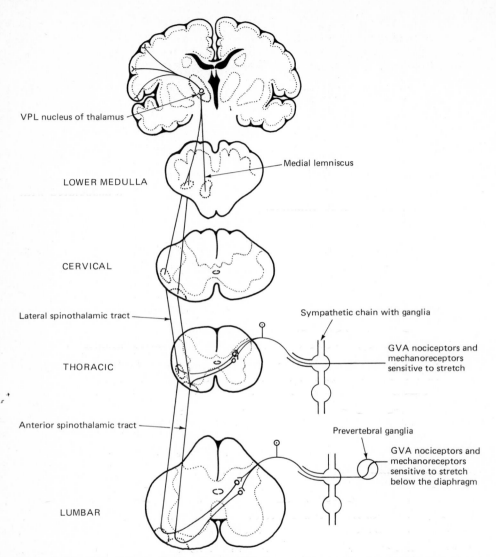

VPL nucleus of thalamus

LOWER MEDULLA

Medial lemniscus

CERVICAL

Lateral spinothalamic tract

Sympathetic chain with ganglia

GVA nociceptors and mechanoreceptors sensitive to stretch

THORACIC

Anterior spinothalamic tract

Prevertebral ganglia

GVA nociceptors and mechanoreceptors sensitive to stretch below the diaphragm

LUMBAR

Figure 8-12 Schematic illustration showing the general visceral afferent (GVA) pathways for visceral pain and pressure sensation from the viscera.

GSA system; however, their peripheral processes reach the visceral receptors via the gray rami communicantes and ganglia of the sympathetic chain (Fig. 8-12). Second-order neurons from the posterior horn cross in the anterior white commissure and ascend to the thalamus in the anterior and lateral spinothalamic tracts. Projections from the VPL of the thalamus relay signals to the sensory cortex.

The localization of visceral pain is relatively poor, making it difficult to tell the exact source of the stimuli. At least a partial explanation of our inability to precisely localize visceral pain relates to its rarity. True visceral pain seldom occurs when compared to the frequency of external pain. An additional compounding factor is the phenomena of _referred pain_. Because true visceral pain is often projected or "referred" by the brain to some area on the surface of the body, its true visceral origin is often confused. The mechanism for referred visceral pain is not fully understood but may result in part from the close proximity in the posterior horn of the central terminals of GVA pain fibers and GSA spinal nerve fibers from the body surface. This is supported by the fact that pain from a visceral origin is referred to a dermatome with which it shares the same posterior root. This is a useful observation, often making it possible to locate the source of a visceral pain from an observation of the surface area to which it is referred. The pain down the inside of the left arm associated with true cardiac pain is a good example.

It is likely that separate second-order neurons relay pain information from GSA and GVA input. If the painful stimulus to the viscera is moderate, the level of activity in the GVA fibers is likely sufficient to stimulate only those second-order neurons which normally relay signals from the viscera. However, if the painful stimulus increases in strength, the increased central synaptic activity of the GVA neurons may "spill over" and raise the central excitatory

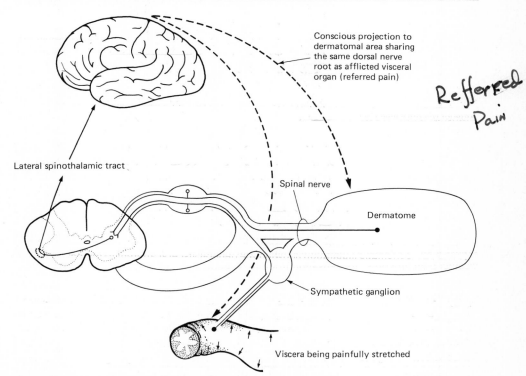

Figure 8-13 Schematic illustration showing how pain originating in a visceral organ is "referred" by the brain to a dermatomal area of the skin in addition to the visceral organ which shares the same dorsal root with it. (Explanation in the text.)

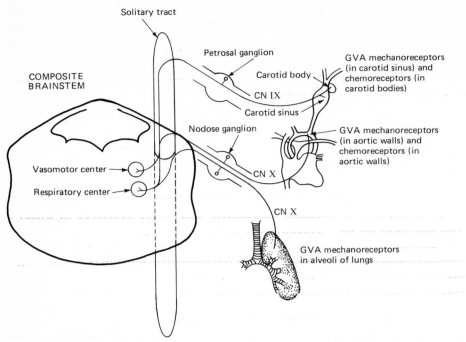

Figure 8-14 Schematic illustration showing the general visceral afferent (GVA) pathways for subconscious reception of visceral mechanoreception and chemoreception via cranial nerves IX and X.

state of those second-order neurons which normally relay information from GSA fibers of the dermatome. If the painful visceral stimulation is very strong, this "spill over" may be sufficient to exceed the threshold of excitation for these neurons, causing them to fire even though no painful stimulus is delivered to the general somatic nociceptors of the dermatome. Thus the brain incorrectly projects the source of the pain to the dermatomal area (Fig. 8-13).

Blood Pressure, Blood Chemistry, and Alveolar Stretch Detection

The walls of the aorta and the carotid sinuses contain special baroreceptors (pressure receptors) which respond to changes in blood pressure. These mechanoreceptors are the peripheral endings of GVA fibers of the glossopharyngeal (IX) and vagus (X) nerves. The GVA fibers from the carotid sinus baroreceptors enter the *solitary tract* of the brainstem and terminate in the vasomotor center of the medulla (Fig. 8-14). This is the CNS control center for cardiovascular activity. The cell bodies of these unipolar neurons are located in the petrosal ganglion. GVA fibers of the vagus nerve conduct signals from the baroreceptors in the walls of the aorta to the solitary tract and on to the vasomotor center. The cell bodies of these unipolar neurons are located in the nodose ganglion.

Stretch receptors in the alveoli of the lungs conduct information concerning rhythmic alveolar inflation and deflation over GVA X fibers to the solitary tract and then to the respiratory center of the brainstem. This route is an important link in the Hering-Breuer reflex, which helps to regulate respiration.

Carotid body chemoreceptors, sensitive to changes in blood Po_2 and, to a lesser extent, Pco_2 and pH, conduct signals to both the vasomotor and respiratory centers over GVA IX nerve fibers. GVA X fibers conduct similar information from the aortic chemoreceptors to both centers. Chemoreceptors were discussed in Chap. 7.

SPECIAL VISCERAL AFFERENT (SVA) PATHWAYS
Taste

The receptors for taste are the taste cells which produce impulses in afferent fibers in response to chemical stimulation. They were described in Chap. 7. The pathways for taste sensation are illustrated in Fig. 8-15.

Special visceral afferent (SVA) fibers of cranial nerves VII, IX, and X conduct signals into the solitary tract of the brainstem, ultimately terminating in the nucleus of the solitary tract on the ipsilateral side. Second-order neurons cross over and ascend through the brainstem in the medial lemniscus to the VPM of the thalamus. Thalamic projections to area 43 (the primary taste area) of the postcentral gyrus complete the relay. SVA VII fibers conduct from the chemoreceptors of taste buds on the anterior two-thirds of the tongue, while

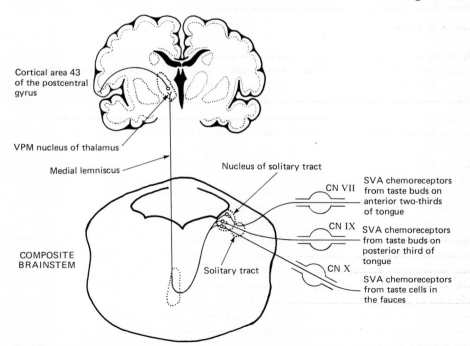

Figure 8-15 Schematic illustration showing the special visceral afferent (SVA) pathways for the sense of taste.

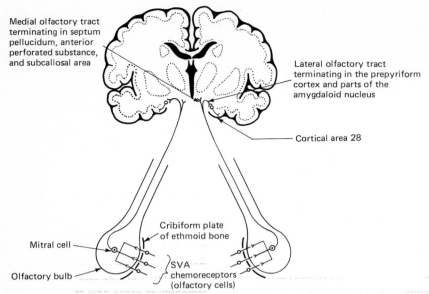

Medial olfactory tract
terminating in septum
pellucidum, anterior
perforated substance,
and subcallosal area

Lateral olfactory tract
terminating in the prepyriform
cortex and parts of the
amygdaloid nucleus

Cortical area 28

Cribiform plate
of ethmoid bone

Mitral cell

Olfactory bulb

SVA
chemoreceptors
(olfactory cells)

Figure 8-16 Schematic illustration showing the special visceral afferent (SVA) pathways for smell.

SVA IX fibers conduct taste information from buds on the posterior one-third of the tongue. SVA X fibers conduct taste signals from those taste cells located throughout the fauces.

Smell

The sense of smell was examined in Chap. 7 and, once again, we will look only at the central pathways here. The smell-sensitive cells (olfactory cells) of the olfactory epithelium project their central processes through the cribiform plate of the ethmoid bone, where they synapse with mitral cells. The central processes of the mitral cells pass from the olfactory bulb through the olfactory tract, which divides into a medial and lateral portion (Fig. 8-16). The *lateral olfactory tract* terminates in the prepyriform cortex and parts of the amygdala of the temporal lobe. These areas represent the *primary olfactory cortex.* Fibers then project from here to area 28, the *secondary olfactory area,* for sensory evaluation. The medial olfactory tract projects to the anterior perforated substance, the septum pellucidum, the subcallosal area, and even the contralateral olfactory tract. Both the medial and lateral olfactory tracts contribute to the visceral reflex pathways, causing the viscerosomatic and viscerovisceral responses described in Chap. 7.

DAMAGE TO THE SPINAL NERVES AND SPINAL CORD

After studying the motor pathways of Chap. 6 and the sensory pathways of Chap. 8, the student should be able to explain why the injuries described in Table 8-1 would be expected to produce the symptoms listed.

Table 8-1 Symptoms of Damage to Spinal Nerves and Spinal Cord

Damage	Possible cause of damage	Symptoms associated with innervated area
Peripheral nerve	Mechanical injury	Loss of muscle tone Loss of reflexes Flaccid paralysis Denervation atrophy Loss of sensation
Posterior root	Tabes dorsalis	Paresthesia Intermittent sharp pains Decreased sensitivity to pain Loss of reflexes Loss of sensation Positive Romberg sign High stepping and slapping of feet
Anterior Horn	Poliomyelitis	Loss of muscle tone Loss of reflexes Flaccid paralysis Denervation atrophy
Lamina X (gray matter)	Syringomyelia	Bilateral loss of pain and temperature sense only at afflicted cord level Sensory dissociation No sensory impairment below afflicted level
Anterior horn and lateral corticospinal tract	Amyotrophic lateral sclerosis	Muscle weakness Muscle atrophy Fasciculations of hand and arm muscles Spastic paralysis
Posterior and lateral funiculi	Subacute combined degeneration	Loss of position sense Loss of vibratory sense Positive Romberg sign Muscle weakness Spasticity Hyperactive tendon reflexes Positive Babinski sign

Hemisection of the spinal cord	Mechanical injury	Brown-Séquard syndrome
		  Below cord level on injured side
		    Flaccid paralysis
		    Hyperactive tendon reflexes
		    Loss of position sense
		    Loss of vibratory sense
		    Tactile impairment
		  Below cord level on opposite side beginning one or two segments below injury
		    Loss of pain and temperature

REVIEW QUESTIONS

1   Pain and temperature signals transmitted over spinal nerves ascend the spinal cord to the brain in the
    a   anterior spinocerebellar tract
    b   lateral spinothalamic tract
    c   anterior spinothalamic tract
    d   trigeminothalamic tract

2   The area of skin supplied by afferent fibers in the posterior root of a single spinal nerve is called a
    a   metamere
    b   neuromere
    c   dermatome
    d   neurotome
    e   none of the above

3   The sensation of touch which implies an awareness of an object's shape, texture, three-dimensional qualities, and other fine points is typically described as
    a   epicritic touch
    b   protopathic touch
    c   discriminating touch
    d   crude touch
    e   simple touch

4   The conscious awareness of body position and movement
    a   is called kinesthesia
    b   involves transmission through thalamic nuclei
    c   is mediated over spinocerebellar tract fibers
    d   is mediated over dorsal column pathways
    e   is mediated over spinothalamic pathways

5   All of the following are signs associated with damage to the dorsal columns, *except*
    a   nystagmus
    b   astereognosis
    c   loss of two-point discrimination
    d   positive Romberg sign
    e   loss of vibratory sense

6   Afferent fibers innervating the organ of Corti hair cells
    a   are bipolar neurons
    b   are SVA fibers
    c   have their cell bodies located in the cochlear nuclei
    d   form two-element receptors with the hair cells
    e   are part of the IXth cranial nerve

7   Fibers from visceral pain receptors
    a   terminate in lamina VII of the spinal cord gray matter
    b   synapse in the peripheral nervous system before entering the spinal cord
    c   give rise to subconscious signals only
    d   pass through autonomic ganglia
    e   none of the above

8   Nerve fibers from carotid sinus baroreceptors
    a   enter the solitary tract of the brainstem
    b   are part of the vagus nerve

    c conduct information to the vasomotor center

    d enter the spinal cord

9 Damage to the posterior roots of spinal nerves

    a is characteristic of poliomyelitis

    b may cause denervation atrophy in the muscles innervated

    c may cause a positive Romberg sign

    d causes flaccid paralysis in the muscles innervated

    e all of the above

10 Lamina X of the spinal cord gray matter is diseased in

    a tabes dorsalis

    b subacute combined degeneration

    c amyotrophic lateral sclerosis

    d syringomyelia

    e none of the above

The Brainstem

The diencephalon along with the midbrain, pons, and medulla oblongata comprise the brainstem. A clear understanding of the importance of this area of the CNS requires that the student be familiar with both its external and internal features. In addition to performing many vitally important regulatory functions (respiratory and cardiovascular, to name two), the brainstem also serves as a central point of relay between the cerebrum, the cerebellum, and the receptors and effectors of the cranial and spinal nerves.

EXTERNAL MORPHOLOGY

The prominent external features of the brainstem are illustrated in Figs. 9-1 through 9-3. The cerebrum and cerebellum have been removed in each drawing in order to afford an unobstructed view of the brainstem from anterior, posterior, and lateral perspectives.

The Midbrain

The most prominent features of the anterior and lateral midbrain are the *cerebral peduncles*. These broad bundles of descending fibers from the cerebrum converge to form a V on the anterior surface, bounded above by the *optic chiasm* and below by the superior border of the pons. The *mammillary bodies*

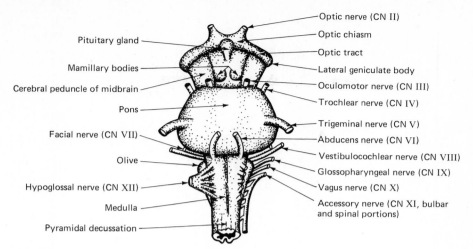

Figure 9-1   Anterior view of the brainstem.

and the *pituitary gland* are framed by the two peduncles. Four prominent enlargements, the *corpora quadrigemina*, can be seen on the posterior surface of the midbrain. The quadrigemina (four bodies) include two *superior colliculi* and two *inferior colliculi*. The *trochlear nerves* (IV) emerge from the posterior surface of the midbrain just below the inferior colliculi, wrapping around the cerebral peduncles to appear anterolaterally at the superior border of the pons. The *oculomotor nerves* (III) also originate in the midbrain, emerging anteriorly at the superior border of the pons.

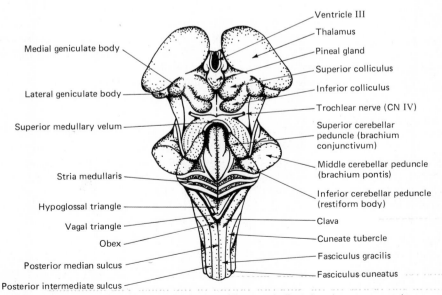

Figure 9-2   Posterior view of the brainstem. The cerebellum has been removed.

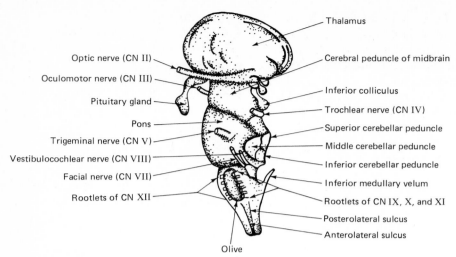

Optic nerve (CN II)
Oculomotor nerve (CN III)
Pituitary gland
Pons
Trigeminal nerve (CN V)
Vestibulocochlear nerve (CN VIII)
Facial nerve (CN VII)
Rootlets of CN XII

Thalamus
Cerebral peduncle of midbrain
Inferior colliculus
Trochlear nerve (CN IV)
Superior cerebellar peduncle
Middle cerebellar peduncle
Inferior cerebellar peduncle
Inferior medullary velum
Rootlets of CN IX, X, and XI
Posterolateral sulcus
Anterolateral sulcus

Olive

Figure 9-3   Lateral view of the brainstem.

The Pons

The pons is a distinctively prominent feature of the brainstem. It appears as a broad band of transversely running fibers when viewed anteriorly and from the side. The fibers extend into the cerebellum behind and appear to be holding it to the brainstem. Those which wrap laterally to the cerebellum form the *middle cerebellar peduncles*.

    The pons is bounded superiorly by the midbrain and inferiorly by the medulla oblongata. The *trigeminal nerves* (V) are prominent lateral projections. The *abducens nerves* (VI) originate in the pons and emerge close together at the anterior inferior border of the pons. The *facial nerves* (VII), originating in the pons, and the *vestibulocochlear nerves* (VIII), originating in the pontomedullary area, emerge at the pontomedullary border.

The Medulla Oblongata

The most prominent anterior features of the medulla oblongata are the *medullary pyramids*. They appear on the anterior surface as two vertically running rounded eminences which emerge from under the pons to become continuous with the spinal cord below. In the lowest portion of the anterior medulla, descending corticospinal (pyramidal) tract fibers cross over in the *pyramidal decussation*. The corticospinal tracts are often called *pyramidal tracts* because of the unique pyramidal shape they give to the anterior medulla as they descend into the spinal cord.

    The *olive* is a lateral feature of the medulla. Emerging from the lateral medulla posterior to the olive in descending order are the *glossopharyngeal nerves* (IX), the *vagus nerves* (X), and the *bulbar accessory nerves* (XI). The *hypoglossal nerves* (XII) emerge from the lateral medulla anterior to the olive.

Three sulci are visible in posterior view, a single *posterior median sulcus* and two laterally placed *posterior intermediate sulci*. Two rounded eminences, the *gracile tubercle* (clava) and the *cuneate tubercle* are observed on either side of the posterior median sulcus. The *fasciculus gracilis* leads to the former while the *fasciculus cuneatus* leads to the latter. The posterior intermediate sulcus separates the fasciculus gracilis and gracile tubercle from the fasciculus cuneatus and cuneate tubercle on either side.

CROSS-SECTIONAL ANATOMY OF THE BRAINSTEM

As pathways ascend and descend through the brainstem they often undergo shifts in position which can only be seen by a careful examination of cross-sec-

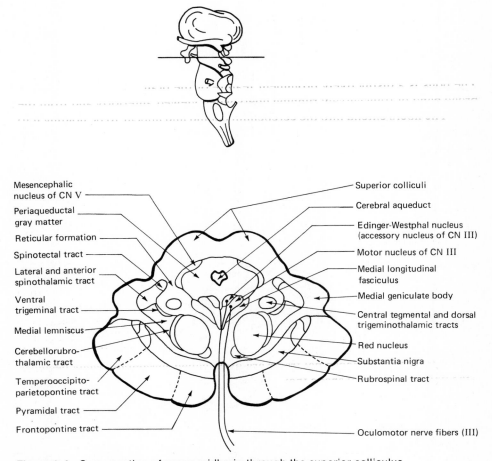

Figure 9-4 Cross section of upper midbrain through the superior colliculus.

tional anatomy. The student can verify this by close examination of the eight representative sections schematically illustrated in Figs. 9-4 through 9-11. There is no real shortcut or alternative to "learning" these cross sections. Indeed, the function of the brainstem as a relay center between the cerebrum above, the cerebellum behind, and the spinal cord below is easier to visualize.

As an academic exercise, it is useful to follow the course of pathways through the brainstem. By doing this it is possible to observe how the tracts change in relative position and size as they descend through the stem. For example, the *corticospinal* tracts enter the brainstem in the middle third of the *basis pedunculi* (ventral portion) of the cerebral peduncles where they are widely separated from each other. As they descend through the pons they move to a deeper position away from the surface. However, upon entering the medulla they begin to converge and once again move to the surface, giving rise to the medullary pyramids. Bundles of crossing fibers of these tracts can be observed in the pyramidal decussation in the lower medulla.

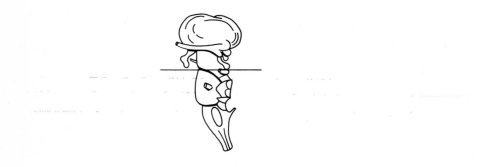

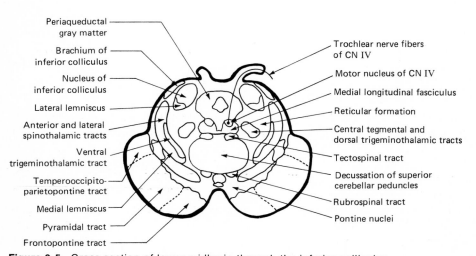

Figure 9-5 Cross section of lower midbrain through the inferior colliculus.

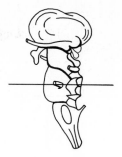

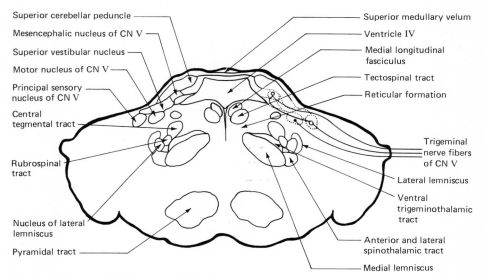

Superior cerebellar peduncle ——————
Mesencephalic nucleus of CN V ——
Superior vestibular nucleus ——
Motor nucleus of CN V ——
Principal sensory —— nucleus of CN V
Central tegmental tract ——
Rubrospinal tract ——
Nucleus of lateral lemniscus ——
Pyramidal tract ——

—————— Superior medullary velum
—————— Ventricle IV
—— Medial longitudinal fasciculus
—— Tectospinal tract
—— Reticular formation
Trigeminal nerve fibers of CN V
Lateral lemniscus
Ventral trigeminothalamic tract
Anterior and lateral spinothalamic tract
Medial lemniscus

Figure 9-6   Cross section of middle pons.

CRANIAL NERVES AND BRAINSTEM NUCLEI

Cranial Nerve Fiber Classification

Cranial nerve fibers are classified as general or special, somatic or visceral, and afferent or efferent. This classification scheme was presented in Chap. 1 and is further amplified here.

Special fibers are those which innervate the special sense organs associated with hearing, seeing, smelling, and tasting. In addition, they innervate the vestibular apparatus and those skeletal muscles derived from the mesoderm of the branchial arches. This latter group includes the muscles of facial expression and mastication as well as laryngeal and pharyngeal muscles. Also included are the sternomastoid and trapezius muscles. All other cranial nerve fibers are classified as *general*.

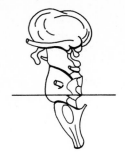

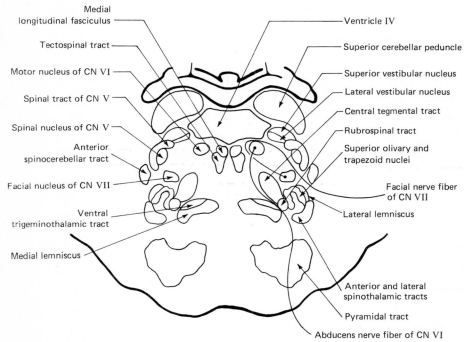

Figure 9-7 Cross section of lower pons.

Fibers are further designated somatic or visceral. *Somatic fibers* innervate those skeletal muscles derived from mesodermal somites as well as innervating structures of ectodermal origin. The latter include the skin, the eye, the vestibular apparatus, and the inner ear. Exceptions are the olfactory epithelium and the taste buds. Even though the olfactory epithelium and taste buds are of ectodermal origin, the cranial nerve fibers innervating them are classified as visceral because of the close functional relationship which the senses of smell and taste have with the truly visceral gastrointestinal tract.

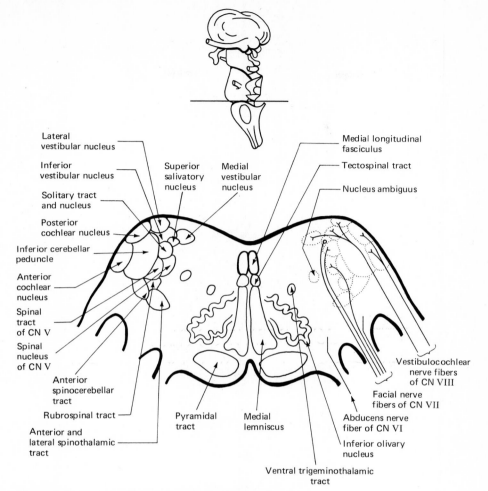

Figure 9-8   Cross section at the pontomedullary border.

Visceral fibers innervate structures of entodermal origin including cardiac muscle, smooth muscle, and glands. Also included here are those skeletal muscles derived from the mesoderm of the branchial arches. As previously noted, cranial nerve fibers mediating smell (I) and taste (VII, IX, and X) are typically included here rather than with the somatic group. Cranial nerve fibers are also classified as afferent or efferent, depending on the direction of their impulse conduction. *Afferent fibers* conduct impulses toward the CNS while *efferent fibers* conduct them away.

An oddity in the classification scheme arises from the practice of classifying all proprioceptors as general somatic regardless of whether they are associ-

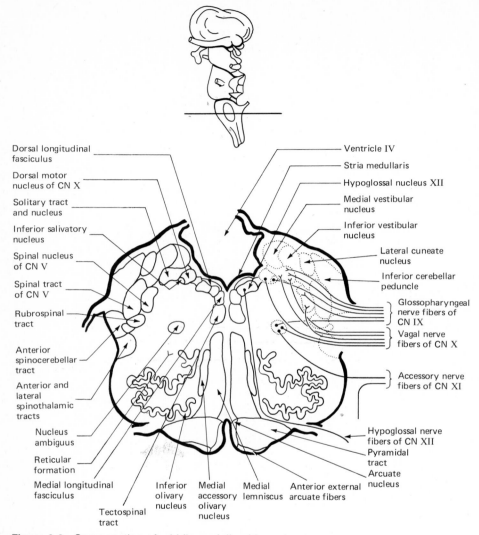

Figure 9-9 Cross section of middle medulla oblongata.

ated with somatic or branchial muscles. This leads to the confusing observation that a muscle can be innervated by both special *visceral* efferent and special *somatic* afferent fibers at the same time. The muscles of mastication are an example (Fig. 9-14). The scheme of cranial nerve fiber classification is presented again in Table 9-1.

Alar and Basal Nuclei

When the embryonic neural tube closes, a groove remains in each lateral wall which separates the posterior from the anterior portions. The former gives rise

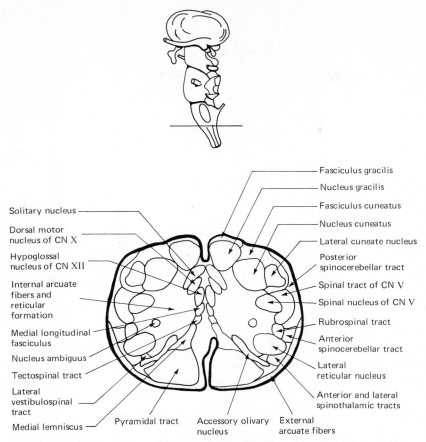

Figure 9-10   Cross section of lower medulla oblongata at sensory decussation.

to the *alar lamina* or *plate*, while the latter forms the *basal lamina* (Fig. 9-12). Brainstem sensory nuclei are found in the alar lamina, while motor nuclei are generally distributed in the basal lamina. Figure 9-12 is a composite sketch of cranial nerve nuclei as found in the brainstem from the midbrain to the medulla oblongata. It is not a sketch of any single brainstem section but instead represents a construct intended to show the relative positions of the nuclei with respect to each other in cross section. Notice that the efferent (motor) nuclei are located in the basal plate, while the afferent (sensory) nuclei are located in the more lateral alar plates. The dividing line is the *sulcus limitans*.

Cranial Nerve Fibers and the Brainstem

It is not too difficult to trace the emergence of each cranial nerve from the brainstem. A more difficult task is to appreciate the distinct fiber types present in each cranial nerve. But unquestionably the most difficult task of all is to trace the efferent origins and afferent terminations of the cranial nerve fibers in the brainstem. These relationships are illustrated in Figs. 9-13 through 9-15.

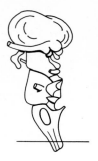

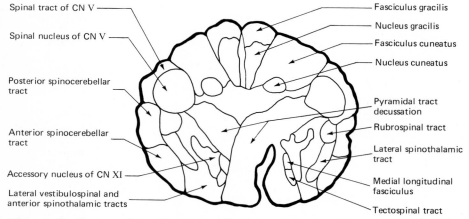

Spinal tract of CN V

Spinal nucleus of CN V

Posterior spinocerebellar tract

Anterior spinocerebellar tract

Accessory nucleus of CN XI

Lateral vestibulospinal and anterior spinothalamic tracts

Fasciculus gracilis

Nucleus gracilis

Fasciculus cuneatus

Nucleus cuneatus

Pyramidal tract decussation

Rubrospinal tract

Lateral spinothalamic tract

Medial longitudinal fasciculus

Tectospinal tract

Figure 9-11   Cross section of lowest medulla oblongata at level of pyramidal decussation.

Olfactory Nerve (I)   The fibers of this nerve are SVA. They carry information pertinent to smell from the olfactory epithelium to the dendritic glomerular zone of the mitral cells in the olfactory bulb. Mitral cell fibers then conduct smell information to the olfactory cortex. Damage to these tracts causes anosmia (loss of the sense of smell).

Optic Nerve (II)   The fibers of this nerve are SSA. They conduct information concerning vision from the ganglion cell layer of the retina primarily to the lateral geniculate bodies. Damage to these fibers causes anopsia (loss of vision).

Oculomotor Nerve (III)   The oculomotor nerve contains GVE and GSE fibers. The GVE fibers originate in the Edinger-Westphal nucleus (an acces-

TABLE 9-1   Classification of Cranial Nerve Fibers

I *General afferent fibers.* The afferent unipolar neurons with cell bodies in the craniospinal ganglia
   A *General somatic afferent* (GSA). From exteroceptors responding to touch, pressure pain, and temperature as well as from the proprioceptors of muscles, tendons, and joints
   B *General visceral afferent* (GVA). From interoceptors of the viscera
II *Special afferent fibers.* The afferent neurons from the special sense organs (eye, ear, nose, and tongue) and the vestibular system
   A *Special somatic afferent* (SSA). Exteroceptors from the eye and ear as well as proprioceptors from the vestibular system
   B *Special visceral afferent* (SVA). Exteroceptors from the olfactory epithelium and the taste buds
III *General efferent fibers.* The efferent neurons originating in brainstem nuclei innervating somatic skeletal muscle as well as those innervating cardiac muscle, smooth muscle, and glands
   A *General somatic efferent* (GSE). To somatic skeletal muscles
   B *General visceral efferent* (GVE). The autonomic fibers to cardiac muscle, smooth muscle, and glands
IV *Special efferent fibers.* The efferent neurons originating in brainstem nuclei innervating branchiomeric skeletal muscle
   A *Special vesceral efferent* (SVE). To branchiomeric skeletal muscles

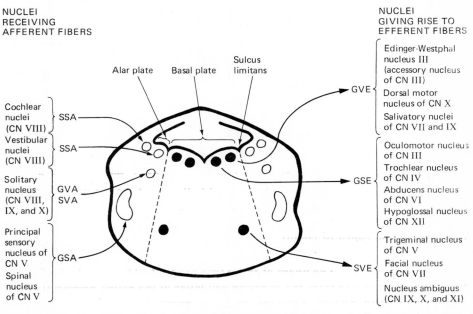

Figure 9-12 Composite sketch of cranial nerve nuclei as seen in the brainstem from midbrain to medulla. This is not a sketch of any single brainstem section but a construct intended to show the relative position of the nuclei with respect to each other in cross section. Notice that the efferent nuclei are confined to the basal plate while the afferent nuclei are located in the more lateral alar plates. The dividing line is the sulcus limitans.

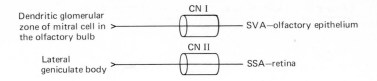

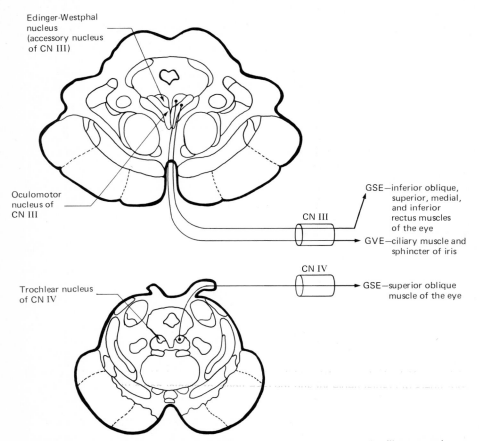

Figure 9-13 Schematic illustration showing the relationship between the fiber types in cranial nerves I, II, III, and IV, brain, and brainstem nuclei, and the various structures innervated.

sory nucleus of III) in the upper midbrain. They represent the preganglionic parasymapthetic fibers to the ciliary ganglion. Postganglionic fibers innervate the ciliary muscles, which control the thickness of the lens, as well as the sphincter muscles of the iris, which control pupil size. Damage to these fibers eliminates the pupillary light reflex and interferes with accommodation reflexes.

The GSE fibers originate in the oculomotor nucleus in the upper midbrain. They innervate the inferior oblique as well as the superior, medial, and inferior

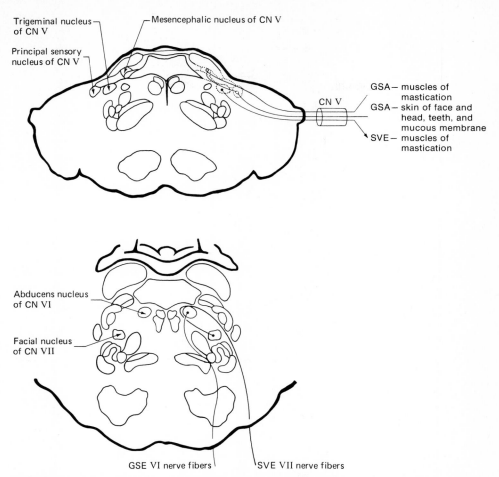

Trigeminal nucleus of CN V

Principal sensory nucleus of CN V

Mesencephalic nucleus of CN V

CN V

GSA— muscles of mastication
GSA— skin of face and head, teeth, and mucous membrane
SVE— muscles of mastication

Abducens nucleus of CN VI

Facial nucleus of CN VII

GSE VI nerve fibers

SVE VII nerve fibers

Figure 9-14 Schematic illustration showing the relationship between the fiber types in cranial nerve V, brainstem nuclei, and the structures innervated. Also shown is the origin of the SVE fibers of cranial nerve VII and the GSE fibers of cranial nerve VI.

rectus muscles of the eye. Damage to these fibers results in external strabismus and ptosis of the eyelid.

Trochlear Nerve (IV)   The fibers of this nerve are GSE. They originate in the trochlear nucleus of the lower midbrain. They innervate the superior oblique muscles of the eye. Damage to these fibers causes the eyes to look slightly upward.

Trigeminal Nerve (V)   The trigeminal nerve contains SVE and GSA fibers. The SVE fibers originate in the trigeminal nucleus located in the middle pons. They innervate the muscles of mastication (branchiomeric origin). Damage to these muscles causes paralysis of the jaws.

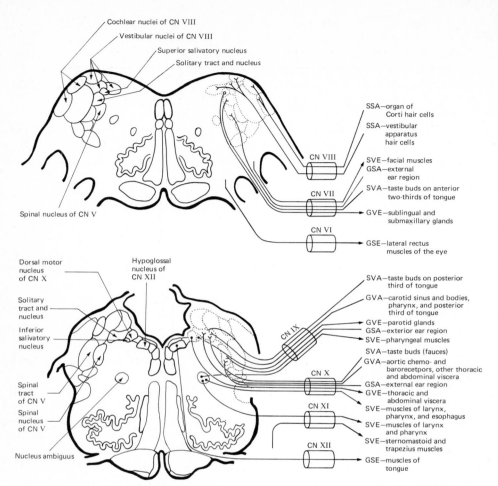

Figure 9-15 Schematic illustration showing the relationship between the fiber types in cranial nerves VI, VII, VIII, IX, X, XI, and XII, brainstem nuclei, and the various structures innervated.

The GSA fibers fall into two groups, those from proprioceptors and those from exteroceptors. Proprioceptive fibers have their cell bodies in the mesencephalic nucleus of V and terminate in the principal sensory nucleus of V in the pons. Exteroceptive fibers from the skin of the face and head as well as the teeth and the mucous membranes conduct information to the principal sensory nucleus of V. Damage to these fibers causes anesthesia in the affected area.

Abducens Nerve (VI)   The fibers of this nerve are GSE. They originate in the abducens nucleus in the lower pons and innervate the lateral rectus muscle of the eye. Damage to these fibers causes internal strabismus and double vision.

Facial Nerve (VII)   The facial nerve is composed of SVE, GVE, GSA, and SVA fibers. The SVE fibers originate in the facial nucleus of the pons and innervate the muscles of facial expression. Damage to these fibers causes facial paralysis. The GVE fibers are the preganglionic parasympathetic fibers to the submaxillary ganglion. They originate in the superior salivatory nucleus of the pontomedullary region. Postganglionic fibers innervate the submaxillary and sublingual salivary glands.

The GSA fibers conduct information from the skin of the external ear region to the spinal tract and nucleus of V. The SVA fibers conduct information from the taste buds on the anterior two-thirds of the tongue to the solitary tract and nucleus.

Vestibulocochlear Nerve (VIII)   The fibers of this nerve are SSA. SSA fibers from the organ of Corti hair cells conduct auditory information to the cochlear nuclei of the pontomedullary region. SSA fibers from the vestibular apparatus hair cells conduct information concerning equilibrium to the vestibular nuclei in the same general region.

Glossopharyngeal Nerve (IX)   The glossopharyngeal nerve is composed of GVE, SVE, GVA, GSA, and SVA fibers. The GVE fibers originate in the inferior salivatory nucleus. These are preganglionic parasympathetic fibers to the otic ganglion. Postganglionic fibers innervate the parotid salivary glands. The SVE fibers originate in the nucleus ambiguus and innervate the pharyngeal muscles (branchiomeric origin). GVA fibers conduct information from the pharynx and posterior third of the tongue. These fibers also innervate the carotid sinus baroreceptors and carotid body chemoreceptors. Signals are conducted to the solitary tract and nucleus.

The GSA fibers conduct information from the skin of the external ear region to the spinal tract and nucleus of V. SVA fibers carry information from the taste buds on the posterior third of the tongue to the solitary tract and nucleus.

Vagus Nerve (X)   The vagus nerve is composed of GVE, SVE, GSA, GVA, and SVA fibers. The GVE fibers originate in the dorsal motor nucleus of X and innervate thoracic and abdominal viscera. These are the parasympathetic fibers of the vagus nerve. The SVE fibers innervate the muscles of the larynx and pharynx (branchiomeric origin) and originate in the nucleus ambiguus. The GSA fibers carry information from the skin of the ear region to the spinal tract and nucleus of V. GVA fibers conduct signals from the aortic baroreceptors and chemoreceptors as well as other thoracic and abdominal viscera to the solitary tract and nucleus. Taste cells in the fauces send signals over SVA fibers to the solitary tract and nucleus.

Accessory Nerve (XI)   The fibers of the accessory nerve are SVE. There are two components to this nerve, a bulbar component arising from nuclei within the brainstem and a spinal component arising from nuclei in upper cervical levels of the spinal cord. The SVE fibers which arise from the nucleus ambiguus of the medulla innervate the muscles of the larynx and pharynx (branchiomeric origin). SVE fibers arising in the spinal accessory nucleus in the upper cervical levels of the cord innervate the sternomastoid and trapezius muscles (also of branchiomeric origin).

Hypoglossal Nerve (XII)   The fibers of this nerve are GSE. They originate in the hypoglossal nucleus of the medulla and innervate the muscles of the tongue.

REVIEW QUESTIONS

1 The brainstem includes all but the
   a diencephalon
   b midbrain
   c pons
   d cerebellum
   e medulla oblongata
2 All of the following cranial nerves originate in nuclei within the midbrain, *except*
   a III
   b IV
   c V
   d VI
3 All of the following cranial nerves contain GSE fibers, *except*
   a IV
   b V
   c VI
   d VII
   e XII
4 Brainstem motor nuclei are generally distributed
   a in the alar lamina
   b in the basal lamina
   c in the lateral portion of the brainstem
   d medial to the sulcus limitans
   e none of the above
5 All of the following are innervated by fibers of the glossopharyngeal nerve, *except*
   a taste buds on the posterior third of the tongue
   b the parotid salivary glands
   c carotid sinus baroreceptors
   d aortic chemoreceptors
   e taste buds on the anterior two-thirds of the tongue
6 Damage to the GSE fibers of the abducens nerve (VI) is likely to cause
   a internal strabismus
   b the eyes to look slightly upward
   c external strabismus
   d ptosis of the eyelid

7 Damage to the SVE fibers of the trigeminal nerve (V) is likely to cause
  a paralysis of the muscles of facial expression
  b paralysis of the jaw
  c paralysis of the sternomastoid muscle
  d paralysis of the tongue
8 All of the following give rise to GVE fibers, *except*
  a nucleus ambiguus
  b Edinger-Westphal nucleus
  c dorsal motor nucleus of X
  d salivatory nuclei
9 The GVA and SVA fibers of cranial nerves terminate in the
  a cochlear nuclei
  b vestibular nuclei
  c solitary nucleus
  d principal sensory nucleus of V
  e nucleus of the spinal tract of V
10 SVA fibers of cranial nerves innervate
  a taste buds
  b proprioceptors in muscles
  c rods and cones
  d olfactory cells
  e none of the above

Sound and Hearing

The ear is the organ and sound is the sensation of hearing. A neurophysiologist might define sound as a change in pressure propagated through an elastic medium (typically air) which is detected by the ear and sensed by the auditory cortex of the brain. An understanding of the characteristics of sound waves as well as the physics of mechanical transduction in the ear are important correlates to the study of hearing by the nervous apparatus. Those parameters of sound which are of particular interest in this regard are frequency, velocity, and amplitude.

CHARACTERISTICS OF SOUND

Frequency

The frequency f of a sound wave is equal to the number of oscillatory cycles it makes per unit time (typically per second). The human ear is sensitive to frequencies in the range between 20 and 20,000 Hz (cycles per second). Actually most people are sensitive to a narrower range between 50 and 10,000 Hz. Most speech is between 60 and 500 Hz and the ear is most sensitive to sounds in the 1200- to 4000-Hz range. The physical characteristics of the human hearing apparatus which favor this very sensitive range will be explained later.

Velocity

The velocity c of a sound wave depends on the medium through which it travels. Typically the greater the density of the medium, the greater the sound velocity. For example, sound travels through air at 331 m/s, water at 1490 m/s, muscle at 1570 m/s, bone at 3360 m/s, and solids at 5000 m/s.

The velocity of a sound wave is independent of its frequency. In other words, changing its frequency doesn't alter its velocity. If this were not the case, low notes from a musical chord might reach the ear at a different time than high notes from the cord, making the appreciation of music considerably less pleasant.

The wavelength λ of a sound wave is equal to its velocity divided by its frequency and is thus expressed in distance per cycle.

$$\lambda = \frac{c}{f}$$

Amplitude

When no sound is disturbing the air, the average pressure P_0 at sea level is 1 atm. This is equivalent to 760 mmHg or 1×10^6 dyn/cm². Sound pressure waves are superimposed on this average pressure. Since sound waves are oscillatory, the instantaneous absolute pressure P periodically varies above and below the average pressure. The sound pressure amplitude p, which is utilized for calculations in sound and hearing studies, is equal to the difference between the average and absolute pressures (Fig. 10-1). The sound pressure amplitude is usually expressed as dynes per square centimeter. The threshold of human hearing for a 1000-Hz pure tone is 2×10^{-4} dyn/cm².

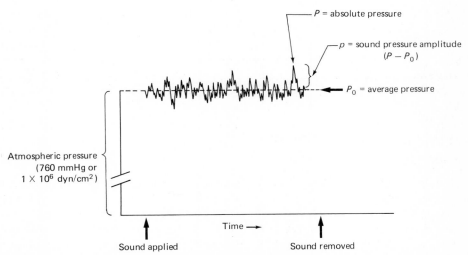

Figure 10-1 Sound pressure waves are superimposed on the average pressure of the atmosphere. In this case, the average pressure is at sea level.

Sound Pressure Level

The sound pressure is usually expressed relative to the threshold of hearing. This relationship, called the *sound pressure level*, is measured in decibels (dB) and is calculated by the following equation:

$$dB = 20 \log \frac{p_i}{p_o}$$

where p_i = actual sound pressure amplitude
  p_o = reference level sound pressure amplitude (typically the hearing threshold)
  dB = sound pressure level in decibels

A factor of 10 change in the sound pressure amplitude represents a 20-dB change in the sound level. For example, a conversational level of sound is about 2×10^{-1} dyn/cm² and is thereby 60 dB greater than the reference threshold level of 2×10^{-4} dyn/cm². The discomfort level is about 2×10^2 dyn/cm² (120 dB). We will deal with this equation again a little later on.

AUDITORY STRUCTURES

The ear is a mechanical transducer which converts the mechanical energy of oscillating air into impulses on the cochlear portion of the vestibulocochlear nerve (VIII). It is composed of an external, middle, and inner portion (Fig. 10-2).

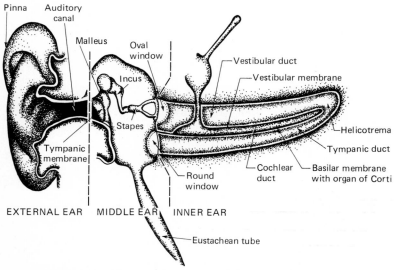

Figure 10-2 Diagrammatic illustration of the external, middle, and inner ear with the cochlea of the inner ear "uncoiled."

The external ear is composed of the part lying outside of the head (the pinna) and the auditory canal. The auditory canal ends at the *tympanic membrane* (eardrum), which separates the external from the middle ear. The middle ear is composed of the bony *ossicles* (malleus, incus, and stapes) along with their muscles and ligaments. It is separated from the inner ear by two thin, flexible membranes, the *oval and round windows*. The pressure in the middle ear is kept atmospheric by adjustments through the *eustachian tube* which opens into the nasopharynx.

The inner ear is composed of the *cochlea*, a spiral fluid-filled tube approximately 3.5 cm long. Actually the cochlea is composed of three fluid-filled compartments. Two of them, the *vestibular duct* (scala vestibuli) and *tympanic duct* (scala tympani) are filled with *perilymph*, a fluid with many of the same ionic constituents as extracellular fluid. The fluid in the two ducts is continuous only at the *helicotrema* at the extreme apical end of the cochlea. The two ducts are separated from each other by a third *cochlear duct* (scala media) for most of the cochlear length (Figs. 10-2 and 10-3). The cochlear duct contains a fluid called *endolymph*, which is similar to intracellular fluid in ionic concentration but is noticeably low in protein. It is separated from the vestibular duct by the *vestibular (Reissner's) membrane* and from the tympanic duct by the *basilar membrane*. Fixed on the basilar membrane is the mechanosensitive portion of the cochlea, the *organ of Corti* (Figs. 10-3 and 10-4).

Figure 10-3 illustrates the cochlea in its normal coiled form. The cochlea

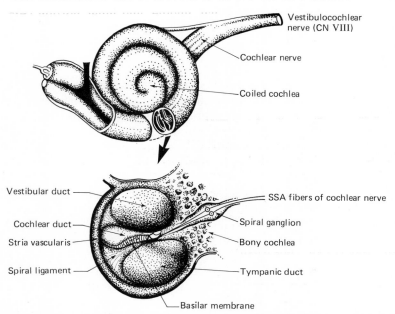

Figure 10-3 Upper illustration shows the coiled cochlea. Lower illustration shows a cross section of the cochlea.

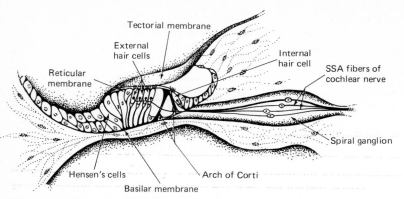

Figure 10-4   Diagrammatic illustration of the organ of Corti.

makes 2 ½ turns in forming its coil. The bottom illustration in Fig. 10-3 shows a cross section of the cochlea, clearly illustrating each of the three ducts. The basilar membrane separating the cochlear from the tympanic duct is narrow (0.04 mm) at its base near the oval window and becomes progressively wider (0.5 mm) at its apex near the helicotrema. The basilar membrane is attached to the outer wall of the cochlea by the fibers of the spiral ligament. Also on the outer wall of the cochlear duct is a secretory structure called the *stria vascularis*. Centrally the membrane is attached to a bony protuberance of the central pillar.

THE ORGAN OF CORTI

The organ of Corti, a sensitive structure resting on the basilar membrane, is responsible for converting mechanical oscillations of sound into impulses on the cochlear nerve. Because of its unique position, the organ of Corti is particularly sensitive to vibrations of the basilar membrane. A stiff but flexible arch of Corti supports a reticular membrane which is penetrated by hair cells. The internal and external spiral tunnels formed by this arch contain a fluid very much like perilymph (Fig. 10-4).

A tectorial membrane makes contact with the individual hair processes of the hair cells. The inner hair cells have 40 to 60 hairs per cell, while the outer hair cells have as many as 80 to 100. While the hairs of the outer cells actually touch the tectorial membrane in the resting state, those of the inner cells apparently contact the membrane only during part of the oscillatory cycle of the basilar membrane. The peripheral endings of SSA fibers of the cochlear neurons make contact with both inner and outer hair cells. Typically one nerve fiber will innervate a single inner hair cell, whereas a single nerve fiber may innervate up to five or ten outer hair cells. The significance of this innervation pattern is not understood.

As the stapes move in and out with the vibrations of middle ear, the oval window and perilymph of the vestibular duct are also set into oscillation. These vibrations are, in turn, transmitted to the endolymph of the cochlear duct through the vestibular membrane. Movement in the cochlear duct, in turn, sets the basilar membrane and organ of Corti into motion. The pressure waves are ultimately absorbed by the perilymph of the tympanic duct and damped at the round window.

Oscillations in the Basilar Membrane

Oscillations in the air are converted into oscillations in the ossicles and ultimately into oscillations of the fluids in the cochlea. The traveling waves which are set up on the basilar membrane near the oval window move outward over the membrane toward its apex near the helicotrema. Each area of the basilar membrane has a natural frequency or resonant point where it responds with maximum amplitude to the passage of the traveling wave. High-frequency sounds cause maximum oscillation of the membrane near the base and then quickly die out. Low-frequency sounds, on the other hand, cause the membrane to oscillate throughout its entire length but with the greatest amplitude near the apex (Fig. 10-5). The natural frequency or resonant point of the basilar membrane decreases steadily from base to apex.

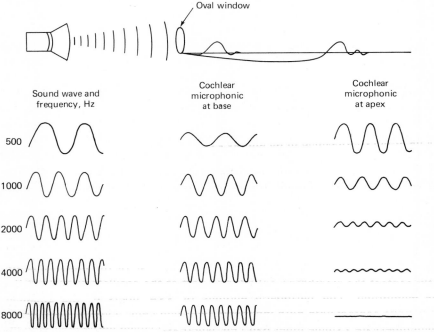

Figure 10-5 High-frequency microphonic potentials are recorded near the base of the basilar membrane, while low-frequency potentials are maximal near the apex. (*Drawn from Tasaki, 1954.*)

Hair Cell Stimulation

The organ of Corti hair cell is mechanosensitive. That is, it responds to the mechanical displacement of its hairs. A stimulated hair cell can initiate impulses in cochlear nerve fibers because the fibers end in tufts around the base of the hair cells. However, the mechanism by which an excited hair cell stimulates and produces impulses in the nerve fibers is still uncertain. To examine this process, let's begin by describing changes in the electrical activity of the cochlea in response to sound.

The stria vascularis secretes K^+ ions into the endolymph of the cochlear duct. This contributes to the establishment of an electrical potential across those membranes separating endolymph from perilymph. It's called the *endocochlear potential* and is typically about 80 mV with the endolymph positive relative to the perilymph. In addition, there is a potential difference across the membrane of the hair cell itself with the inside about 80 mV negative with respect to the outside. Thus there is a total potential difference of approximately 160 mV between the endolymph in contact with the hair cells and the cytoplasm of the cells.

When the basilar membrane is stimulated by sound pressure waves propagated through the cochlear fluids, it alternately moves up and down in response to the frequency of the sound wave. Even though this displacement is small (about 3 μm at the resonant point), it is sufficient to excite the hair cells by altering the potential difference across their membranes. As the basilar membrane goes through its upward half-cycle, the reticular membrane with its hair cells moves upward and backward. Alternatively, as the membrane goes through its second half-cycle it moves downward and forward. Because the hairs are in contact with the tectorial membrane, they bend one way on the up cycle and the opposite way on the downward cycle.

If a recording electrode is placed in the endolymph of the cochlear duct and a reference eletrode placed in the perilymph, an oscillating potential called the *cochlear microphonic potential* (CMP) can be recorded when a sound is presented to the ear. This potential has both a positive and negative component. As might be expected, low-frequency sounds produce higher amplitude CMPs near the apex of the basilar membrane, while those produced by high-frequency sounds are larger near the base (Fig. 10-5). If the cochlear microphonic potential plays any role in impulse production in the cochlear nerve fibers, it has not yet been established.

The positive and negative components of the CMP vary with the upward and downward movements of the basilar membrane. As the membrane moves upward, the hair cell membranes are thought to depolarize and impulses are generated in the cochlear nerve fibers tufted around their bases. Alternately, as the basilar membrane moves downward the hair cell membranes hyperpolarize, decreasing impulse production in the nerve fibers. When no sound is presented to the ear, the basilar membrane is quiet. Nevertheless, there is a small but basal firing rate of about 50 impulses per second on the nerve fibers which alternately increases and decreases during oscillations of the membrane. A single cochlear nerve fiber has a maximum firing rate of about 1000 impulses per second.

SOUND AMPLIFICATION THROUGH THE OUTER AND MIDDLE EAR

A sound wave approaching the ear must displace the tympanic membrane, the ossicles, and the fluid of the vestibular duct before it can displace the basilar membrane and organ of Corti, generating impulses in the cochlear nerve. During this transfer from an air pressure wave to a fluid pressure wave, the sound loses about 40 dB at the oval window. This is due to the fact that the vestibular perilymph has greater inertia than the air. To compensate for this loss of intensity, the auditory canal and the ossicular system ordinarily amplify the incoming sound pressure wave by about 35 dB. Because of this amplification, little or no loss in sound intensity occurs as the wave is transferred from the air to the fluid medium. This is an example of *impedance matching*. In other words, the loss in intensity due to the fluid inertia is compensated for by an equally strong previous amplification.

What is the Source of the 35-dB Gain through the Outer and Middle Ear?

As an example, assume that a 1000-Hz pure tone with a sound pressure amplitude of 2×10^{-1} dyn/cm^2 is presented to the ear. A sound with these characteristics will be amplified about 10 dB as it travels through the auditory canal of the outer ear and another 25 dB as it travels through the ossicular system of the middle ear. The 10-dB gain through the auditory canal can be explained because it behaves exactly like sound in a closed tube. The sound pressure is about 3 times greater at the closed end than at the open end. This translates to a 10-dB gain as follows:

$$dB = 20 \log \frac{\text{sound pressure at eardrum}}{\text{sound pressure entering canal}}$$

$$= 20 \log \frac{6 \times 10^{-1} \text{ dyn/cm}^2}{2 \times 10^{-1} \text{ dyn/cm}^2}$$

$$= 10\text{-dB gain through the auditory canal}$$

A more complex problem is explaining the 25-dB gain through the ossicular system as several factors are involved. Three initial physical characteristics of the ear are required: the surface areas of the tympanic membrane, that portion of the membrane in contact with the manubrium, and faceplate of the stapes in contact with the oval window.

0.66 cm^2 = surface area of tympanic membrane
0.55 cm^2 = surface area of membrane in contact with manubrium
0.032 cm^2 = surface area of faceplate of stapes

Because of the threefold increase in amplitude gained through the auditory canal, the sound pressure on the tympanum is 6×10^{-1} dyn/cm². Since only 0.55 cm² of the membrane is actually in contact with the manubrium of the malleus, the force produced on the malleus can be calculated as follows:

$$\text{Force (on malleus)} = \text{area (of malleus)} \times \text{pressure (on tympanum)}$$
$$= (0.55 \text{ cm}^2)(6 \times 10^{-1} \text{ dyn/cm}^2)$$
$$= 3.3 \times 10^{-1} \text{ dyn}$$

Experimental models indicate that the vesicles have a theoretical mechanical advantage of 1.3. Therefore, the force on the stapes can be calculated as follows:

$$\text{Force (on stapes)} = 1.3 \times \text{force (on malleus)}$$
$$= 1.3 (3.3 \times 10^{-1} \text{ dyn})$$
$$= 4.29 \times 10^{-1} \text{ dyn}$$

Given that the area of the faceplate of the stapes is 0.032 cm² and knowing the force on the stapes, the pressure on the oval window can be calculated as follows:

$$\text{Sound pressure (on oval window)} = \frac{\text{force (on stapes)}}{\text{area (of stapes)}}$$
$$= \frac{4.29 \times 10^{-1} \text{ dyn}}{0.032 \text{ cm}^2}$$
$$= 1.34 \times 10^{1} \text{ dyn/cm}^2$$

Using the pressure on the tympanum as the reference level, the gain through the ossicular system can now be calculated.

$$\text{dB} = 20 \log \frac{\text{pressure (on oval window)}}{\text{pressure (on tympanum)}}$$
$$= 20 \log \frac{1.34 \times 10^{1} \text{ dyn/cm}^2}{6 \times 10^{-1} \text{ dyn/cm}^2}$$
$$= 27\text{-dB gain through the ossicles}$$

The 27-dB gain calculated above ignores friction and damping, however. Thus the actual recorded experimental value is closer to 25 dB. Consequently the total gain through the outer and middle ear is approximately 35 dB. This is certainly important as the air-fluid interface at the oval window reflects about 99 percent of the sound energy back to the air. This represents a 40-dB loss in transmission and is calculated as follows:

$$\text{dB} = 20 \log \frac{\text{pressure (in perilymph)}}{\text{pressure (on oval window)}}$$
$$= 20 \log \frac{1.34 \times 10^{-3} \text{ dyn/cm}^2}{1.34 \times 10^{-1} \text{ dyn/cm}^2}$$
$$= -40\text{-dB loss at oval window}$$

It is important to realize that impedance matching is never perfect. It is probably 50 to 90 percent perfect for sound waves in the 300- to 3000-Hz range. This allows almost full utilization of the energy in the incoming sound wave. However, at very high and very low frequencies, the impedance becomes higher and thus the impedance matching becomes poorer. Consequently a higher threshold for hearing is observed in these ranges.

The natural resonating frequency of the ossicular system is between 700 and 1400 Hz. However, due to the action of ligaments and muscles in the middle ear, the system is slightly damped, causing sound waves of 1200 Hz to be transmitted through the ossicular system with slightly greater ease than sound waves of any other frequency.

The natural resonating frequency of the auditory canal is about 4000 Hz and thus selectively favors waves of this frequency. Therefore, combining the resonating effects of the auditory canal and the ossicular system, the best transmission of sound waves from air to the inner ear is for sound waves in the 1200- to 4000-Hz range. Transmission is not as good above and below this range.

Pure Tone Threshold Curve

The threshold of hearing is a function of sound frequency and intensity (Fig. 10-6). Under ideal laboratory conditions, the threshold of hearing for a 1000-Hz pure tone is 2×10^{-4} dyn/cm². However, as the sound frequency decreases, the threshold for hearing increases. For example, the sound intensity would have to be 2×10^{-2} dyn/cm² in order to just be able to hear a 100-Hz pure tone. This is 40 dB greater than would be required to just hear a 1000-Hz pure tone. Notice that the most sensitive range is between 1200 and 4000 Hz. Points on

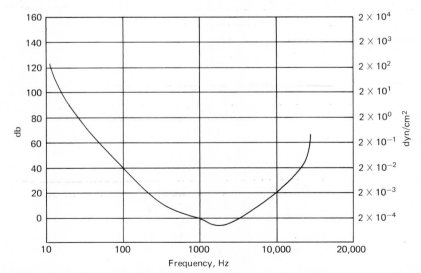

Figure 10-6 Pure tone threshold curve. This curve shows the relationship between sound frequency and intensity and the threshold of hearing. Points on the curve represent combinations of coordinates which produce sound just barely audible to the human ear under ideal laboratory conditions.

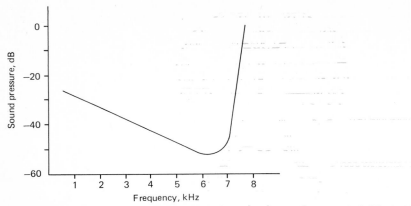

Figure 10-7 Response of a single auditory nerve fiber to tone "pips" of different frequencies and intensities. Notice that the fiber has a characteristic "best" frequency at about 6.5 kHz. At this frequency, the fiber responds to the least intense signal. (*Drawn from Tasaki, 1954.*)

the curve represent the threshold of hearing for each combination of frequency and intensity. A threshold point is established when the subject hears the tone 50 percent of the time it is presented. A 130-dB sound is felt as well as heard and eardrum rupture is a real possibility at 160 dB.

Response of a Single Cochlear Nerve Fiber to Tone "Pips"

When sounds of different frequencies are presented to the ear and responses are recorded from a single cochlear nerve fiber, it can be seen that the fiber has a characteristic or "best" frequency. This is the frequency to which the fiber responds with the least intensity (Fig. 10-7). Notice that as the frequency is increased or decreased from the best frequency the intensity of the sound required to fire the fiber increases. The best frequency of the nerve fiber illustrated is about 6.5 kHz. Thus while it is apparently true that each area of the basilar membrane responds maximally to a relatively narrow band of frequencies, it will respond, although with less sensitivity, to a broader range as well.

Auditory Efferents and Attention Control

We ordinarily pay very little attention to the background noise in our immediate environment. However, if we wish to single out a particular sound from all others we can often do it by the conscious effort of directing our attention to that sound to the exclusion of all others. While the mechanisms by which this is done are not known, one intriguing possibility is based on the discovery of auditory efferents. While their origin is largely unknown, the possibility exists that they may function by inhibiting the basilar membrane to tones on either side of the desired frequency. This would in effect "sharpen" or add "contrast" to the desired frequency range.

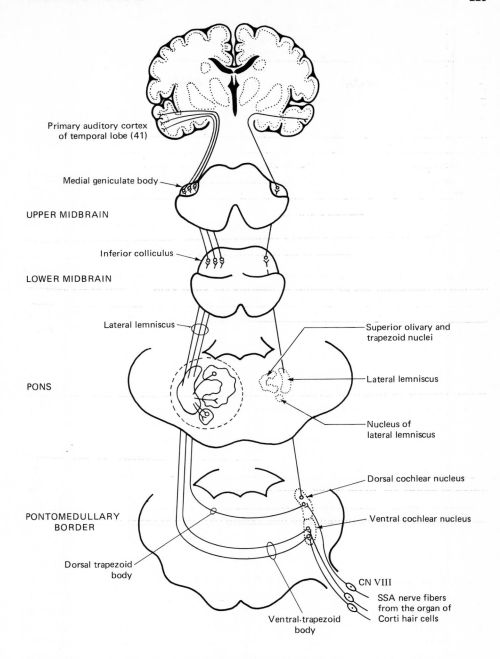

Figure 10-8 Schematic illustration showing the special somatic afferent (SSA) pathway for hearing. In addition to those fibers which cross in the trapezoid body, some fibers cross the midline in between the nuclei of the lateral lemnisci and between the two inferior colliculis (not pictured). Still others remain uncrossed and ascend in the ipsilateral lateral lemniscus.

THE CONSCIOUS AUDITORY PATHWAY

Special somatic nerve fibers of the cochlear nerve conduct sound information from the organ of Corti hair cells to the cochlear nuclei of the brainstem. These are bipolar neurons with cell bodies in the spiral ganglia of the cochlea with central processes terminating in the dorsal and ventral cochlear nuclei on the ipsilateral side of the brainstem (Fig. 10-8). Their fibers are *tonotopically organized.* This means that fibers from each part of the basilar membrane terminate in specific areas of the cochlear nuclei. In this way the frequency characteristics of the membrane are preserved in the brainstem.

Most of the second-order neurons arising in the cochlear nuclei cross over in the trapezoid body and turn upward in the *lateral lemniscus* to terminate in the inferior colliculus of the midbrain. Along the way collaterals are sent to the nucleus of the trapezoid body, the superior olivary nucleus, the nucleus of the lateral lemniscus, and the brainstem reticular formation. In return, fibers from these nuclei enter the ascending lateral lemniscus. Fibers from the cochlear nuclei which don't cross over in the trapezoid body ascend in the lateral lemniscus of the same side to the ipsilateral inferior colliculus. Bilateral connections between each inferior colliculus and each lemniscal nucleus further convey sound information from one side to the other. Consequently each individual lateral lemniscus conveys sound information from both ears, which helps to explain why damage to a lateral lemniscus produces no appreciable hearing loss other than problems with sound localization.

From the inferior colliculus, signals are relayed to the ipsilateral medial geniculate body. Terminal neurons project from here to the *primary auditory area* of the temporal lobe (area 41). The adjacent cortical area (areas 22 and 42) is the auditory *association area,* which is apparently necessary to make "sense" out of the sound signals arriving at the primary area. The two areas have extensive neural connections. The auditory pathways are tonotopically organized all the way from the basilar membrane, through the brainstem relay centers, to the auditory cortex. Thus the selectivity afforded by the location of cochlear nerve fibers and their "best frequencies" throughout the basilar membrane are preserved in the transmission of signals to the brain.

AUDITORY REFLEXES

In addition to the conscious awareness of sound, which is mediated over the conscious pathways just described, humans are also subject to a variety of auditory reflexes. A sudden, loud, unexpected sound can cause reflex quickening of the pulse, increased blood pressure, and sudden movements of the eyes, head, neck, and the whole body. Cardiovascular and other visceral responses are mediated over the autonomic nervous system. While the exact relationship between the auditory system and the autonomic nervous system is not known, the second-order neurons from the cochlear nuclei do send some collateral fibers to the brainstem reticular formation in addition to the other routes previously described. The relationship between the reticular formation and the autonomic nervous system is well documented and probably plays some role in the cardiovascular and visceral reflexes in response to sound.

Reflex eye movements are mediated by input from the cochlear nuclei to both ipsilateral and contralateral motor nuclei of cranial nerves III, IV, and VI via the medial longitudinal fasciculus. Reflex movements of the head, neck, and body in response to sound are probably mediated over reflex pathways from the cochlear nuclei to the midbrain tegmental nuclei. Descending signals over the tectospinal tracts from these nuclei then produce the appropriate movements.

DETERMINATION OF SOUND DIRECTION

If the head of a person with normal hearing is fixed in a restrainer so that it can't be moved in any direction, that person will probably have little difficulty in determining the direction from which a sound is coming. However, a person totally deaf in one ear will have great difficulty in localizing the sound. The implication is that input to both ears (binaural input) is necessary for sound localization. Similarly, a person with damage to the auditory cortex will also have difficulty with sound localization. Thus it appears that central interaction of the auditory input is also a necessary component of the process.

Time Lag and Intensity Difference

Figure 10-9 illustrates how the location of a sound with respect to the head causes a time lag and intensity difference between both ears. When a sound source is directly in front of the head, the sound reaches each ear at exactly the same time (no time lag) and with the same intensity (no intensity difference). Of course the same is true if the sound source is directly behind the head. Moving the head slightly to the left or right creates a time lag and intensity difference which provide clues needed for sound localization. For example, if the sound source is directly in front and the head is turned to the right, the sound reaches the left ear earlier and with greater intensity than it does the right. The intensity difference is caused primarily by the fact that the head itself serves as somewhat of a sound shield. Of course if the sound source were directly behind the head, moving the head to the right would produce just the opposite effects in time lag and intensity difference. Thus it is important to recognize that sound localization is aided by moving the head, a response most of us perform automatically when localizing sounds without even thinking. Obviously, sound localization when the head is fixed in space is much more difficult.

If a sound source starts directly in front of the head and then moves to the right in a circle around the head, time lag and intensity differences will constantly be changing (Fig. 10-10). As it moves through the first 90° quadrant, the time lag and intensity difference increase to a maximum. As the sound source continues to move around the fixed head, through the remaining 270° of the circle, predictable changes in time lag and intensity difference occur.

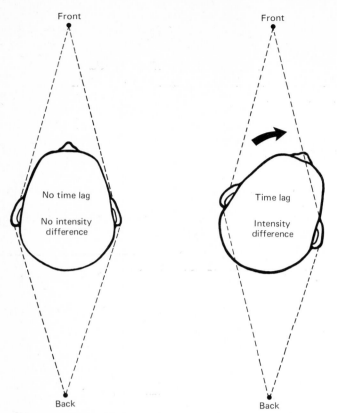

Figure 10-9 How movement of the head helps to localize a sound. When a sound source is directly in front of the head, the sound reaches each ear at exactly the same time (no time lag) and with the same intensity (no intensity difference). The same is true if the sound source is directly behind the head. Moving the head to the left or the right creates a time lag and intensity difference which provide clues needed for localization.

Moving the head is necessary for quadrant localization. Notice that the time lag and intensity difference are essentially the same when the sound source is at the 30 and 160° positions. Consequently these two clues are not enough to tell the brain from which direction the sound is coming. The additional clue necessary for localization is provided by moving the head. When the head is turned slightly to the right, there will be a *decrease* in the time lag and intensity difference if the sound source is at the 30° position, and an *increase* in both of these parameters if the source is in the 160° position.

The Central Neural Mechanism for Sound Localization

The central neural mechanisms for detecting sound direction are unknown. The following is a hypothesis based on observed available evidence. When recording electrodes are placed on certain projection neurons of the medial superior

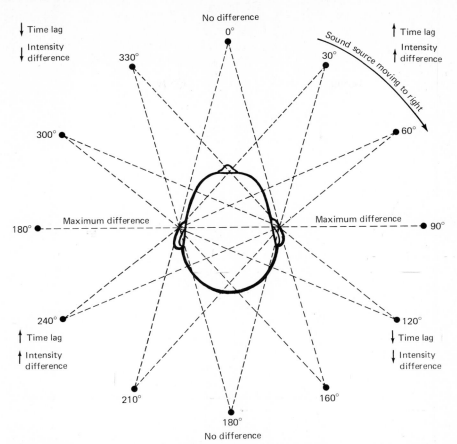

Figure 10-10 Changes in time lag and intensity difference as a sound source moves from directly in front of the head around a 360°circle to the right. The time lag and intensity clues are use to localize the source of the sound.

olivary nucleus of the cat, a lateral source of sound causes a net increase in activity in the contralateral nucleus and a net decrease in the ipsilateral nucleus. In other words, if the sound source were in the left frontal quadrant of the cat, the right lateral lemniscal fibers from the medial superior olivary nucleus to the inferior colliculus would show a relative increase in firing rate, while the left lemniscal pathway would show a decrease. This net "weighting" of activity toward the contralateral side provides the signal for sound *lateralization.*

Figure 10-11 illustrates a possible mechanism for this weighting. Certain neurons and neuronal circuits in the auditory pathway are specifically designed for sound localization. The cochlear nuclei project inhibitory fibers to this group of neurons in the ipsilateral medial superior olivary nucleus and excitatory fibers to those in the contralateral nucleus. Now if the sound source is directly in front of the head, the sound localization neurons in both nuclei receive

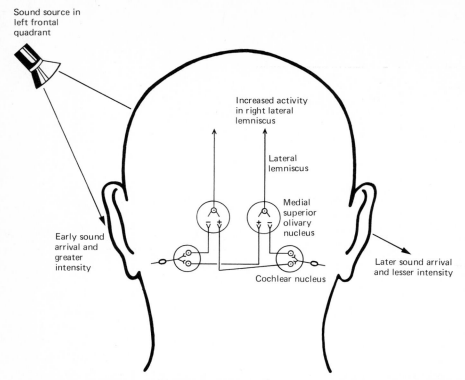

Sound source in
left frontal
quadrant

Increased activity
in right lateral
lemniscus

Lateral
lemniscus

Medial
superior
olivary
nucleus

Early sound
arrival and
greater
intensity

Later sound arrival
and lesser intensity

Cochlear nucleus

Figure 10-11 Medial superior olivary neurons are ipsilaterally inhibited and contralaterally stimulated by neurons from the cochlear nuclei. Thus, a sound source in the left quadrant causes a proportionately greater increase in activity in the contralateral lateral lemniscus, and in this way provides a clue for lateralization of a sound source. (*Drawn from Van Bergeiyk, 1962.*)

identical levels of ipsilateral inhibitory and contralateral excitatory input, producing similar central excitatory states and firing rates in each. Thus the brain receives the message "no difference" over the neural pathways and interprets this as a sound source directly in front of (or directly behind) the head. Which of these two conditions it is can be determined by a slight movement of the head in either direction as previously explained.

If the sound source is moved to the left as illustrated in Fig. 10-11, a net weighting of activity toward the contralateral (right) side is produced. This occurs because the sound wave reaches the left ear a few microseconds before the right. Sound localization neurons in the inferior colliculus respond to different time delays, referred to as the *characteristic delay* of the neuron.

Characteristic Delay and Sound Localization

Figure 10-12 illustrates the response of a single collicular neuron to tones of three different frequencies in the cat when the sound source arriving at the right ear is increasingly delayed with respect to the left ear. Notice that as the sound

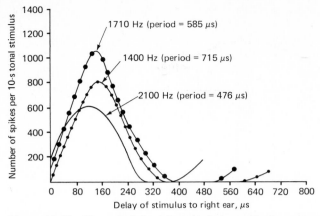

Figure 10-12 Characteristic delay of inferior collicular neurons in the cat. Discharge curves are generated by a single collicular neuron to tones of three different frequencies when the sound arrival at the right ear is increasingly delayed with respect to the left ear. (*Drawn from Rose, 1966.*)

source moves from a position directly in front of the head (zero delay) progressively to the left, the delay of stimulus to the right ear produces a characteristic pattern of impulse firing in the collicular neuron. The firing rate increases to a maximum at about 140 μs and then decreases again. The delay time which produces the greatest firing rate is the *characteristic delay* of that neuron. Thus the characteristic delay in this case is 140 μs. Notice that the actual value of the maximum firing rate varies with the frequency of the tone, but the characteristic delay remains the same. Since different sound-delay neurons respond maximally to different time lags, the brain interprets the location of a sound by a combination of which sound location neurons are maximally firing. An assumption is made that the maximum signal a neuron can produce is an important message for the brain with the sound-delay neurons providing the signal for localization.

Summary of the Neural Role in Sound Lateralization and Localization

It is likely that the right auditory cortex recognizes that when certain sound localization neurons fire at their maximum rate, the sound is at a particular location in the left auditory field. A possible mechanism for sound localization is the following. Assume that a sound is located at a particular point in the left auditory field so that the sound delay is 120 μs. Those contralateral inferior collicular neurons with characteristic delays of 120 μs will respond with their maximum firing rate. Presumably the right auditory cortex "recognizes" that when this particular group of neurons is firing maximally, the sound is at a particular location in the left auditory field. Now if the sound were to move even further to the left, the sound delay would increase and a group of neurons with characteristic delays equal to this new time lag would begin to fire maximally.

This would signal the new position of the sound to the auditory cortex. The left auditory cortex is no doubt also involved in this process.

Sound lateralization (determining whether the sound is coming from the left or the right) is probably based on a different mechanism. The relative weighting of activity to the contralateral lateral lemniscus, and thus ultimately to the contralateral auditory cortex, may be the clue for lateralization. If the brain detects a net increase in firing in the left lateral lemniscus, it "knows" that the sound is coming from the right auditory field, and vice versa.

REVIEW QUESTIONS

1 Sound travels with the greatest velocity through
   a air
   b water
   c muscle
   d bone

2 The threshold of human hearing for a 1000-Hz pure tone is
   a 2×10^{-10} dyn/cm²
   b 4×10^{-4} dyn/cm²
   c 2×10^{-4} dyn/cm²
   d 20 dB

3 A change by a factor of 10 in the sound pressure amplitude p represents
   a a 10-dB change in the sound level
   b a 20-dB change in the sound level
   c a 100-dB change in the sound level
   d a 0.1-dB change in the sound level

4 The natural resonating frequency of the human ossicular system falls in a range between
   a 100 and 400 Hz
   b 400 and 700 Hz
   c 700 and 1400 Hz
   d 1400 and 1700 Hz

5 The principal ascending tract which carries auditory information from the cochlear nuclei through the brainstem is
   a the solitary tract
   b the medial lemniscus
   c the cuneocerebellar tract
   d the reticular formation
   e the lateral lemniscus

6 A sound source in the left auditory field produces all of the following, *except* that it
   a causes a net increase in activity in the right lateral lemniscus and a decrease in the left
   b causes a net increase in activity in the left lateral lemniscus and a decrease in the right
   c causes cochlear nuclei on the left side to project inhibitory fibers to the left superior olivary nucleus
   d causes cochlear nuclei on the left side to project excitatory fibers to the right superior olivary nucleus

7 Cochlear microphonic potentials (CMPs)
   a have both a positive and negative component
   b produced by low-frequency sounds have highest amplitudes near the base of the
      basilar membrane
   c are recorded between the endolymph of the cochlear duct and the perilymph
      when a sound is presented to the ear
   d are resting potentials

8 Neurons from the medial geniculate body project to the primary auditory area,
   which is
   a located in the parietal lobe
   b roughly equivalent to Brodmann's area 22
   c able to make "sense" out of the sound
   d roughly equivalent to Brodmann's area 41 and 42

9 The sound frequency to which a single cochlear nerve fiber is most sensitive is
   described as
   a the characteristic delay
   b the best frequency
   c the adequate frequency
   d the sensitive frequency

10 The ossicular system has been estimated to have a mechanical advantage of nearly
    a 1
    b 3
    c 5
    d 7
    e none of the above

Chapter 11

The Vestibular System

The vestibulocochlear nerve (VIII) has the dual function of serving both the sense of hearing (via cochlear fibers) and proprioception (via vestibular fibers). In Chap. 10 we examined the cochlear portion of the nerve and now we will look at the vestibular fibers and their functional relationship with the vestibular apparatus.

THE VESTIBULAR APPARATUS

A cavernous network called the *bony labyrinth* exists within the temporal bone on either side of the head. Within this bony labyrinth is a *membranous labyrinth* of roughly the same shape filled with endolymph, the same fluid present in the cochlear duct of the inner ear (Fig. 11-1). The endolymph in both the vestibular and cochlear systems is continuous, and is formed in the *endolymphatic sac*, which makes contact with the fluid of the temporal dura. The space between the membranous and bony labyrinths is filled with perilymph.

The membranous labyrinth is composed of three *semicircular canals*. Each canal is twice connected to the *utriculus*, a large endolymph-containing sac. The endolymph of each canal is continuous with that in the utriculus at one

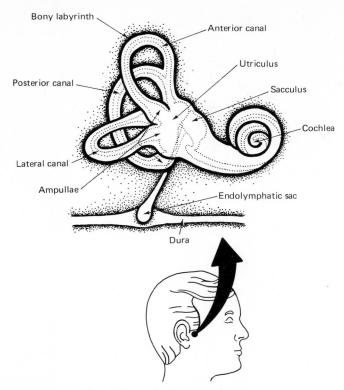

Bony labyrinth

Anterior canal

Utriculus

Posterior canal

Sacculus

Cochlea

Lateral canal

Ampullae

Endolymphatic sac

Dura

Figure 11-1 The right vestibular apparatus.

end, and separated from it at the other end by a flexible mechanosensitive barrier called the *crista ampullaris*. The crista is located in the enlarged end of each canal known as the *ampulla*. The *anterior* and *posterior canals* are essentially vertical when a person holds his head erect and they are at right angles to each other. The *lateral canal* is almost horizontal (actually elevated 23° anteriorly) and forms a plane at right angles to the other two. This geometric arrangement provides the vestibular system with the capability of detecting movements of the head in all directions.

The utriculus is continuous with a second endolymphatic enlargement, the *sacculus*. A mechanosensitive structure, the *macula acustica*, is located in the wall of the utriculus with a second macula located in the saccular wall. The three cristae and two maculae are the actual proprioceptive units in each vestibular apparatus. The cristae and maculae are in neural contact with the central nervous system through SSA VIII nerve fibers. Mechanosensitive *hair cells* in the cristae and maculae form two-element receptors with these fibers.

Figure 11-2 illustrates the distribution of the vestibular nerve fibers to the membranous labyrinth. Notice that one branch of the nerve is distributed to each ampulla, where it distributes to the crista ampullaris hair cells. Separate

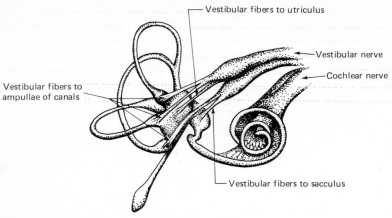

Vestibular fibers to utriculus

Vestibular nerve

Cochlear nerve

Vestibular fibers to
ampullae of canals

Vestibular fibers to sacculus

Figure 11-2 The distribution of vestibular nerve fibers to the ampullae, the utriculus, and the sacculus of the membranous labyrinth on the right side.

branches of the nerve are also distributed to the maculae of the utriculus and sacculus, where they form two-element receptors with the macular hair cells.

The Crista Ampullaris

The *crista ampullaris* is a mechanosensitive flexible barrier to the flow of endolymph between one end of the semicircular canal and the utriculus (Fig. 11-3). A number of sensitive hair cells are interposed with supporting cells at

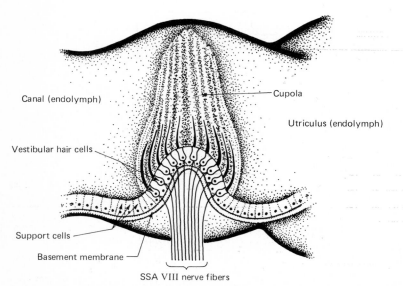

Canal (endolymph)

Cupola

Utriculus (endolymph)

Vestibular hair cells

Support cells

Basement membrane

SSA VIII nerve fibers

Figure 11-3 Diagrammatic illustration showing the crista ampullaris of a semicircular canal.

the base of the crista within the ampulla. The hair cell hairs project into a gelatinous mass, the *cupola*, which projects upward to form a flexible barrier across the space of the ampulla. Recent evidence indicates that the cupola behaves like an elastic diaphragm rather than like a swinging door, as was originally supposed. Angular movements of the head cause the endolymph to push against the cupola so that it bows in one direction or the other. Deflection toward the utriculus is *utriculopetal* deflection, while deflection away from the utriculus is *utriculofugal* deflection. Deflecting the cupola bends the hairs, excites the hair cells, and produces impulses in the SSA VIII nerve fibers. In this way the CNS is informed of movements of the head.

There are two types of hair cells in the vestibular apparatus. *Type I hair cells* are somewhat spherical in shape with 60 to 70 small hairs (*stereocilia*) emerging from the cuticle (Fig. 11-4). A particularly long hair process, the *kinocilium*, stands at one end of the stereocilia. *Type II hair cells* are more cylindrical in shape but their stereocilia and kinocilia are identical with type I cells.

SSA VIII nerve fibers are in close contact with both types of cells, although they form more extensive processes around the base of type I cells. In addition to the SSA fibers, there is evidence that small-diameter efferent fibers of unknown origin also innervate the hair cells. They form direct synaptic contacts with the type II cells but appear instead to terminate on SSA fibers of the type I cells. The origin and function of these efferent fibers is unknown. It seems likely that they may in some way influence the excitability of the hair cells and their potential for producing impulses in the SSA VIII nerve fibers.

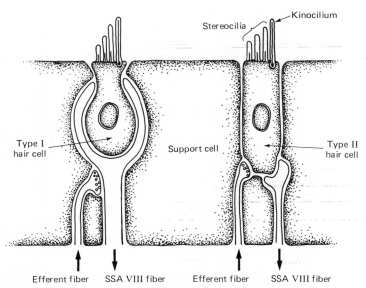

Figure 11-4 Diagrammatic illustration showing the two types of vestibular hair cells. (*Drawn from Wersall, 1975.*)

Hair Cell Stimulation and Cochlear Nerve Discharge

The stereocilia and kinocilium of each hair cell project up into the gelatinous cupola. Consequently, whenever the cupola is displaced, either toward the utriculus or away from it, the hairs are also deflected. Deflection of the hairs toward the kinocilium produces a change in the hair cell sufficient to increase the firing rate in the SSA VIII nerve fibers. Conversely, deflection away from the kinocilium decreases the firing rate (Fig. 11-5).

The hair cells in a given crista ampullaris are all orientated in the same direction so that deflection of the cupola either bends *all* the hairs toward the kinocilia or away from it. Thus deflection of the cupola either increases or decreases the firing rate of the SSA VIII nerve fibers.

In the lateral canals, the kinocilia all face the utriculus. In the vertical canals they all face away from the utriculus, toward the canal. Thus, utriculopetal deflection in the lateral canals produces an increase in the firing rate, while utriculofugal deflection produces a decrease. However, just the opposite is true concerning the vertical canals. Here the hair cell kinocilia are oriented in the opposite direction so that utriculopetal deflection causes a decrease while utriculofugal deflection produces an increase in the firing rate.

Coplanar Canals are Functional Units The anterior canal on one side of the head and the posterior canal on the opposite side are in the same plane. Thus the two canals are a functional unit since any head movement which

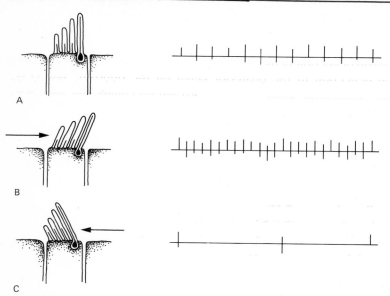

Figure 11-5 Illustration showing that deflection of the hair cell stereocilia toward the kinocilium increases the firing rate along the SSA VIII nerve fiber. Similarly, deflection of the stereocilia away from the kinocilium decreases the firing rate along the nerve fiber. A, basal rate; B, deflection toward kinocilium; C, deflection away from kinocilium.

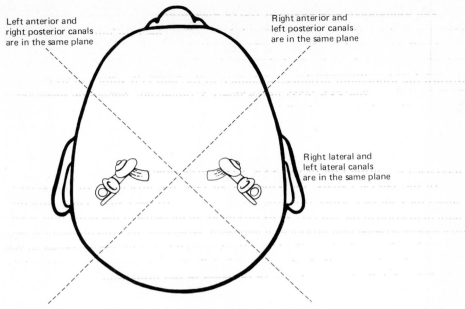

Left anterior and
right posterior canals
are in the same plane

Right anterior and
left posterior canals
are in the same plane

Right lateral and
left lateral canals
are in the same plane

Figure 11-6   Illustration showing that the anterior canal on one side of the head is in the same plane as the posterior canal on the opposite side of the head. This arrangement makes the two canals a functional unit since utriculofugal deflection in the anterior canal on one side is matched by utriculopetal deflection in the posterior canal on the opposite side, and vice versa. Similarly, the two lateral canals are also in the same plane and are a functional unit with utriculofugal deflection on one side matched by utriculopetal deflection on the opposite side.

causes utriculofugal deflection in the anterior canal on one side will be matched by utriculopetal deflection in the posterior canal on the opposite side (Fig. 11-6). A similar relationship exists with the two lateral canals and they also form a functional unit (Fig. 11-7).

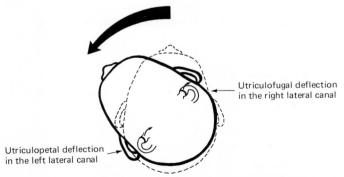

Utriculofugal deflection
in the right lateral canal

Utriculopetal deflection
in the left lateral canal

Figure 11-7   Illustration showing that as the head turns to the left in the horizontal plane, inertia of the endolymph causes utriculofugal deflection in the right lateral canal and utriculopetal deflection in the left lateral canal.

Evidence suggests that hair cells stimulate SSA VIII nerve fibers via chemical synapses. Because a fairly steady resting discharge of 40 to 60 impulses per second can be recorded in the nerve fibers, it is assumed that a small amount of transmitter chemical (possibly a catecholamine) is constantly being released. It has been proposed that displacement of the hairs toward the kinocilium increases the firing rate by increasing the rate or amount of transmitter released by the hair cell. Likewise, displacement of the hairs in the opposite direction decreases the firing rate by lowering the rate or amount of release.

In contrast to the stereocilia, which are embedded in the cuticle, the base of the kinocilium is in direct contact with the hair cell cytoplasm. The kinocilium plunging inward (with the aid of the stereocilia leaning against it) may depolarize the hair cell membrane and establish a receptor potential, which in turn causes transmitter release. Alternatively, deflection of the stereocilia away from the kinocilium pulls the kinocilium outward, hyperpolarizing the membrane and decreasing transmitter release.

The cristae are particularly sensitive to changes in angular acceleration and deceleration of the head. The greatest change in firing rate along nerve fibers from the cristae occur at the beginning and end of angular movements of the head. As Fig. 11-7 shows, the inertia of the endolymph when the head first starts rotating to the left produces utriculopetal deflection in the left canal and utriculofugal deflection in the right canal. Thus we see a large initial change in firing rate from each canal at the beginning of the movement. However, if the rotation of the head to the left continues, we see no further change in firing rates until the rotation begins to slow down (decelerate). At this point, the inertia of the endolymph causes the cupola to deflect in the opposite direction, once again causing a change in the firing rate. This time, however, there is a decrease in the left canal and an increase in the right canal. Thus one can see that the canal system is particularly adept at signaling changes in acceleration and deceleration of the head's angular movements. Further, because the canals are arranged in three planes, angular movements in all directions are easily detected by the canal system. No doubt angular movements which are not exactly parallel with a single coplanar canal system are detected by the brain through some "weighted" input from two or more coplanar functional units.

The Macula Acustica

The *macula acustica* is a mechanosensitive structure in the utriculus and sacculus. It is similar to the crista in that the base of the structure is composed of type I and type II hair cells (Fig. 11-8). Likewise, the base of the hair cells forms contacts with SSA VIII nerve fibers. Maculae are also called *otolith receptors* because the hair processes project into a low-lying gelatinous structure which is impregnated with dense calcareous formations called *otoliths* or *otoconia*. The otolith receptors respond to static gravitational pull and are therefore well equipped to signal the position of the head in space at any given time. A basal discharge rate of the SSA VIII fibers from the utriculus is observed when the head is in the normal erect position. This rate increases to a

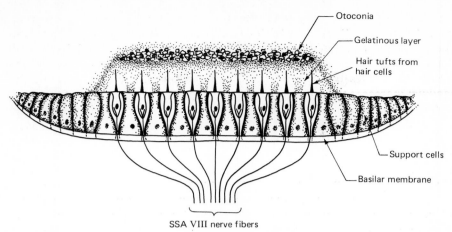

Figure 11-8   Diagrammatic illustration showing the macula acustica of the utriculus and sacculus.

maximum when the head is moved to a position 90° from normal (i.e., 90° forward, backward, or to either side).

In addition to their gravitational or static response, utricular otolith receptors also respond to linear acceleration and deceleration of the head, thus exhibiting a dynamic response characteristic as well. Saccular otolith receptors respond only to the static position of the head in space and demonstrate no appreciable dynamic response.

VESTIBULAR SYSTEM INTERACTIONS
Vestibular Control of Eye Movements

An interesting cooperative relationship exists between the vestibular system and the extraocular muscles of the eye. Those eye movements caused by vestibular stimulation are generally compensatory in nature, attempting to keep to the visual axis relatively fixed when the head is moved in space. This aids both vision and the maintenance of posture. As an example, a cooperative relationship exists between the lateral canals on both sides of the head that is designed to keep the eyes directed toward a reference point in the visual field as the head is moved in a lateral plane (Fig. 11-9). Unless consciously overridden, the eyes move slowly to the left as the head is turned slowly to the right, maintaining a constant reference point in the visual field.

These reflex conjugate eye movements are produced by changes in activity of the extraocular eye muscles in response to vestibular activity. A close examination of Fig. 11-9 shows that when the head is turned to the right, the endolymph in the right lateral canal deflects the cupola toward the utriculus (utriculopetal), while the endolymph of the left lateral canal deflects its cupola away from the utriculus (utriculofugal). Now if we remember that utriculopetal

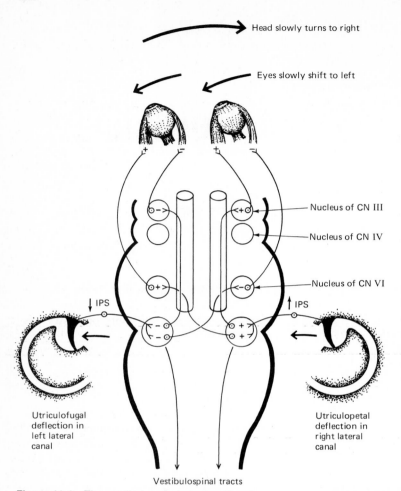

Head slowly turns to right

Eyes slowly shift to left

Nucleus of CN III

Nucleus of CN IV

Nucleus of CN VI

↓ IPS

↑ IPS

Utriculofugal
deflection in
left lateral
canal

Utriculopetal
deflection in
right lateral
canal

Vestibulospinal tracts

Figure 11-9   The vestibular control of conjugate eye movements. Utriculopetal deflection in a lateral canal increases the firing rate of the SSA VIII nerve fibers, while utriculofugal deflection decreases the firing rate. Unless consciously overridden by the brain, the eyes reflexly turn in a direction opposite to the slow movement of the head. In the above example, one can see how the lateral canals are a functional unit capable of producing a conjugate slow shift of both eyes to the left as the head is slowly turned to the right.

deflection in the lateral canals increases the firing rate while utriculofugal deflection decreases it, an examination of the neural circuitry in Fig. 11-9 explains the slow shift of the eyes to the left. The lateral rectus muscle of the left eye and medial rectus of the right eye both contract, while their antagonists relax, pulling the eyes slowly to the left. A similar cooperative relationship exists between the anterior canal on one side and the posterior canal on the other. The anterior canals are able to produce stimulation of the ipsilateral superior rectus muscle and the contralateral inferior oblique. The posterior canals produce stimulation of the ipsilateral superior oblique and the contralateral inferior rectus muscle. In this way the eyes can maintain their reference point when the head is moved through any plane.

The Vestibulospinal System

While the vestibular system responds primarily to movements of the head, it is able to produce far-reaching postural changes throughout the body. The vestibular system can regulate alpha and gamma motor neuron activity in the spinal cord through the lateral and medial vestibulospinal tracts (Fig. 6-7). The vestibulospinal tracts originate in the vestibular nuclei of the brainstem. Those fibers which originate in the lateral vestibular (Deiter's) nucleus descend ipsilaterally in the anterior funiculus and form the *lateral vestibulospinal tract*. The fibers of this tract terminate in laminae VII, VIII, and IX at all levels of the cord. Arising from the medial vestibular nucleus are the fibers of the *medial vestibulospinal tract*. While there is a small crossed component, most of its fibers descend ipsilaterally only as far as the midthoracic level, where they too synapse in laminae VII, VIII, and IX.

The vestibulospinal tracts facilitate extensor and inhibit flexor alpha and gamma motor neurons. Input to the vestibular nuclei via fibers of cranial nerve VIII from the vestibular apparatus presupposes an antigravity or postural role for the vestibulospinal tracts. Activity in these tracts is also influenced by input to the vestibular nuclei from the cerebellum, and through it, the peripheral proprioceptors of muscles, tendons, and joints.

The Vestibular System and the Cerebellum

Because of the role the vestibular system plays in the maintenance of posture and muscle control, it is not surprising to find that the system has a close relationship with the cerebellum. Both first- and second-order vestibulocerebellar fibers end as mossy fibers on the granular cells of the cerebellar cortex of the flocculonodular lobe. In addition, the fastigial and dentate cerebellar nuclei also receive vestibular input. Presumably the cerebellar cortex integrates the vestibular input with other proprioceptive input from all parts of the body. The cerebellum is then in a position to exert influence on the postural musculature via output to the vestibular, reticular, and red nuclei. Vestibulospinal, reticulospinal, and rubrospinal fibers influence muscle activity at the spinal cord level, while cerebellar output through the thalamus to the cerebral cortex modifies motor activity at the cortical source.

Vestibulocortical Projections

In order to be consciously aware of position and movements of the head in space, it is necessary that vestibular information reach the cerebral cortex. The kinesthetic sense (conscious awareness of body position and movement) requires cortical input from peripheral proprioceptors as well as from the vestibular system. The cortical area which receives this information is located in the postcentral gyrus near the somatosensory projection of the mouth. Vestibulocortical projections appear to be primarily contralateral with intermediate synapses in the ipsilateral vestibular nuclei and the contralateral thalamus.

Vestibular System and Autonomic Effects

The effects of vestibular activity on autonomic function are well known and are grouped under the heading "motion sickness." They include effects on the vasomotor system (typically a vasodepressor action with a blood pressure drop), an increase in the rate and depth of respiration, decreased salivation, increased sweating, pupillary dilation, and disturbances of the gastrointestinal tract. Most of these effects are mediated through the sympathetic nervous system.

Tests for the Integrity of the Semicircular Canals

Certain bodily responses to vestibular stimulation are reflexly predictable, such as conjugate movements of the eyes and other postural adjustments of the body. The integrity of the various canals can be tested by their capacity to produce the expected responses. The rotation (swivel chair) test and the caloric test are both designed to do this.

The *rotation test* allows maximum stimulation of the horizontal and vertical canals. Maximum deflection of the cupola of a particular canal occurs when the movement of the head is in the same plane as the canal which contains that cupola. This is accomplished in the swivel chair by placing the head in various positions and then rotating the chair. Recall that maximum deflection in a canal on one side of the head is accompanied by maximum deflection in its functional counterpart on the opposite side.

Predictable responses observed with rotation tests are *nystagmus, vertigo*, and *past pointing*. Nystagmus refers to rapid to-and-fro movements of the eyes. As previously noted, the eyes slowly shift to the left as the head is turned slowly to the right. Of course there is a limit to how far left the eyes can shift if the head continues turning to the right. When they have pulled as far left as possible, they suddenly "snap" back to the right and "fix" on a new reference point in the visual field. This alternating slow phase to the left followed by a fast phase to the right continues as the head keeps rotating to the right unless consciously overridden. While nystagmus technically refers to the eye shifts in both directions, neuroscientists typically refer to nystagmus as the direction of the fast phase. For example, nystagmus is to the right in the case just described.

Because cupola deflection directly controls eye movements, and because this deflection is in one direction during the acceleration phase of the angular rotation and in the opposite direction during the deceleration phase, it follows that nystagmus is in one direction during rotation (perrotation) and in the opposite direction after rotation (postrotation). *Perrotational nystagmus is in the same direction as the* rotation. However, if the rotating chair is suddenly stopped, the canals cease to rotate but the inertia of the endolymph is not so easily overcome. Consequently the cupolae are deflected in the opposite direction for a brief period of time, producing a *postrotational nystagmus in the direction opposite the rotation*.

Vertigo and past pointing are also predictably observed following rotation in a normal individual. Vertigo is the sensation of a movement when no such movement exists. This is caused by the fact that once the actual turning stops, the inertia of the endolymph remains for a while, deflecting the cupolae and sending signals to the brain that turning is still occurring. Normally the *vertigo (false sense of movement) is in the same direction as the postrotational nystagmus*. The body will ordinarily attempt to reflexly make postural adjustments for the vertigo just as it would for a real movement. Thus, predictable leaning of the whole body (a reflex attempt to correct for the false movement) is typically observed following a period of rotation. Specifically, *the body leans in the direction opposite the postrotational nystagmus*. An extended arm also points in the direction opposite the post rotational nystagmus. This is *past pointing*.

The rotation test has the disadvantage of not allowing the canals on each side of the head to be tested separately. However, *caloric tests*, which involve the introduction of hot or cold solutions into the auditory canal, allow the clinician to test each side of the head separately. A hot water solution introduced into the auditory canal causes the endolymph to expand, deflecting the cupola in a predictable direction. This is later followed by the use of a cold water solution which cools the endolymph, producing deflection in the opposite direction. Like the rotation test, predictable changes in nystagmus, vertigo, and past pointing can be observed.

REVIEW QUESTIONS

1 The enlarged end of each semicircular canal where it contacts the utriculus is
   a the cupola
   b the sacculus
   c the macula acustica
   d the ampulla
2 Deflection of the hair cell hairs toward the utriculus in a single lateral canal
   a is called utriculopetal deflection
   b increases the firing rate in the SSA VIII nerve fibers
   c is matched by deflection toward the utriculus in the other lateral canal
   d causes no change in the nerve fiber firing rates
3 The vestibular apparatus on each side of the head contains
   a three cristae and three maculae
   b two cristae and two maculae
   c three cristae and two maculae
   d two cristae and two maculae
4 The numerous small hairs which project from the cuticle of vestibular hair cells are called
   a kinocilia
   b type I hairs

  c type II hairs
  d stereocilia
  e vestibulocilia

5 All of the following statements concerning the macula acustica are true, *except:*
  a The maculae are located in the utriculus and sacculus.
  b The maculae are also called otolith receptors.
  c The maculae can signal the static position of the head in space.
  d The maculae respond to angular movements of acceleration and deceleration of the head.

6 All of the following statements concerning testing the integrity of the semicircular canals are true, *except:*
  a Caloric tests are able to examine the canals on each side of the head separately.
  b Rotation tests examine the canals on both sides of the head simultaneously.
  c Rotation tests can only examine the integrity of the lateral canals.
  d Vertigo is not experienced with the caloric tests.

7 The following is (are) true concerning the results of rotation tests of the vestibular system:
  a Perrotational nystagmus is in the direction opposite rotation.
  b Postrotational nystagmus is in the same direction as the rotation.
  c Vertigo is in the same direction as postrotational nystagmus.
  d The body tends to lean in the direction opposite the postrotational nystagmus.

8 All of the following statements concerning the crista ampullaris are true, *except:*
  a Angular acceleration and deceleration cause the greatest change in firing rates from the cristae.
  b Rotation of the head to the left causes utriculopetal deflection in the left lateral canal and utriculofugal deflection in the right lateral canal.
  c The cristae contain both type I and type II hair cells.
  d The cristae are associated with the utriculus and sacculus as well as the ampullae.
  e The hair cells in a given crista ampullaris are all oriented in the same direction.

9 All of the following are true concerning the vestibular system hair cells, *except:*
  a Type II cells are more spherical than type I cells.
  b SSA VIII nerve fibers form more extensive processes around the base of type I cells than around type II cells.
  c Deflection of the small hairs toward the kinocilium produces an increase in the firing rate of a cell's SSA VIII fibers.
  d Small efferent fibers appear to directly synapse on type II cells.

10 All of the following statements concerning the membranous labyrinth are true, *except:*
  a The membranous labyrinth of the vestibular apparatus is filled with perilymph.
  b The membranous labyrinth is located in the temporal bone on either side of the skull.
  c The membranous labyrinth is located within the bony labyrinth.
  d The fluid in the membranous labyrinth is continuous with that in the cochlea.

Vision and Optic Reflexes

The eyes are truly remarkable organs. Their light-sensitive retinas are able to convert light rays from objects in the visual field to impulses on the optic nerves, which ultimately give rise to images in the visual cortex of the brain. Thses images are usually sharp and clear because of the focusing power of the lens. As if the ability to perceive images isn't enough, the eyes are also able to function under widely varying conditions. For example, they are able to adjust to viewing near and far objects, large and small objects, moving and stationary objects as well as objects in bright daylight and under the poor light conditions of night vision. A number of optic reflexes enable the eyes to make these adjustments. In this chapter we will examine the physiology of vision and its attendant reflexes.

THE EYE AND THE PATH OF LIGHT

Light from an object in the visual field must pass through the cornea, the aqueous humor, the pupillary aperture, the lens, and the vitreous humor before reaching the light-sensitive retina (Fig. 12-1). When we look directly at an object, the light rays from that object are focused on an especially sensitive area of the retina, the *fovea*. Items in the peripheral visual field are focused on the

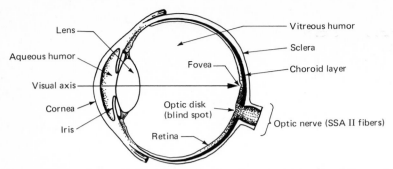

Figure 12-1 Schematic illustration showing the principal parts of the eyeball.

remainder of the retina. Both kinds of photoreceptors (rods and cones) are located throughout the peripheral retina, while the fovea contains only cones. The *optic disk,* formed by the confluence of the optic nerve fibers from the nasal (medial) and temporal (lateral) portions of the retina, is devoid of any photoreceptors and is called the *blind spot.*

Refractive Power and Accommodation of the Lens

Light rays entering the eyes are selectively bent as they pass through the cornea, aqueous humor, lens, and vitreous humor on their way to the retina. While each of these contributes somewhat to bending the entering light rays, it is nevertheless the lens which is responsible for bending the rays sufficiently to focus them on the retina since it is the only refractive surface which can change its light bending (refractive) capability. The other three are all fixed values which give rise to the same amount of bending whether the eye is focused for distant or near vision.

The refractive power L of the lens is measured in diopters and is equal to the reciprocal of the focal length F expressed in meters. The natural tendency for the lens is to assume a curved shape, giving it a high refractive power and dioptric strength. Now when the eye is focused for distant vision (any distance greater than about 20 ft), the lens is pulled relatively flat and has only minimal refractive power. Nevertheless, even in this condition it does bend light and has a refractive power equal to 18 diopters. When the eye focuses on objects closer than 20 ft, the refractive power of the lens increases in order to focus the light rays on the retina. This increase in refractive power is caused by increasing the curvature (and hence the dioptric strength) of the lens. When very young children focus on an extremely close object they can increase their dioptric strength from 18 to nearly 32 diopters. This represents an accommodation of 14 diopters in adjusting from distant to near vision.

Accommodation is accomplished by contraction of the ciliary muscles of the eye. When they contract, the suspensory ligaments to which the lens is attached begin to slacken. This allows the lens to assume its more naturally curved (and hence more refractively powerful) shape (Fig, 12-2).

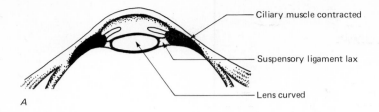

Ciliary muscle contracted

Suspensory ligament lax

Lens curved

A

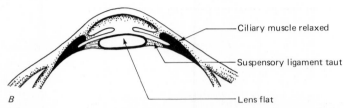

Ciliary muscle relaxed

Suspensory ligament taut

B Lens flat

Figure 12-2 *A.* Lens working, accommodating for near vision, L-32 diopters. *B.* Lens resting, accommodating for distant vision, L-18 diapters. Diagrammatic illustration showing that contraction of the ciliary muscle partially removes tension from the suspensory ligament. This allows the lens to assume its naturally more spherical shape. The lens has more refractive power *L* in the curved condition than it does when it is relatively flat, as happens when the eye is at rest.

With advancing age our ability to accommodate begins to deteriorate. The lens begins to take on an inelastic and somewhat permanently flattened shape. Consequently the eye is less able to focus on near objects. Accordingly, the nearest point in front of the eye at which an object can be brought into focus (the *near point*) begins to increase. These relationships are illustrated in Figs. 12-3 and 12-4.

Notice that accommodation is greatest in the very young child (about 14 diopters), decreases to about 11.5 in the young adult, and is not much better than 2 or 3 in the elderly. Accordingly, the near point increases with age. It is typically about 12 cm in the young adult and often reaches 100 cm in the elderly. Thus we see the familiar pattern of the aging person holding reading material farther and farther away from the eyes in order to be able to focus on it. Of course since 100 cm is beyond the reach of the arms, reading glasses are often required.

Emmetropia, Hypermetropia, and Myopia In normal vision (*emmetropia*) parallel light rays from a viewed object are brought to a focus exactly on the retina. The individual perceives the image as sharp, clear, and in focus. However, if the refractive surfaces of the eye can't focus the parallel rays on the retina, the image is blurred and corrective glasses or contact lenses are required. If insufficient light bending occurs, parallel rays aren't sufficiently refracted to be brought to a focus on the retina. This condition is called *hypermetropia* and the

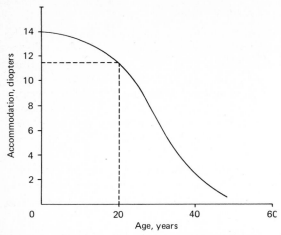

Figure 12-3 Graph showing the relationship between age and the maximum number of diopters the eye can accommodate. (*Drawn from Duane, 1922.*)

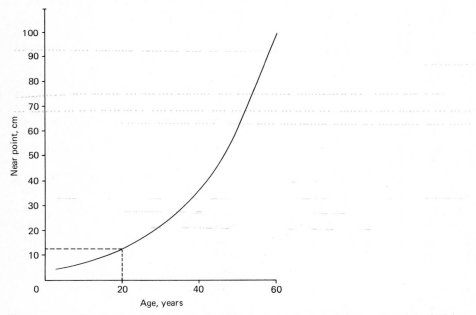

Figure 12-4 Graph showing the relationship between age and the near point of vision. (*Drawn from Duane, 1922.*)

individual is said to be far-sighted. That is, he can focus well on distant objects which don't require much light bending, but can't focus well on objects up close. On the other hand, if the refractive power of the eye is so great as to focus parallel rays in front of the retina, the image is also blurred and the condition is called *myopia* (near-sightedness).

Neural Control and Accommodation of the Lens

The ciliary muscle is innervated by both the somatic and autonomic nervous systems. Through the former, we are able to voluntarily change the focus from near to far vision by altering the thickness and curvature of the lens. The geometric orientation of the ciliary muscle is such that when it is relaxed, the suspensory ligament is taut and the lens is pulled flat, setting it for distant vision (Fig. 12-2). Since the eyes are set for distant vision most of the time, it follows that the ciliary muscle is usually relaxed. Contraction causes the suspensory ligament to become less taut and allows the lens to assume the more spherical (and hence more powerful) shape.

The shape of the lens is also automatically adjusted as the gaze shifts between near and far vision. The autonomic nervous system regulates automatic adjustments. Parasympathetic stimulation contracts the ciliary muscle and thereby increases the refractive power of the lens. Sympathetic stimulation appears to relax the muscle, decreasing the strength of the lens (Fig. 12-5).

Depth of Focus and Accommodation of the Pupil

Further examination of Fig. 12-5 will show that pupil diameter is also under autonomic control. GVE fibers of the oculomotor nerve (III) supply parasympathetic innervation to the sphincter muscle of the iris, while sympathetic fibers innervate the radial muscles. Contraction of the former causes the pupils to constrict, while contraction of the latter produces pupillary dilation.

The amount of ambient light to a large extent determines the size of the pupillary aperture. In low-light situations the pupils dilate to allow the available light to reach the retina. In bright daylight the pupils are constricted in order to limit the amount of light entering the eyes. The pupils also automatically con-

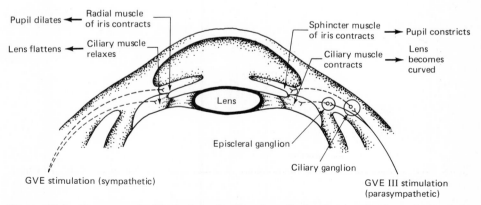

Figure 12-5 Diagrammatic illustration showing the effects of sympathetic and parasympathetic stimulation on pupil size and lens thickness (strength). Parasympathetic stimulation contracts the sphincter muscle of the iris, constricting the pupil, and contracts the ciliary muscle, which allows the lens to assume the more curved and powerful shape. Sympathetic stimulation contracts the radial muscles of the iris, dilating the pupil, and also relaxes the ciliary muscle, producing tension in the suspensory ligament and causing the lens to flatten and become less refractive.

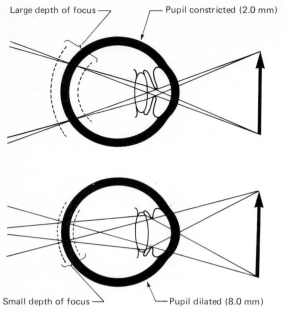

Large depth of focus ⌐   ⌐ Pupil constricted (2.0 mm)

Small depth of focus ⌐   └─Pupil dilated (8.0 mm)

Figure 12-6   Schematic illustration showing that the pupillary aperture determines the depth of focus. In the top illustration, the pupil is constricted and the depth of focus is very large. This means that if the object moved slightly closer or farther away from the eye it would still be in focus on the retina, requiring no additional accommodation by the lens. In the bottom illustration, the pupil is dilated and the depth of focus is small. In this case, even small shifts of the object would give an out-of-focus image on the retina.

strict when viewing objects at very close range and dilate when the gaze shifts to distant vision. The *depth of focus* is greatest in bright light when the pupillary aperture is small (i.e., 2 mm). On the other hand, it is minimum in dim light when the aperture is large (i.e., 8 mm). All things being equal, a large depth of focus means that a viewed object can move back and forth a slight distance without going out of focus. On the other hand, if the depth of focus is very small, even the slightest movement will put the object out of focus (Fig. 12-6).

OPTIC REFLEXES

Pupillary Light Reflex

This is the well-known response in which the pupils constrict in bright light. The reflex arc employed in this response is illustrated in Fig. 12-7. If an equal amount of light shines into both eyes, the degree of constriction is generally equal. However, if the light is directed primarily into one eye (i.e., with a flashlight), the pupil of that eye greatly constricts (*direct reflex*) while the pupil of the other eye shows a much smaller degree of constriction (*consensual reflex*).

Notice that some of the fibers of the optic tracts pass to the colliculi of the

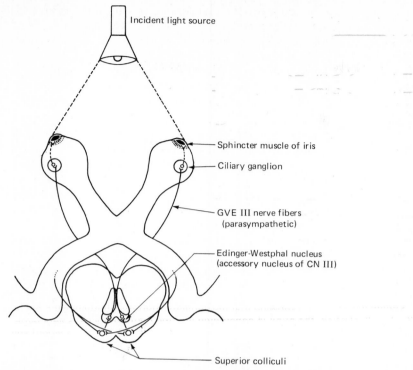

Incident light source

Sphincter muscle of iris

Ciliary ganglion

GVE III nerve fibers
(parasympathetic)

Edinger-Westphal nucleus
(accessory nucleus of CN III)

Superior colliculi

Figure 12-7 The pupillary light reflex. As a light is shined into the eyes, collaterals from the optic tract project to nuclei in the superior colliculi of the upper midbrain. Short interneurons then conduct impulses into the Edinger-Westphal nucleus (an accessory nucleus of III). From here preganglionic GVE III fibers emerge to synapse in the ciliary ganglia. Short postganglionic fibers then cause the sphincter muscles of the iris to contract, thus causing the pupils to constrict.

upper midbrain rather than continuing on to the lateral geniculate bodies. These fibers project to both the ipsilateral and contralateral superior colliculi. Short neurons project from the colliculi to the Edinger-Westphal nucleus (an accessory nucleus of III) in the midbrain, which serves as the origin of preganglionic parasympathetic fibers (GVE) of the oculomotor nerves (III). The GVE III fibers, in turn, project to the ciliary ganglia from which postganglionic fibers innervate the sphincter muscles of the iris. If the light is directed evenly into both eyes, the pupillary change is uniform. However, if it is directed primarily into one eye, the neural firing is "weighted" toward that side and the greatest constriction is observed on that side.

Accommodation Reflexes As an Object Is Brought Closer to the Eyes

When an object is brought closer to the eyes we must make visual adjustments (accommodations) in order to keep it in sharp focus. These accommodations include (1) convergence of the eyes, (2) thickening of the lenses, and (3) pupillary constriction. Convergence is necessary in order to keep the viewed object lined up with the visual axis of each eye. This keeps the object focused on the fovea for maximum visual acuity. As a viewed object is brought closer, light rays from any single point source on the object become less parallel, and the refractive power of the lens must be increased in order to focus the image on the retina. The lens accomplishes this by becoming thicker and more spherical, thereby increasing its refractive power. Finally, in order to increase the depth of focus (always a problem at short distances), the pupils constrict. It should be pointed out that one can consciously "override" the accommodation reflexes and prevent their occurrence. However, lacking such conscious effort, they proceed automatically.

Convergence of the eyes is brought about by the following reflex pathway. GSE fibers of the oculomotor nerves (III) in the nucleus of III in the midbrain tegmentum become stimulated via an undefined route from the visual cortex. These fibers then project to the medial rectus muscles of the eyeballs, causing them to contract. This produces an inward turning of the eyes, keeping the viewed object focused on the fovea for maximum visual acuity. The oculomotor nerves also innervate the superior oblique and superior and inferior rectus muscles of the eyes as well. Thus, by selective stimulation of the appropriate GSE III fibers, specific muscles can be activated, causing appropriate degrees and angles of convergence.

Thickening of the lens and constriction of the pupils are both produced through reflex pathways involving the parasympathetic (GVE) fibers of the oculomotor nerve. The pathway for pupillary constriction is identical to that of the pupillary light reflex, starting from the Edinger-Westphal nucleus. However, it appears likely that signals are relayed to this nucleus via undefined routes from the visual cortex in the occipital lobe. Some of the GVE III fibers which enter the ciliary ganglia pass right through without synapsing to enter the episcleral ganglia (Fig. 12-5). Postganglionic fibers project from here to the ciliary muscle, causing it to contract, thereby thickening the lens and increasing its refractive power.

THE CONSCIOUS VISUAL PATHWAY

We previously mentioned that impulses on the optic nerve give rise to both conscious visual images and a variety of purposeful optic reflexes. The conscious visual pathway, which we will examine now, is illustrated in Fig. 12-8. In order to give rise to a conscious image, impulses generated by light stimulation of the retina must be transmitted to areas 17, 18, and 19 of the optic lobe. Area 17 is the primary visual area and initially receives the signals from the optic radiations. However, the visual association area (areas 18 and 19) helps to "make sense" out of the signals reaching area 17.

The retina of each eye is divided into a medial half, the *nasal retina,* and a lateral half is called the *temporal retina*. Optic nerve fibers from the nasal retina

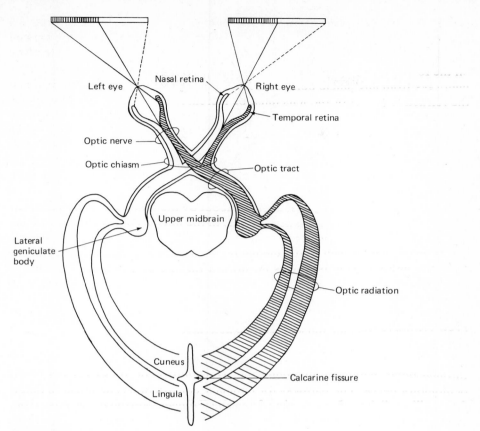

Figure 12-8 The conscious pathway for vision.

of each eye cross over in the *optic chiasm* and terminate in the lateral geniculate body on the contralateral side (Fig. 12-8). Those from the temporal retina do not cross over in the chiasm but continue instead on the same side, terminating in the ipsilateral lateral geniculate body. The *optic nerve* is composed of that portion of nerve fibers between the eye and the optic chiasm. The continuation of the fibers from the optic chiasm to the lateral geniculate bodies are collectively called the *optic tracts*. Thus the optic nerves contain fibers from only one eye, while the optic tracts are composed of fibers from both eyes. The optic chiasm lies just anterior to the pituitary gland.

Fibers carrying visual signals from each lateral geniculate body project posteriorly as the *optic radiations*, terminating in the visual cortex of each occipital lobe. Some of these fibers terminate in the *cuneus* above the calcarine fissure, and some terminate below it in the *lingula*. Figure 12-9 illustrates the conscious visual pathway when a single quadrant of the retina is stimulated. Notice that light from the left visual field of each eye stimulates the nasal retina of the left eye and the temporal retina of the right eye. Further, light from the

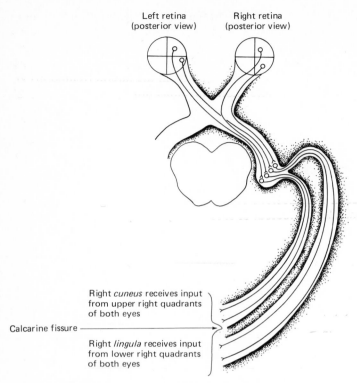

Left retina
(posterior view)

Right retina
(posterior view)

Right *cuneus* receives input
from upper right quadrants
of both eyes

Calcarine fissure —————————————

Right *lingula* receives input
from lower right quadrants
of both eyes

Figure 12-9 Diagrammatic illustration showing that the right cuneus of the optic lobe receives input from the upper right quadrant of the retina of both eyes. Conversely, the right lingula of the optic lobe receives input from the lower right quadrants of the retina of both eyes.

lower left visual field of both eyes stimulates the upper right quadrants of the nasal retina of the left eye and the temporal retina of the right eye. A little thoughtful examination of Fig. 12-9 will enable you to appreciate the relationships between a point source of light in the visual field and the retinal quadrant which it stimulates.

The image focused on each retinal quadrant is represented on a specific area of the visual cortex. The upper right quadrant of each eye projects to the right cuneus while the upper left quadrant of each eye projects to the left cuneus. Similarly, the lower right quadrant of each eye projects to the right lingula while the lower left quadrants project to the left lingula. Thus the fibers of the optic radiation are spatially oriented with the more superior half of the radiation projecting to the cuneus, while the inferior half projects to the lingula.

Injury to the Conscious Visual Pathway

Figure 12-10 illustrates the defects in viewing the visual field associated with lesions to several specific locations in the conscious visual pathway. A complete lesion in a single optic nerve causes total anopsia (blindness) in that eye. Vision in the opposite eye is unaffected. An interior-posterior lesion through the middle of the optic chiasm interrupts only the crossing fibers (those from the nasal retinae) while leaving those from the temporal retinae intact. Now because the nasal retinae are stimulated by light from the lateral (temporal) visual fields, the visual field loss is called *heteronymous bitemporal hemianopia.* Hemianopia means that the loss is to one-half of the visual field. Heteronymous means that the loss is to different visual fields for each eye. However, a lesion to the optic tract eliminates visual signals from the nasal retina of the contralateral eye as well as the temporal retina of the ipsilateral eye. This condition is also described as hemianopia since one-half of the visual field is eliminated from each eye, However, the hemianopia is *homonymous* as the loss is to the same visual field of each eye. Lesions of the optic radiation might cause either hemianopia (entire radiation affected) or loss in only one quadrant if cuneal or lingular radiation fibers are selectively damaged. Of course partial loss can

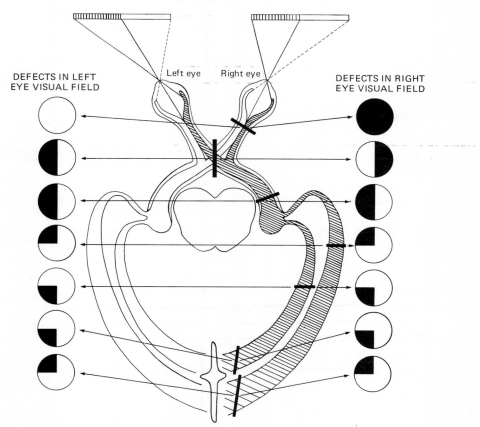

DEFECTS IN LEFT EYE VISUAL FIELD

Left eye   Right eye

DEFECTS IN RIGHT EYE VISUAL FIELD

Figure 12-10   Schematic illustration showing defects in the visual fields of each eye which are associated with seven individual lesions in the visual pathway.

occur if the damage to the superior or inferior part of the radiation is only partial.

THE RETINA: THE LIGHT-SENSITIVE PORTION OF THE EYE

Photons of light entering the eye must reach the light-sensitive rods and cones of the retina before neural signals are generated in the visual system. Figure 12-11 diagrammatically illustrates the 10 characteristic layers of the retina. Notice that the direction of light is opposite to the direction of the generated impulses.

Light first reaches the retina by passing through the inner limiting membrane. The impinging light rays next encounter the optic nerve layer which is composed of the fibers of the ganglion cells (optic nerve cells), whose cell bodies comprise the ganglion cell layer. Deeper bipolar neurons synapse with these cells in large dendritic arborizations forming the inner plexiform layer. The peripheral processes of these bipolar neurons receive synaptic input from the rods and cones in the outer plexiform layer. The cell body region of the bipolar neurons makes up the inner nuclear layer. The outer nuclear layer is the region of rod and cone cell bodies. The outer limiting membrane separates the outer nuclear layer from the enlarged photosensitive ends of the rods and cones in the rod and cone layer. Finally, the rods and cones are in close functional contact with pigmented epithelial cells, which comprise the tenth layer of the retina.

Photoreceptor Stimulation and Impulse Production

Light passing through the retinal layers stimulates the enlarged photosensitive portion of the rods and cones before being absorbed by the pigmented epithelium. Once activated, the rods and cones stimulate the bipolar neurons, which in turn excite ganglion cells, producing impulses in the optic nerve. It is likely that a receptor potential is generated on the photoreceptor cell membrane, which then generates impulses in the bipolar and ganglion cells. No impulses have actually been recorded in the rods and cones themselves.

The absorption of light by the pigmented epithelium is important for visual acuity as it prevents reflected light from stimulating rods and cones in other areas of the retina. By minimizing reflected light, the optical quality of the image detected by the array of photoreceptors in the retina is improved. The fovea is capable of generating higher visual acuity than any other part of the retina partly because it has more pigment in its tenth layer. Also, the cones in the fovea are more slender than elsewhere in the retina and thus produce a finer "grain" to their image.

The visual signals generated in the rods and cones converge considerably upon reaching the ganglion cells. Figure 12-11 gives the impression that each ganglion cell is in direct contact with a single bipolar neuron which is stimulated by a single rod or cone cell. Actually there are many more rods and cones than bipolar neurons, and many more bipolar neurons than ganglion cells. Each retina contains approximately 125 million rods and 5.5 million cones. Thus an

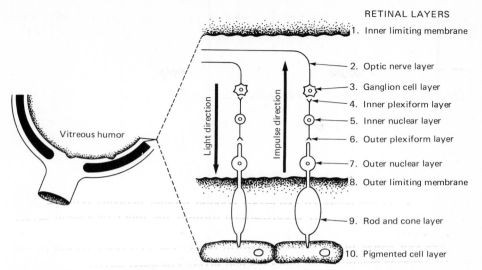

RETINAL LAYERS

1. Inner limiting membrane
2. Optic nerve layer
3. Ganglion cell layer
4. Inner plexiform layer
5. Inner nuclear layer
6. Outer plexiform layer
7. Outer nuclear layer
8. Outer limiting membrane
9. Rod and cone layer
10. Pigmented cell layer

Vitreous humor

Light direction

Impulse direction

Figure 12-11 Diagrammatic illustration showing the 10 layers of the retina. Notice that the direction of light and the direction of the visual signal are opposite to each other in the retina.

average of 140 rods and 6 cones feed visual information into a single ganglion cell. This considerable convergence of the visual signal may possibly add "sharpness" to the visual image.

RHODOPSIN: THE PHOTOSENSITIVE CHEMICAL IN RODS AND CONES

Both rods and cones contain a photosensitive pigment, rhodopsin, which decomposes on exposure to light, releasing sufficient energy to establish a receptor potential on the photoreceptor cell membrane. Rods and cones appear to stimulate the bipolar neurons through chemical transmission. Whether the central state of the bipolar neurons is raised above the excitation threshold is probably a function of the quantity of chemical transmitter released, which itself is probably a function of the magnitude of the receptor potential developed on the photoreceptor.

Rods and cones have different characteristics. Rods are usually narrower (4 to 5 μm) than cones (5 to 8 μm). The photochemicals in the two kinds of photoreceptors are slightly different. Their functional capabilities are also different. Cones function best at high intensities of light such as that associated with daylight vision. Further, they are responsible for color vision and are characterized by high visual acuity. Rods, on the other hand, have higher sensitivity and are more suited for vision at night, when light intensity is low. They don't mediate color vision nor are they able to resolve fine detail. Most of the research on photoreceptor cells has been done on rods because of their relatively great number. Consequently, most of the functional information we have about the chemistry of rhodopsin has been obtained from rod studies. Nevertheless, there is evidence that cones probably function in a similar manner.

Rhodopsin is a complex chemical with a protein portion complexed with a caratinoid pigment, *cis*-retinine. The difference between rod rhodopsin and cone rhodopsin is in the protein portion. Rod rhodopsin (scotopsin) differs from cone rhodopsin (photopsin) by the number, type, and sequence of its amino acids. In either case, exposure of rhodopsin to light causes it to decompose with the release of sufficient energy to establish a receptor potential on the cell membrane.

The Rhodopsin Cycle

When rhodopsin is decomposed by light, releasing energy, the breakdown products of this decomposition subsequently recombine to synthesize more rhodopsin. The sequence is called the *rhodopsin cycle* (Fig. 12-12).

Rhodopsin is a stable molecule. However, once exposed to light, it undergoes a configurational change becoming first lumirhodopsin and then *meta*-rhodopsin. *meta*-Rhodopsin is quite unstable and quickly decomposes to *trans*-retinine and scotopsin. This latter decomposition is accompanied by the release of sufficient energy to produce a receptor potential on the cell membrane. Most of the *trans*-retinine undergoes enzymatically catalyzed isomerization, becoming *cis*-retinine. Once formed, *cis*-retinine combines with scotopsin, reforming rhodopsin.

In dim light it is important that sufficient amounts of rhodopsin are available for decomposition so that the rods are maximally sensitive to any light which is present. On the other hand, when plenty of light is available, much of the *trans*-retinine is shunted into the pigmented epithelial cells which are in close contact with the photoreceptor cells (Fig. 12-12). Here it undergoes conversion to *trans*-vitamin A. Of course, shunting *trans*-retinine into the pigment cells decreases the amount of rhodopsin available for decomposition by light, thus decreasing the sensitivity of the retina. This is certainly a desirable feature when abundant light is available.

trans-Vitamin A in the pigmented epithelial cells is in chemical equilibrium with its isomer, *cis*-vitamin A. The *trans*-retinine-*trans*-vitamin A and *cis*-retinine-*cis*-vitamin A interconversions are oxidation-reduction reactions. A constant supply of vitamin A is made available to the epithelial cells by capillaries of the choroid plexus, the vascular layer between the retina and the sclera (Fig. 12-1).

Light Adaptation

A person in the dark for up to 30 min is said to be *dark-adapted*. That is, retinal sensitivity has increased to a sufficiently high level so that the eyes are sensitive to whatever minimal light is available. When the person subsequently moves into a well-lighted environment, everything is initially very bright due to the high sensitivity of the retina, and visual acuity is initially quite poor. So much

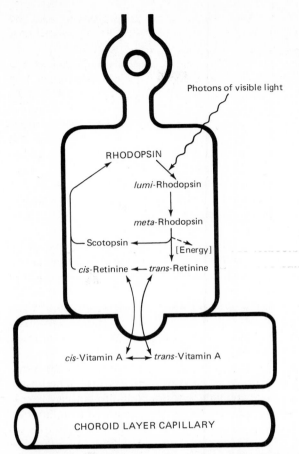

Photons of visible light

RHODOPSIN

lumi-Rhodopsin

meta-Rhodopsin

Scotopsin

[Energy]

cis-Retinine ◄── *trans*-Retinine

cis-Vitamin A ◄──► *trans*-Vitamin A

CHOROID LAYER CAPILLARY

Figure 12-12 Diagrammatic illustration of the rhodopsin cycle. The energy released from the breakdown of rhodopsin is used to generate a receptor potential on the rod.

rhodopsin is being decomposed that a "flash" of light rather than any fine detail is experienced. After a few seconds to a minute, the eyes adapt to the light and the retinal sensitivity is decreased. This is *light adaptation*. It is caused by the conversion of retinine to vitamin A and its subsequent storage in the pigment cells. Since the rate-limiting step for the reformation of rhodopsin is the availability of retinine, this effectively reduces the stores of rhodopsin in the photoreceptors and decreases their sensitivity.

Dark Adaptation

A light-adapted person has low retinal sensitivity. That is, rod and cone rhodopsin stores have been reduced to a relatively low level by the conversion of retinine to vitamin A and its subsequent storage in the pigment cells. Now when the light-adapted person suddenly enters a very dark room, the available

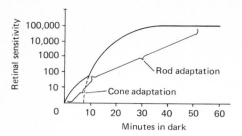

Figure 12-13 Graph showing the increase in retinal sensitivity during dark adaptation. Retinal sensitivity increases with time in the dark. Most of the initial increase in sensitivity is due to cone adaptation. Nevertheless, the greatest increase in sensitivity is due to rod adaptation. Resynthesis of pigment is slower in rods than in cones, but they are much more numerous. (*Drawn from Guyton, 1976.*)

light is drastically reduced and it becomes necessary to increase the sensitivity of the retina in order to see. This process is called *dark adaptation*. Dark adaptation is a slower process than light adaptation. The adaptation occurs as stored vitamin A is converted to retinine, which immediately complexes with scotopsin to reform more rhodopsin. This obviously increases the rhodopsin stores and hence the sensitivity of the retina.

Insufficient dietary vitamin A intake can produce chronic low retinal sensitivity since it is a necessary precursor for rhodopsin production. The effects are more severe at night when high retinal sensitivity is necessary. The condition is called *night blindness* and is directly related to the lack of vitamin A. It takes weeks for a dietary deficiency to bring on symptoms, however, as the liver is capable of storing large amounts of vitamin A.

Figure 12-13 illustrates the increase in retinal sensitivity as dark adaptation progresses. The bimodal characteristic of the curve is due to the differences in rod and cone adaptability. Cones adapt more quickly than rods. That is, they resynthesize retinine from vitamin A at a greater rate. The initial small increase in sensitivity upon entering a dark room is due to activity in the cones, which start to adapt immediately. However, because of the relatively few cones compared to rods, the overall increase in retinal sensitivity due to cone adaptation is quite small. On the other hand, while rods adapt more slowly, they contribute much more to the overall increase in retinal sensitivity because of their relatively great numbers. Three-quarters of an hour is often required for full adaptation to the dark.

Color Vision

While only one type of rod is found in the vertebrate retina, there are three types of cones. Each has its own color-sensitive pigment, making cones the photoreceptors responsible for color vision. The difference in the pigments of each type of cone probably lies in the opsin (protein) portion of the cone rhodopsin. Each type of cone responds maximally to a different wavelength of light. These three types are illustrated in Fig. 12-14. *Blue cones* respond maximally to light of 430 nm (nanometers) wavelength, *green cones* to 535 nm, and *red cones* to 575 nm. Figure 12-14 is a spectral sensitivity curve for each of the three types of cones. Notice that while each cone is maximally sensitive to a specific wavelength, it nevertheless will respond (though to a lesser extent) to

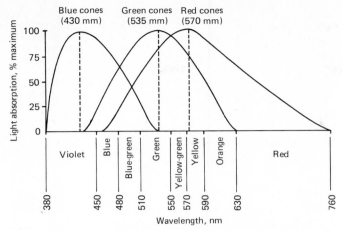

Figure 12-14 The spectral sensitivities of the three types of cones found in the retina. (*Drawn from Marks, American Association for the Advancement of Science, 1964.*)

other wavelengths as well. Notice also that the response curves of the three types of cones significantly overlap.

The Young-Helmholtz theory of color vision states, in part, that the ratio of the relative responses of each different type of cone stimulated determines the color we see. If monochromatic light of 575-nm wavelength is presented to the eye and is focused on the retina, the response of the cone types in this area of the retina will be different. Examination of Fig. 12-14 shows that the red cones will be maximally stimulated, the green cones will be stimulated to 50 percent maximum, and the blue cones will not be stimulated at all. Therefore the response ratio of the cones (red:green:blue) is 100:50:0. The brain decodes this signal and interprets it as the color yellow. Similarly, a monochromatic light of 535 nm would produce the ratio 65:100:0 and be interpreted as green. A light of 502 nm would give rise to the response ratio 30:60:30 and would be seen as blue-green, and so on.

REVIEW QUESTIONS

1   The refractive power of the human lens
    a   increases when focusing for near vision
    b   is fixed and unchangeable
    c   can change by 32 diopters in the very young child
    d   is the single refractive surface in the eye
2   Sympathetic stimulation of appropriate GVE III fibers
    a   contracts the radial muscles of the iris
    b   relaxes the ciliary muscles
    c   dilates the pupils
    d   adjusts the lens for distant vision
    e   none of the above

3   The visual depth of focus
    a   is increased by pupillary dilation
    b   should be maximum for good near vision
    c   is decreased by contraction of the sphincter muscles of the iris
    d   all of the above
4   Compared to a person of age 40, a 20-year-old
    a   is capable of greater accommodation with the lens
    b   has a greater near point
    c   has a less flexible lens
    d   typically has the same accommodative ability
5   Complete severing of the right optic tract causes all of the following, *except*
    a   complete blindness in the right eye
    b   homonymous hemianopia
    c   a visual defect in the left visual field of each eye
    d   no permanent damage to the right visual field of each eye
6   All of the following statements about photoreceptors are true, *except:*
    a   Cones are more abundant than rods in the retina.
    b   Cones dark adapt more quickly than rods.
    c   Rod rhodopsin incorporates the protein scotopsin.
    d   Impulses have been recorded on the photoreceptor cell membrane.
7   The following occur(s) when a dark-adapted person suddenly enters a very bright
    environment:
    a   Retinal sensitivity begins to increase.
    b   Retinine conversion to vitamin A increases.
    c   The rate of rhodopsin synthesis increases.
    d   Rod sensitivity is unaffected.
    e   None of the above.
8   The following statements about cones are true, *except:*
    a   Blue cones respond maximally to light of a shorter wavelength than red cones
          do.
    b   Cones in the fovea are narrower than those elsewhere.
    c   Cones are particularly important for daylight vision.
    d   There are basically two types of cones in the retina, each with its own color-sen-
          sitive pigment.
9   When parallel light rays from a viewed object are brought to a focus in front of the
    retina, the condition is called
    a   myopia
    b   hypermetropia
    c   emmetropia
    d   far-sightedness
10 The accommodation reflexes which are acitvated as we focus on an object which is
    brought closer to the eyes include all of the following, *except*
    a   convergence of the eyes
    b   thickening of the lens
    c   pupillary constriction
    d   dark adaptation

Chapter 13

The Cerebellum

One way to fully appreciate the role of the cerebellum in normal function is to examine those signs associated with its dysfunction. These include muscle weakness (asthenia), a decrease in muscle tone (hypotonia), to-and-fro movements of the eyes (nystagmus), muscle tremor while performing a voluntary task (intention tremor), and a general loss of muscle coordination (ataxia). Ataxia is apparent through problems with posture and gait and is further evidenced by dysmetria, asynergia, and adiadochokinesia.

THE CEREBELLUM AS A COMPARATOR

The cerebellum appears to function as a comparator, at least with respect to its role in muscle control. A sample of the motor command from the cerebral cortex to the skeletal muscles is relayed to the cerebellar cortex for evaluation (Fig. 13-1). Once the motor act begins, the cerebellar cortex begins to receive input (via spinocerebellar tracts) from the proprioceptors in those muscles, tendons, and joints involved in the movement. In this way the cerebellum is in a position to compare the actual performance of a given movement with the original "intent" of the brain. Of course this comparing only has functional value if the cerebellum is capable of making adjustments when the actual performance

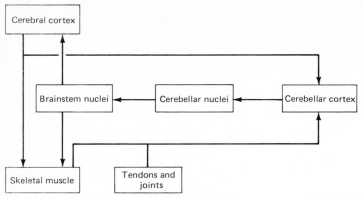

Figure 13-1 Diagrammatic illustration of the interrelationship between the cerebellum, the cerebral cortex, and activity in the skeletal muscles. Details explained in text.

doesn't equal the intent. As illustrated in Fig. 13-1, the cerebellar cortex, through the cerebellar and brainstem nuclei, can direct corrective action both at the cortical source through ascending pathways, as well as at the spinal cord level through descending pathways. It is important to recognize that this simplistic mechanism is by no means intended to fully explain the role of the cerebellum in motor control, but is probably a good starting point from which to launch our discussion of cerebellar function.

CEREBELLAR STRUCTURE

The cerebellum is the largest part of the metencephalon. It lies posterior to the pons, from which it is separated by the fourth ventricle. It is separated from the cerebrum above by a bony covering, the tentorium cerebelli. It weighs about 150 g in the adult male and the ratio of cerebellar to cerebral mass is greater in the adult than in the child.

Like the cerebrum, the cerebellum is composed of cortical gray matter surrounding a large area of subcortical white matter. Similarly, the cerebellar surface is regular and grooved, forming *folia* (folds). Some of the grooves are particularly deep, forming *fissures,* which separate the cerebral mass into *lobules.* Also, the cerebellum is composed of two hemispheres separated (in this case) by the *vermis* (Fig. 13-2). The cerebellum is held firmly to the brainstem by the *cerebellar peduncles.* In Fig. 13-2, the peduncles are illustrated with the cerebellum removed.

Figure 13-3 shows a midsagittal section of the cerebellum through the vermis. The vermis is divided by short, deep fissures into the *lingula, central lobule, culmen, declive, folium, tuber, pyramid, uvula,* and *nodule.* Figure 13-4 shows a somewhat artificial "opened" view of the cerebellum as seen from the rear. It can be seen here that each vermal division, with the single exception of the lingula, is continuous laterally with a lobule of the cerebellar hemisphere.

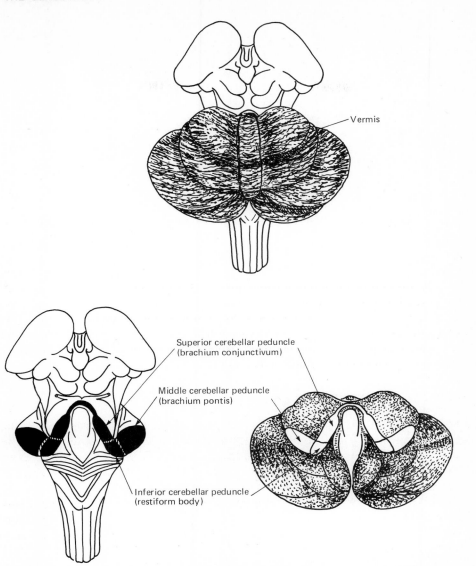

Figure 13-2 Posterior view of the brainstem with the cerebellum in place (above) and removed (below).

These include the central lobule with the *ala of the central lobule*, the culmen with the *quadrangular lobule*, the declive with the *lobulus simplex*, the folium with the *superior semilunar lobule*, the tuber with the *inferior semilunar lobule and gracilis*, the pyramid with the *biventral lobule*, the uvula with the *tonsil*, and the nodule with the *flocculus*.

Phylogenetically, the lingula along with the flocculonodular lobe (nodule and flocculi) are called the *archicerebellum* and represent the cerebellum's

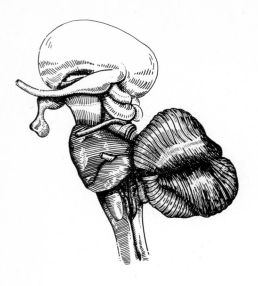

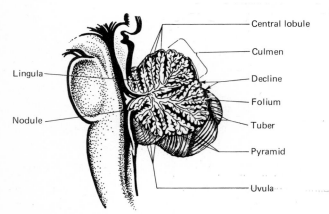

Lingula

Nodule

Central lobule

Culmen

Decline

Folium

Tuber

Pyramid

Uvula

Figure 13-3 Lateral view of the cerebellum (above) and a midsagital section through the vermis (below).

most primitive component. Because of its close functional relationship with the vestibular system, it is also sometimes called the vestibulocerebellum (stippled area of Fig. 13-4). The central lobule with its alae, the culmen with its quadrangles, as well as the pyramid and uvula, comprise a somewhat more recent phylogenetic development of the cerebellum called the *paleocerebellum* or spinocerebellum, because of the large input it receives from the spinal cord. The most recent addition to the cerebellum is the *neocerebellum,* composed of the declive, folium, and tuber along with their lateral hemispheric extensions.

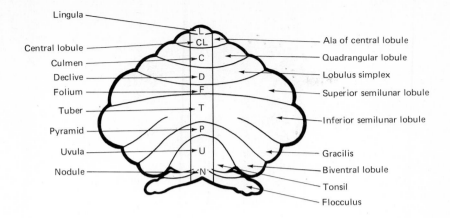

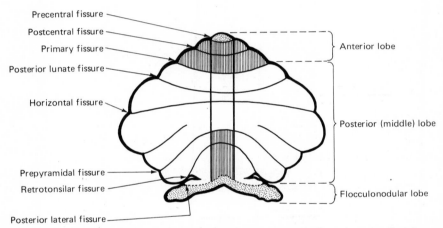

Figure 13-4 Schematic illustrations of the "opened" cerebellum. Imagine that the cerebellum is approached from the rear and the lingula and flocculonodular lobe are pulled backward, opening the cerebellum. In the lower illustration, the stippled area represents the archicerebellum, the lined area represents the paleocerebellum, and the remainder represents the neocerebellum.

Also included are the biventral lobules and tonsils. The neocerebellum is also called the *pontocerebellum* because most of its afferent input is via the pontocerebellar tracts.

Intracerebellar Nuclei

Another similarity between the cerebellum and the cerebrum is the presence of nuclei in the subcortical white matter. These are respectively called *intracerebellar nuclei* in the cerebellum and *basal nuclei* in the cerebrum. The in-

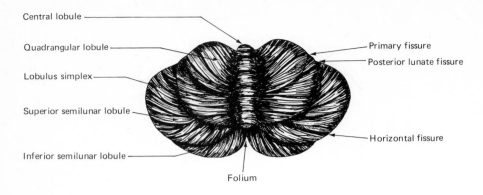

Central lobule

Quadrangular lobule

Lobulus simplex

Superior semilunar lobule

Inferior semilunar lobule

Primary fissure

Posterior lunate fissure

Horizontal fissure

Folium

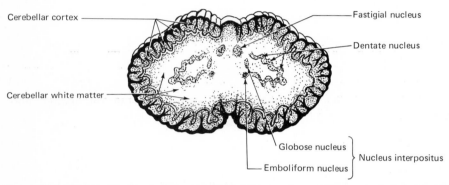

Cerebellar cortex

Cerebellar white matter

Fastigial nucleus

Dentate nucleus

Globose nucleus

Emboliform nucleus

Nucleus interpositus

Figure 13-5   Schematic illustration showing a superior view of the cerebellum (upper). The lower illustration is a horizontal section through the cerebellum. The deep cerebellar nuclei are labeled on the right.

tracerebellar nuclei are paired and located on either side of the midline. The largest and most lateral is the _dentate nucleus_ (Fig. 13-5). Medial to this in order approaching the midline are the _emboliform, globose_, and _fastigial nuclei_. The emboliform and globose nuclei are known collectively as the _nucleus inter-positus._ The intercerebellar nuclei function as important relay centers between the cerebellar cortex and other parts of the brain, brainstem, and spinal cord.

CEREBELLAR INPUT AND OUTPUT

Considering the importance of the cerebellum in motor control, it is not surprising to find that there are numerous neural pathways connecting it with the cerebral cortex, brainstem nuclei, spinal cord proprioceptive tracts, and the vestibular system. The information-conducting fibers entering and leaving the cerebellum pass through the superior, middle, and inferior cerebellar peduncles.

The Inferior Cerebellar Peduncle (Restiform Body)

The inferior cerebellar peduncles (restiform bodies) are thick bundles of afferent and efferent fibers which diverge as they ascend from the posterior aspect of the medulla oblongata. As they arch backward to enter the cerebellar hemispheres, they converge medially and are bounded laterally by the middle cerebellar peduncles (Fig. 13-2). Most of the inferior cerebellar pedunclular fibers are afferent, although there are some efferent routes as well. The names of these tracts or fiber bundles, as well as the location of the cell bodies of their fibers and their distribution, are summarized in Table 13-1.

The afferent tracts include the olivocerebellar, paraolivocerebellar, vestibulocerebellar, reticulocerebellar, posterior spinocerebellar, cuneocerebellar, and trigeminocerebellar. Also included are the anterior external arcuate fibers and the striae medullares. The efferent fibers include the cerebelloolivary, cerebellovestibular, and cerebelloreticular tracts.

The Middle Cerebellar Peduncle (Brachium Pontis)

The middle cerebellar peduncles (brachie pontes), the largest of the peduncles, are composed chiefly of fibers of the pontocerebellar tracts. These fibers originate in the contralateral pontine nuclei, sweep across the anterior aspect of the pons, and then project posteriorly through the peduncles to terminate in the cortex of the cerebellar hemispheres and vermis, except the lingula and flocculonodular lobe.

The Superior Cerebellar Peduncle (Brachium Conjunctivum)

The superior cerebellar peduncles (brachia conjunctiva) emerge from the cerebellum and ascend to form the lateral portion of the roof of the fourth ventricle, where they enter the brainstem below the inferior colliculi. They are bridged by the superior medullary velum. The superior cerebellar peduncles represent the main output route from the cerebellum, and as such, most of their fibers are efferent. However, some afferent input utilizes this route as well. Again, the names of these tracts or fiber bundles and their distributions are summarized in Table 13-1.

The efferent pathways include cerebellorubral, dentatothalamic, and fastigioreticular fibers. All of them emerge from cerebellar nuclei; the cerebellorubral fibers from the globose and emboliform nuclei, the dentatothalamic fibers from the dentate nucleus, and the fastigioreticular fibers from the fastigial nucleus. They emerge together from the various nuclei to ascend in the roof of the fourth ventricle and proceed anteriorly to the midbrain tegmental area medial to the lateral lemniscus. The cerebellorubral fibers cross over at this point to enter the contralateral red nucleus. The dentatothalamic fibers also cross over and ascend to synapse in the ventral intermediate (VI) and ventral anterior (VA) nuclei of the thalamus. The fastigioreticular fibers enter the reticular formation of the midbrain, pons, and medulla oblongata.

Afferent pathways include the anterior spinocerebellar and tectocerebellar

Table 13-1 Cerebellar Connections

Tracts or fiber bundles	Distribution	Location of cell bodies
	Inferior cerebellar peduncle	
Afferent paths		
Olivocerebellar tract	Lateral hemispheres and cerebellar nucleus	Contralateral inferior olivary nucleus
Paraolivocerebellar tract	Vermis, paravermis, and cerebellar nucleus	Contralateral accessory olivary nucleus
Vestibulocerebellar tract	Fastigial nucleus, flocculonodular lobe, and uvula	Ipsilateral vestibular nucleus and vestibular ganglion
Reticulocerebellar tract	Spinal region of cerebellar vermis	Ipsilateral lateral reticular nucleus
Posterior sinocerebellar tract	Hind limb region of cerebellar cortex	Ipsilateral Clarke's column
Trigeminocerebellar tract	Dentate and emboliform nucleus	Bilateral principal sensory and spinal nucleus
Cuneocerebellar tract	Forelimb and upper trunk region of cerebellar cortex	Ipsilateral accessory cuneate nucleus
Anterior exterior arcuate fibers	Flocculus	Bilateral arcuate nucleus
Arcuatocerebellar fibers (striae medullares)	Flocculus	Bilateral arcuate nucleus
Efferent paths		
Cerebelloolivary tract	Inferior olivary nucleus	Fastigial nucleus
Cerebellovestibular tract	Vestibular nucleus	Fastigial nucleus and direct axons of Purkinje cells in flocculus, nodule, anterior and posterior vermis
Cerebelloreticular tract	Pontine and medullary reticular nucleus	Fastigial nucleus
	Middle cerebellar peduncle	
Afferent paths		
Pontocerebellar tract	Neocerebellar cortex	Contralateral pontine nucleus

Table 13-1 Cerebellar Connections (Continued)

Tracts or fiber bundles	Distribution	Location of cell bodies
	Superior cerebellar peduncle	
Afferent paths		
Anterior spinocerebellar tract	Hind limb region of cerebellar cortex	Ipsilateral Clarke's column
Tectocerebellar tract	Intermediate vermis and lobulus simplex	Bilateral superior and inferior colliculi
Efferent paths		
Cerebellorubral fibers	Red nucleus	Contralateral globose and emboliform nucleus
Dentatothalamic fibers	Ventral intermediate (VI) and ventral anterior (VA) nucleus of thalamus	Contralateral dentate nucleus
Fastigioreticular fibers	Reticular nucleus of midbrain, pons, and medulla oblongata	Ipsilateral fastigial nucleus

tracts. You will recall that the fibers of the anterior spinocerebellar tract originate in Clarke's column of the spinal cord and cross in the anterior white commissure to the lateral funiculus, where they ascend to upper pontine levels before crossing back to enter the cerebellum through the superior peduncle. They terminate in the hind limb region of the cerebellar cortex. The tectocerebellar tracts emerge from the superior and inferior colliculi on both sides, terminating in the intermediate vermis (culmen, declive, folium, tuber, pyramid) and the lobulus simplex. The function of the tectocerebellar tract is not known, but it is widely believed to mediate visual and auditory reflexes.

CIRCUIT FUNCTIONING IN THE CEREBELLAR CORTEX

In recent years a good deal of experimental work has helped to illuminate the roles of individual cell types in the cerebellar cortex. Such work has led to the development of a generally accepted model of the interrelationships between these cells, as well as to some elementary hypotheses of how the cerebellum performs its role in motor control.

Unlike the cerebral cortex, the cellular makeup of the cerebellar cortex is quite uniform throughout. A "plug" of cortex from one area is very much like that from any other area. Five types of excitable cells are found in the cortex, forming three distinct layers. Four of the five cell types are inhibitory, including Golgi cells, stellate cells, basket cells, and Purkinje cells. The fifth type, granular cells, represent the only excitatory cells in the cerebellar cortex. Each of these cells, their interactions with one another, and their relative positions in the three cortical layers are schematically illustrated in Fig. 13-6.

The deepest (*granular*) *layer* is made up of granular and Golgi cells. While the cell bodies and dendritic processes of the granular cells are located in this layer, they project long axons up into and through the Purkinje cell layer to ultimately reach the most superficial (molecular) layer. Here the axons run horizontally through the molecular layer as *parallel fibers*. Collaterals from these parallel fibers synapse upon and excite the dendrites of the other four cortical cell types. Golgi cells represent the other cell type found in the granular layer. Axons from these cells project to and inhibit the granular cells. Golgi cells typically project a large dendritic apparatus up through the two higher cortical layers.

The *molecular layer* contains both stellate and basket cells. These relatively small cells are inhibitory to the large Purkinje cells of the middle layer. Typically, the stellate cell axonal endings are inhibitory to the Purkinje cell dendrites, while basket cells inhibit Purkinje cell bodies.

The *Purkinje cell layer* (middle layer) is characterized by the presence of the Purkinje cell bodies. These large inhibitory cells represent the only output from the cerebellar cortex. They project flat broad dendritic trees (Fig. 13-9) up into the molecular layer. Most of the Purkinje cell axons descend through the granular layer to leave the cortex and synapse in the cerebellar nuclei. Nevertheless, some of them from the flocculus and nodule, as well as the anterior and

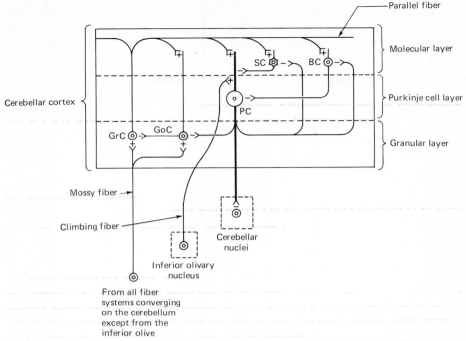

Figure 13-6 Diagrammatic illustration of the cells in the cerebellar cortex. The Purkinje cells represent the only efferent output from the cortex, and they are inhibitory to the cerebellar nuclei. Collaterals from the Purkinje cells (PC) are also inhibitory to three other cortical cell types: Golgi cells (GoC), stellate cells (SC), and basket cells (BC). Granular cells (GrC) project long axons up into the molecular layer where they run laterally as parallel fibers, exciting the dendrites of Golgi cells, Purkinje cells, stellate cells, and basket cells. Afferent input to the cortex is via two types of fibers. Climbing fibers, arising from the contralateral inferior olivary nuclei make multiple excitatory synaptic contacts with the extensive dendritic tree of a single Purkinje cell. Mossy fibers arising from all other fiber systems entering the cerebellum make excitatory contacts with granular and Golgi cells.

posterior vermis, project directly to the vestibular nuclei of the brainstem. Collaterals from these axons project to and synaptically inhibit the Golgi, stellate, and basket cells.

Two kinds of fibers are afferent to the cerebellar cortex. These are the so-called *climbing fibers* from the inferior olivary nucleus, and the *mossy fibers* from all other sources afferent to the cortex. Each climbing fiber enters the cortex and makes numerous synaptic contacts with the dendritic tree of a single Purkinje cell. By contrast, each mossy fiber synapses with several granular and Golgi cells. Both climbing and mossy fibers are excitatory to the cells they synapse with.

Leaving aside for the moment a hypothesis of how the cortical cells integrate motor activity, let's have another look at the cerebellum as a comparator. Recall that the cerebellum is in a position to compare the actual performance of a motor action with the intended command signal and then subsequently initi-

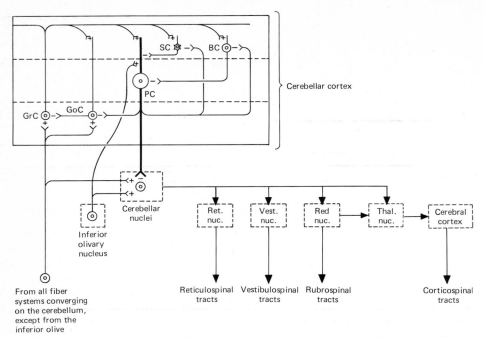

Figure 13-7 Diagrammatic illustration showing the afferent input and functional output of the cerebellum. SC, stellate cell; BC, basket cell; PC, purkinje cell; GrC, granular cell; GoC, Golgi cell; ret. nuc., reticular nucleus; vest. nuc., vestibular nucleus; thlm. nuc., thalomic nucleus.

ate whatever corrective action is necessary through its efferent output. We now know that this output is a two-link process: first from the cortex to the cerebellar nuclei via the axons of Purkinje cells, and then from the cerebellar nuclei through the peduncles to the various brainstem nuclei (Fig. 13-7).

Through such output from the brainstem nuclei, the cerebellum can influence motor activity both at the cortical source as well as at the spinal cord level. Fibers leave the cerebellum via the superior cerebellar peduncle, projecting first to the ventral anterior (VA) and ventral intermediate (VI) nuclei of the thalamus, to ultimately modify cerebrocortical motor neurons through thalamocortical projections. Similarly, through cerebellar projections to the reticular, vestibular, and red nuclei, the cerebellum can modify spinal cord alpha and gamma motor neurons through the reticulospinal, vestibulospinal, and rubrospinal tracts.

A small basal firing rate is generally observed in the efferent fibers from the cerebellar nuclei. This is apparently due to the excitatory collateral input of the mossy and climbing fibers. One can see from Fig. 13-7 that the cerebellar cortex is in an ideal position to modify the firing of cerebellar nuclear fibers by varying the firing of the inhibitory axons of Purkinje cells which also synapse

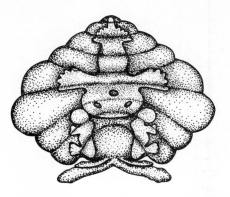

Figure 13-8 Somatotopic map of cerebellar cortex, representing the areas of evoked responses produced by cutaneous stimulation.

on these neurons. Recall that the firing rate of a neuron is a function of its central excitatory state, which is itself a function of the "integration" of the cell's excitatory and inhibitory input.

NEURAL "SHARPENING" OF CEREBELLAR CORTICAL INPUT

We must recognize that even with the most recent information concerning the functional histology of the cerebellar cortex, little is still known about the way in which the cortex utilizes mossy and climbing fiber input. Because of the absence of long association fibers such as are found in the cerebral cortex, it is assumed that small discrete regions of the cerebellar cortex handle the full integration of their "own" climbing and mossy fibers, and can thereby direct appropriate output over their own Purkinje cell axons. The cerebellar cortex has been "mapped," and a homunculus for sensory cutaneous stimulation is illustrated in Fig. 13-8. The homunculus represents points on the cerebellar cortex where cutaneous electrical stimulation produces evoked responses. While it is probably naive to suspect that proprioceptors from a given muscle project to the same region of cortex which modifies (through brainstem nuclei and descending tracts) the motor neurons to that same muscle, the possibility is intriguing and undoubtedly partly true.

Evidence suggests that the cerebellar cortex "sharpens" the input from its afferent fibers so that it is constantly dealing with the strongest (and presumably most important) input at all times. A possible mechanism for this sharpening is presented here. As Fig. 13-9 illustrates, the dendritic trees of the Purkinje cells are relatively flat and run in a plane transverse to the folds of the cortical surface. The parallel fibers of the granular cells pass through these trees much like telephone wires on a series of poles. Because the parallel fibers run parallel to the long axis of the folia (folds), they cross the dendritic trees at right angles. Consequently, when a discrete cluster of granular cells are stimulated, a narrow strip of excited Purkinje cells is produced down a limited length of the folium. These same parallel fibers also make excitatory contacts with basket, stellate,

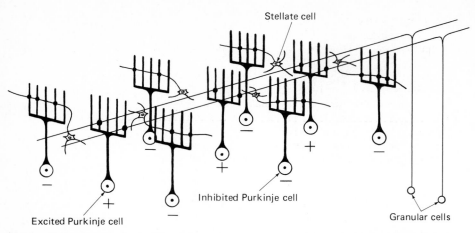

Figure 13-9 Diagrammatic illustration of the "inhibitory surround". The parallel fibers of granular cells excite a narrow strip of Purkinje cells through excitatory synapses. The same parallel fibers also excite laterally projecting stellate cells which inhibit a surrounding area of Purkinje cells.

and Golgi cells. Now recall that each of the latter are inhibitory neurons. The stellate and basket cells are relatively small and hence have low excitation thresholds, rendering them easily stimulated by the parallel fibers. Their axons are directed at more or less right angles to the parallel fibers and make synaptic contacts with the dendritic trees of Purkinje cells on either side of the narrow excited strip. Because basket and stellate cells are inhibitory, the result is the production of a narrow inhibited zone (inhibitory surround) of Purkinje cells on either side of the narrow excited strip. It has been postulated that these ever-changing patterns of excited strips flanked by the inhibitory surround provide neural sharpening which enables the cortex to deal only with the strongest input at all times.

If the mossy fiber input to the cerebellar cortex is sufficient to excite a great number of granular cells in a particular locus, it follows that the width of the excited strip would increase. Theoretically, this could cause the degree of neural sharpening to decrease. Current thinking holds that this is prevented by inhibitory action of the Golgi cells. These cells have very extensive dendritic projections which are not limited to a single transverse plane like the Purkinje cells, but rather extend through the molecular layer to share space with the dendritic trees of as many as 10 Purkinje cells. Now the Golgi cells aren't as easily excited as Purkinje cells because a proportionately smaller number of their dendritic branches receive excitatory input from the parallel fibers. However, if the number of granular cells firing increases, the strip of excited Purkinje cells becomes wider also. Nevertheless, at some point the Golgi cells will become sufficiently stimulated by the increased number of activated parallel fibers to inhibit the granular cells, preventing the widening of the excitatory strip to a point where its sharp focus is lost.

REVIEW QUESTIONS

1 That portion of the cerebellum phylogenetically called the neocerebellum
   a is also called the pontocerebellum
   b receives most of its input from the spinal cord
   c represents the largest part of this organ
   d includes the pyramid and uvula

2 The cerebellorubral fibers project from the contralateral globose and emboliform nuclei to the red nucleus via the
   a superior cerebellar peduncle
   b restiform body
   c brachium conjunctivum
   d middle cerebellar peduncle
   e inferior cerebellar peduncle

3 All of the following cerebellar cortical cells are thought to be inhibitory, *except*
   a Golgi cells
   b stellate cells
   c basket cells
   d Purkinje cells
   e granular cells

4 The "climbing fibers" which enter the cerebellar cortex
   a synapse primarily with Purkinje cells
   b orginate in the inferior olivary nucleus
   c synapse with granular and Golgi cells
   d are thought to be inhibitory
   e none of the above

5 The parallel fibers of granular cells are located in
   a the granular layer of the cerebellar cortex
   b the molecular layer of the cerebellar cortex
   c the Purkinje cell layer of the cerebellar cortex
   d the emboliform nucleus

6 The largest and most lateral of the deep cerebellar nuclei are the
   a emboliform nuclei
   b globose nuclei
   c fastigial nuclei
   d dentate nuclei

7 All of the following statements about the cerebellum are true, *except:*
   a The cerebellum is the largest part of the metencephalon.
   b The ratio of cerebellar to cerebral mass is greater in the adult than in the child.
   c The cerebellum weighs about 300 g in the adult male.
   d The cerebellum has two hemispheres.

8 Efferent fibers from the cerebellar cortex
   a primarily project directly to brainstem nuclei
   b are excitatory
   c have cell bodies located in all three cerebellar cortical layers
   d receive direct synaptic input from mossy fibers
   e none of the above

9 All of the following statements concerning the deep cerebellar nuclei are true, *except:*
   a They project fibers to the cerebellar cortex primarily.
   b The nuclei are not paired.
   c They receive input from the climbing and mossy fibers.
   d They project fibers to the reticular, vestibular, and red nuclei.
10 The following is (are) true concerning the functional relationships between cells in the cerebellar cortex:
   a Granular cells excite all other cortical neurons.
   b Stellate and basket cells excite Purkinje cells.
   c Stellate, basket, and Golgi cells are inhibited by Purkinje cells.
   d The "inhibitory surround" refers to a narrow inhibited zone of Purkinje cells on either side of a narrow excited strip of these cells.

The Autonomic Nervous System

Fortunately the body's vital functions are regulated automatically and require no conscious effort on our part. The *autonomic nervous system* (ANS) is to a large extent responsible for automatically and subconsciously regulating the cardiovascular, renal, gastrointestinal, thermoregulatory, and other systems, in order to enable the body to meet the continual and ever-changing stresses to which it is exposed.

Autonomic nerve fibers innervate cardiac muscle, smooth muscle, and glands. Through these fibers the ANS plays a role in regulating (1) blood pressure and flow, (2) gastrointestinal movements and secretions, (3) body temperature, (4) bronchial dilation, (5) blood glucose levels, (6) metabolism, (7) micturition and defecation, (8) pupillary light and accommodation reflexes, and (9) glandular secretions, just to name a few.

A muscle or gland innervated by autonomic fibers is called an *effector organ*. If the autonomic nerve fibers to an effector organ are cut, the organ may continue to function, but will lack the capability of adjusting to changing conditions. If the autonomic nerve fibers to the heart are cut, the heart will continue to beat and pump blood normally, but its ability to increase cardiac output under stress will be seriously limited. In a very real sense, the ANS bestows on the vital functions of the body the capability of adjusting activity levels to meet ever-changing needs.

Anatomically and functionally, the autonomic nervous system is made up of two subdivisions: the *sympathetic system* with long-lasting and diffuse effects, and the *parasympathetic system* with more transient and specific effects. In either case the nerve fibers of the ANS are motor only, and represent the general visceral efferent (GVE) fibers of the cranial and spinal nerves.

THE SYMPATHETIC OUTFLOW

The nerve fibers which comprise the sympathetic system originate in the intermediolateral horn (lamina VII) of the gray matter in all twelve thoracic and the first two lumbar segments of the spinal cord. The axons of these GVE fibers travel through the anterior horn and exit the cord in the anterior root before entering the spinal nerve. While the general somatic efferent (GSE) fibers (alpha and gamma motor neurons of the anterior horn) continue in the spinal nerve trunks to innervate skeletal muscle fibers and muscle spindles, almost all of the GVE fibers leave the spinal nerve trunks to enter *sympathetic ganglia* via a thin arm, the *white ramus* (Figs. 14-1, 14-2, and 14-3).

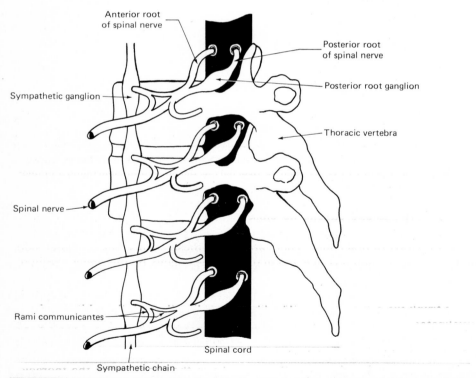

Figure 14-1   The relationship of the sympathetic chain to the spinal nerves. The sympathetic ganglia associated with spinal nerves T1 through L2 are connected to the nerve by two arms, the rami communicantes.

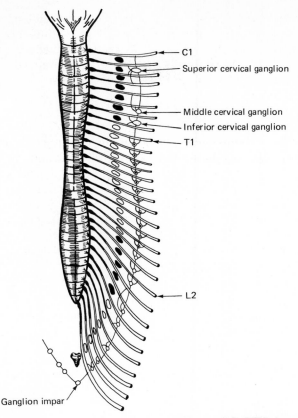

C1
Superior cervical ganglion
Middle cervical ganglion
Inferior cervical ganglion
T1
L2
Ganglion impar

Figure 14-2 The relationship between the ganglia of the sympathetic chain and the 31 pairs of spinal nerves. Notice that those ganglia associated with spinal nerves T1 through L2 contact the nerve through two rami (white and gray) . The superior, middle, and inferior cervical ganglia send gray rami only to the eight cervical nerves. Similarly, a variable number of ganglia (4 to 8) below L2, send gray rami only to the spinal nerves in this area.

The sympathetic ganglia lie close to the vertebral bodies and are also known as *paravertebral ganglia*. They are strung together to form a sympathetic or paravertebral *chain*. There are two of these chains, one on either side of the vertebral column connected in front of the coccyx by the single *ganglion impar* (Fig. 14-2).

Some of the fibers from nerve cells within the ganglia return to the spinal nerve trunk via a *gray ramus*. The fibers traveling through the white rami are myelinated while those in the gray rami are not, and this fact is responsible for their respective names. Each of the twelve thoracic and first two lumbar nerves is in contact with a paravertebral ganglion via a white and gray ramus. You will notice, however, that there are three ganglia in the chain above the thoracic region as well as several below L2 (Fig. 14-2). Each of these additional ganglia is connected to a spinal nerve by a single gray ramus.

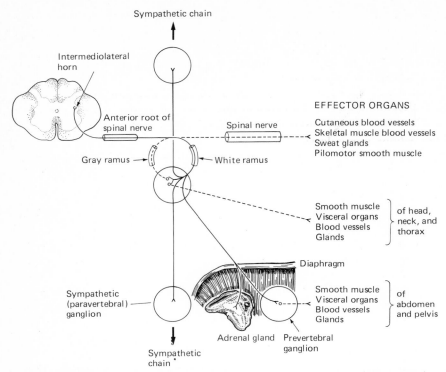

Figure 14-3 Schematic illustration showing the sympathetic outflow. Preganglionic neurons (solid lines) originate in the intermediolateral horn of the spinal cord between T1 and L2. The fibers leave the spinal nerve in the white ramus and enter the sympathetic ganglia where they take one of five divergent routes: (1) terminate by synapsing, (2) leave the ganglion and pass up the sympathetic chain to synapse in ganglia at a higher level, (3) leave the ganglion and pass down the chain, (4) leave the ganglion and penetrate the diaphragm to terminate in the adrenal medulla, (5) leave the ganglion and penetrate the diaphragm to terminate in the prevertebral ganglia. Postganglionic fibers (dashed lines) innervate the effector organs.

The superior, middle, and inferior cervical ganglia probably represent the fusion of smaller individual cervical ganglia. These three send gray rami to all eight cervical spinal nerves. The superior cervical ganglion sends to the first four cervical nerves, the smaller middle cervical ganglion supplies the next two, and the large inferior cervical ganglion projects a gray ramus to the seventh and eighth cervical nerves. Similarly, a variable number of ganglia (four to eight) below L2 send gray rami to all of the spinal nerves below this level. Consequently, all 31 pairs of spinal nerves are in contact with the sympathetic chain and carry fibers of the sympathetic system. This is an important feature, enabling those effector organs which are innervated only by spinal nerves (cutaneous and skeletal muscle blood vessels, sweat glands, and pilomotor smooth muscle) to receive sympathetic input.

In addition to the paired paravertebral ganglia, there are several unpaired *prevertebral ganglia* in the abdomen and pelvis. They also play a role in the sympathetic outflow. Figure 14-3 illustrates the many possible ways by which the sympathetic system innervates its effector organs.

There is always a two-neuron link to each effector organ innervated, with the single exception of the adrenal medulla. The first is the *preganglionic neuron* and the second is the *postganglionic neuron*. The four possible routes of the preganglionic and postganglionic fibers, as illustrated in Fig. 14-3, are summarized below. After entering the sympathetic ganglia via the white rami, the preganglionic fibers may:

1 Pass without synapsing up or down the sympathetic chain to ultimately synapse in a higher or lower ganglion. By passing up the chain, the first four or five thoracic cord levels contribute all of the preganglionic fibers to the superior, middle, and inferior cervical ganglia. Similarly by passing down the chain, the lower thoracic and upper lumbar cord levels contribute all of the preganglionic fibers to the ganglia in the chain below L2. Postganglionic fibers then leave the ganglia via their gray rami to enter their respective spinal nerves for distribution to their effector organs (cutaneous and skeletal muscle blood vessels, sweat glands, and pilomotor smooth muscle).

2 Synapse in the ganglia and subsequently stimulate postganglionic fibers which leave the ganglia to reenter the spinal nerves via the gray rami. The postganglionic fibers are then distributed with the spinal nerves to their effector organs (cutaneous and skeletal muscle blood vessels, sweat glands, and pilomotor smooth muscle).

3 Synapse in the ganglia and subsequently stimulate postganglionic fibers which leave the ganglia and are directly distributed to their effector organs (smooth muscle, visceral organs, blood vessels, and glands of the head, neck, and thorax).

4 Pass without synapsing into the abdomen to synapse in one of the prevertebral ganglia or the adrenal medulla. Postganglionic fibers leave the prevertebral ganglia to innervate their effector organs (smooth muscle, visceral organs, blood vessels, and glands of the abdomen and pelvis).

THE PARASYMPATHETIC OUTFLOW

The nerve fibers which comprise the parasympathetic system originate in two quite distant regions, the brainstem and the sacral portion of the spinal cord. For this reason it is often called the *craniosacral outflow* to distinguish it from the thoracolumbar outflow of the sympathetic system. Those GVE fibers which make up the cranial portion of the system originate in specific brainstem nuclei and are distributed with cranial nerves III, VII, IX, and X. Those which comprise the sacral portion originate in lamina VII of sacral cord segments 2 to 4 and are distributed as the GVE fibers of the pelvic nerves (nervi erigentes).

As with the sympathetic system, there are always two neurons in the pathway to the effector organ supplied. Thus, there are pre- and postganglionic

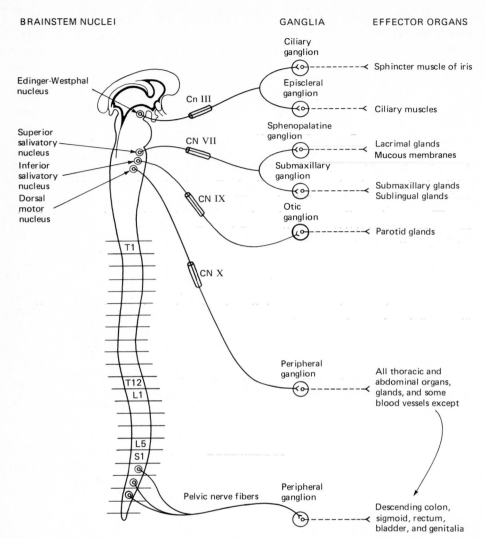

BRAINSTEM NUCLEI   GANGLIA   EFFECTOR ORGANS

Figure 14-4   Schematic illustration showing the parasympathetic outflow. Preganglionic neurons (solid lines) emerge from brainstem nuclei and from the intermediolateral region of the gray matter in sacral segments 2 to 4. GVE fibers of cranial nerves III, VII, IX, and X compose the cranial portion of the parasympathetic system. The GVE fibers of the pelvic nerve comprise the sacral portion. Postganglionic fibers (dashed lines) innervate the effector organs shown.

fibers in the parasympathetic system also. However, unlike those in the sympathetic system, parasympathetic ganglia are quite distant from the brainstem and cord, often located directly on the effector organ itself. Thus the postganglionic fibers are much shorter in the parasympathetic system than they are in the sympathetic system.

It should be noted here that <u>autonomic effector organs typically receive</u> <u>both sympathetic and parasympathetic innervation,</u> though some receive input from one system only. The effects of sympathetic and parasympathetic stimulation of the autonomic effector organs are summarized in Table 14-1. The effects are often but not always opposite, as will be described later.

Figure 14-4 illustrates the parasympathetic outflow. The Edinger-Westphal nucleus (an accessory nucleus of III) in the tegmentum of the midbrain gives rise to the preganglionic parasympathetic fibers of the oculomotor (III) nerve. <u>Some of these fibers terminate in the ciliary ganglion and</u> <u>others in the episcleral ganglion.</u> The former stimulate postganglionic fibers innervating the sphincter muscles of the iris, which control pupillary diameter, while the latter stimulate postganglionic fibers innervating the ciliary muscle controlling the curvature of the lens (Fig. 12-5).

The <u>superior salivatory nucleus in the pons gives rise to the preganglionic</u> <u>fibers of the facial (VII) nerve.</u> Some of these fibers terminate in the <u>sphenopalatine ganglion</u> and others in the <u>submandibular (submaxillary) ganglion.</u> Postganglionic fibers from the former innervate the lacrimal gland and mucous membranes in the head and neck region while postganglionic fibers from the latter innervate the submaxillary and sublingual salivary glands. The <u>inferior</u> <u>salivatory nucleus at the pontomedullary border gives rise to the preganglionic</u> <u>fibers of the glossopharyngeal nerve (IX).</u> These fibers terminate in the otic ganglion, from which postganglionic fibers innervate the parotid gland.

The overwhelming majority of cranial preganglionic fibers are distributed within the vagus (X) nerve. They originate in the <u>dorsal motor nucleus of X in</u> the medulla and terminate in unnamed peripheral ganglia on thoracic and abdominal organs, glands, and some blood vessels. Short postganglionic fibers run from these ganglia to receptor sites on the effector organ cells.

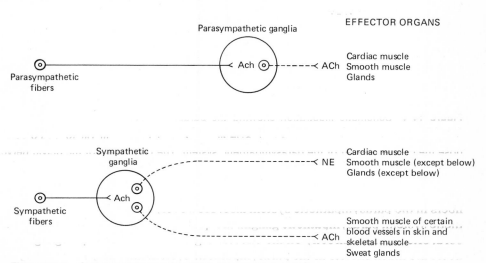

Figure 14-5   General scheme of autonomic neurotransmitters.

Table 14-1   Autonomic Effects on Various Organs of the Body

Effector organs	Effects of sympathetic stimulation	Effects of parasympathetic stimulation
Eye		
Radial muscle of iris	(α) Contraction (mydriasis)	
Sphincter muscle of iris		Contraction (miosis)
Ciliary muscle of lens	(β) Relaxation (lens flattens)	Contraction (lens curves)
Heart		
SA node	(β) ↑ heart rate	↓ heart rate
Atria	(β) ↑ heart rate and force	↓ heart force
AV node	(β) ↑ conduction velocity	↓ conduction velocity
Purkinje system	(β) ↑ conduction velocity	
Ventricles	(β) ↑ heart rate and force	
Blood vessels		
Coronary	(α) Constriction	Dilatation
	(β) Dilatation	
Cutaneous	(α) Constriction	
	(ACh) Dilatation	
Skeletal muscle	(α) Constriction	
	(β) Dilatation	
	(ACh) Dilatation	
Abdominal visceral	(α) Constriction	
	(β) Dilatation	
Renal	(α) Constriction	
Salivary glands	(α) Constriction	Dilatation
Stomach		
Motility and tone	(β) Decrease (usually)	Increase
Sphincters	(α) Contraction (usually)	Relaxation (usually)
Secretion	Inhibition (?)	Stimulation
Intestine		
Motility and tone	(α, β) Decrease	Increase
Sphincters	(α) Contraction (usually)	Relaxation (usually)
Secretion	Inhibition (?)	Stimulation
Gallbladder and ducts	Relaxation	Contraction
Urinary bladder		
Detrusor	(β) Relaxation (usually)	Contraction
Trigone and sphincter	(α) Contraction	Relaxation
Ureter		
Motility and tone	Increase (usually)	Increase (?)
Male sex organs	Ejaculation	Erection
Skin		
Pilomotor muscles	(α) Contraction	
Sweat glands	(α) Slight, localized secretions	
	(ACh) Generalized secretions	
Spleen capsule	(α) Contraction	

Table 14-1   Autonomic Effects on Various Organs of the Body *(Continued)*

Effector organs	Effects of sympathetic stimulation	Effects of parasympathetic stimulation
Lung (bronchial muscles)	(β) Relaxation	Contraction
Adrenal medulla		Secretion of epinephrine and norepinephrine
Liver	(β) Glycogenolysis	
Pancreas		
Acinar cells	↓ secretion	Secretion
Islet cells	(α) Inhibition of insulin and glucagon secretion (β) Insulin and glucagon secretion	Insulin and glucagon secretion
Salivary glands	(α) Thick, sparse secretion	Profuse, watery secretion
Lacrimal glands		Secretion
Nasopharyngeal glands		Secretion
Adipose tissue	(β) Lipolysis	
Juxtaglomerular cells	(β) Renin secretion	
Pineal gland	(β) Melatonin synthesis and secretion	

Source: Modified from Goodman L. S., and A. Gilman: *The Pharmacological Basis of Therapeutics,* 5th ed., Macmillan, 1975.

The sacral parasympathetic outflow supplies the organs and glands in part of the lower abdomen and all of the pelvis. Included are the descending colon, sigmoid, rectum, bladder, and external genitalia. As noted earlier, the preganglionic fibers originate in lamina VII of the sacral cord between S2 and S4. These fibers travel with the pelvic nerve and terminate in peripheral ganglia on the effector organs themselves.

AUTONOMIC NEUROTRANSMITTERS

Both sympathetic and parasympathetic preganglionic neurons are *cholinergic;* that is, the preganglionic fibers of both systems release acetylcholine (ACh) at the synapse in the ganglion. Thus ACh is the principal transmitter in the autonomic ganglia. There are also some dopaminergic (dopamine releasing) interneurons present, but their function is still unknown. Nevertheless, the preganglionic fibers themselves are all cholinergic.

All postganglionic fibers of the parasympathetic system are cholinergic, but postganglionic sympathetic fibers are more diverse. The overwhelming majority are *adrenergic* [release norepinephrine (NE)], but a few are cholinergic. The few which are known to be cholinergic are those which innervate the sweat glands and some cutaneous and skeletal muscle blood vessels (Fig. 14-5).

Acetylcholine Synthesis, Release, and Inactivation

Figure 14-6 illustrates the general scheme of activity at the cholinergic synapse. Synthesis of ACh occurs in the cytoplasm of cholinergic presynaptic terminals. Coenzyme A (CoA) combines with acetate to form acetyl coenzyme A (acetyl CoA). Energy for this reaction is supplied by ATP. Once formed, the acetyl CoA combines with choline in the presence of the enzyme choline acetyltransferase to form acetylcholine (ACh). Once synthesized, ACh is taken up by the synaptic vesicles and held there in a bound form until its released.

When an impulse reaches the presynaptic terminal, several synaptic vesicles release ACh into the synaptic cleft. ACh then diffuses across the cleft to activate cholinergic receptor sites on the postsynaptic membrane. In order to allow the presynaptic terminal to effectively control the postsynaptic membrane, the released ACh must be quickly degraded (within microseconds) by the enzyme acetylcholinesterase (AChE) to acetate and choline, which are then reabsorbed into the presynaptic terminal for resynthesis to ACh. A small fraction is reabsorbed intact into the presynaptic terminal while an even smaller fraction diffuses out of the synaptic cleft before it can be degraded or reabsorbed. AChE is abundantly available in the cholinergic synaptic cleft. And

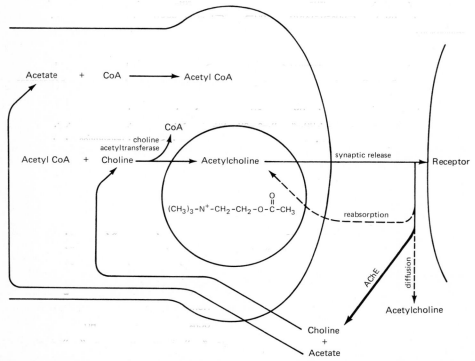

Figure 14-6 Schematic illustration of the synthesis and fate of synaptically released acetylcholine at the cholinergic synapse.

even though the enzyme can degrade ACh within microseconds, there is adequate time for the ACh to activate receptor sites.

Norepinephrine Synthesis, Release, and Inactivation

Figure 14-7 illustrates the synthesis and fate of synaptically released norepinephrine at adrenergic synapses. Norepinephrine is synthesized in the presynaptic terminal by a series of enzymatically catalyzed reactions typically starting with the amino acid tyrosine. The sequence can also start with phenylalanine, which can be enzymatically converted to tyrosine. In either case tyrosine is converted to dihydroxyphenylalanine (dopa), dopamine, and finally to norepinephrine. The final synthetic step from dopamine to norepinephrine occurs in the synaptic vesicle where the norepinephrine is held in a bound form. The for-

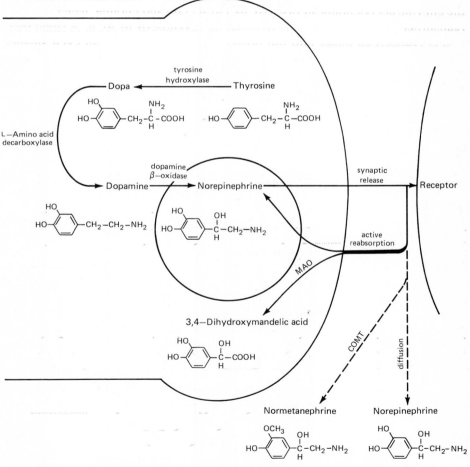

Figure 14-7 Schematic illustration of the synthesis and fate of synaptically released norepinephrine at the adrenergic synapse.

mation of dopa is apparently the rate-limiting step in the synthesis of norepi-nephrine.

When an impulse reaches the presynaptic terminal, several vesicles release norepinephrine into the synaptic cleft, where it diffuses to activate receptor sites on the postsynaptic membrane. Within a few milliseconds, the norepi-nephrine is subject to one of three fates. A small amount is methylated by the enzyme *catechol-o-methyl transferase* (COMT), which is present in the cleft, and thereby rendered inactive. An even smaller fraction diffuses out of the cleft and away from receptor sites. But certainly the greatest amount of norepi-nephrine is reabsorbed by active transport into the presynaptic terminal. If norepinephrine stores in the synaptic vesicles are low, as might be the case in a rapidly firing fiber, the reabsorbed norepinephrine may be taken up by the vesicles for subsequent rerelease. If adequate stores of the transmitter are available, the reabsorbed norepinephrine is subjected to oxidative deamination by mitochondrial *monoamine oxidase* (MAO).

AUTONOMIC TONE

Table 14-1 shows the effects of sympathetic and parasympathetic stimulation on autonomic effector organs. The sympathetic and parasympathetic systems are continually active and the level of activity at a given rate of firing is known as *autonomic tone*.

Sympathetic Tone

To illustrate sympathetic tone, consider this example. Most arteries are nor-mally in a state of partial constriction. That is, they are neither fully constricted nor fully dilated. Since most blood vessels receive only sympathetic innerva-tion, it is the only system that need be considered. If the normal partially con-stricted state of an artery is maintained by a basal firing rate of 1 impulse per second, we can describe the artery as displaying a basal sympathetic tone. Now if the firing rate should increase to say 50 impulses per second, the artery would constrict further, showing an increase in sympathetic tone. Conversely, if the firing rate were to decrease, the smooth muscle of the blood vessel would relax, causing the artery to vasodilate with a decrease in sympathetic tone.

The adrenal medulla is also an important contributor to sympathetic tone throughout the body. Each time the sympathetic system is activated, the adre-nal medullae are also sufficiently stimulated via the splanchnic nerves, to increase their output of epinephrine and norepinephrine to the general circula-tion. These two catecholamines then travel to all parts of the body stimulating sympathetic effector organs. It is easy to see how the increased release of these two chemicals by the adrenal medulla can cause a general increase in sympa-thetic tone throughout the body. In fact, this increased output by the adrenal gland with sympathetic stimulation is the principal reason why the effects of sympathetic stimulation are longer lasting and more diffuse than those associ-ated with the parasympathetic system.

Parasympathetic Tone

An example of parasympathetic tone is the control of peristalsis in the GI tract. Gastrointestinal smooth muscle receives both sympathetic and parasympathetic innervation. Increasing the firing rate of parasympathetic fibers to the gut causes an increase in intestinal motility and peristalsis, and hence, an increase in parasympathetic tone. Decreasing the firing rate produces a decrease in peristaltic activity, and hence, parasympathetic tone. Table 14-1 shows parasympathetic stimulation increases peristalsis while sympathetic stimulation decreases it. Thus, the GI musculature is an example of the often true observation that the effects of sympathetic and parasympathetic stimulation are opposite and tend to balance each other. Further examination of Table 14-1, however, will show that this is not always true. Unfortunately for first-time students, there is no substitute for learning this table.

Alpha and Beta Receptors

The action of catecholamines on adrenergic effector organs varies with the organs. Catecholamines excite some effectors and inhibit others. Experiments with a series of sympathetic drugs have shown there are at least two types of adrenergic receptors. They are called *alpha* and *beta*. Blocking agents were later developed for each receptor which further confirmed their existence. The response of an effector to a catecholamine is then partly a function of the type of receptor it has. Epinephrine excites both alpha and beta receptors quite equally, while norepinephrine excites mainly alpha receptors. Nevertheless, norepinephrine will also excite beta receptors, but only to a slight extent. This explains why epinephrine has a much stronger effect on the heart (which has only beta receptors) than norepinephrine does. To further confuse the picture, some effectors have only alpha receptors, others have only beta receptors, and still others have both. Thus the specific response of an effector is both a function of the relative ratio of receptor types and the kind of transmitter involved. A partial list of the effects of alpha and beta stimulation is given in Table 14-2.

   Notice that some alpha functions are inhibitory while others are excitatory. The same is true for certain beta effects. Therefore it is not possible to refer to one receptor as excitatory and the other as inhibitory, as is sometimes true. Beta receptors have also been divided into two types: beta$_1$ and beta$_2$, ac-

Table 14-2   Effects of Alpha and Beta Stimulation

Alpha receptor	Beta receptor
Vasoconstriction	Vasodilation
Mydriasis (pupil dilation)	Cardioacceleration
Intestinal relaxation	Bronchial relaxation
	Increased cardiac strength
	Intestinal relaxation
	Glycogenolysis
	Lipolysis

cording to their responses to various drugs. *Beta$_1$ receptors* are those responsible for the inotropic (strength) and chronotopic (rate) responses of the heart, as well as lipolysis. *Beta$_2$ receptors* bring about vasodilation and bronchial relaxation. This is a distinction useful to the pharmacologist, who can then use a beta$_2$ agonist to treat asthma and produce bronchial relaxation with very little cardiac stimulation.

AUTONOMIC AND RELATED DRUGS

A large number of drugs have been developed which are active at various sites in the autonomic nervous system. Figure 14-8 schematically illustrates the action and site of action of several of these.

Drugs Acting on Autonomic Effector Organs

Acetylcholine, pilocarpine, and methacholine all directly stimulate cholinergic receptors on autonomic effector organs. Physostigmine and neostigmine also potentiate activity at these receptors, but do it by the indirect action of inhibiting cholinesterase (AChE). Conversely, atropine is a potent antagonist at these receptors, inhibiting the action of endogenously released ACh as well as administered cholinomimetic drugs.

A variety of drugs are also active at adrenergic receptors on autonomic effector organs. Norepinephrine, epinephrine, isoproterenol (a beta agonist) and

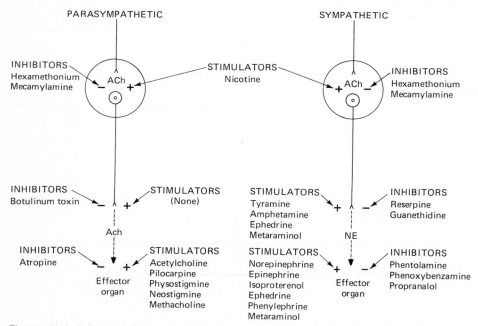

Figure 14-8 Schematic illustration of the action of various drugs on the autonomic nervous system. Mechanisms of action for several of the drugs are explained in the text.

phenylephrine (an alpha agonist) are all capable of directly stimulating these receptors. In addition, ephedrine and metaraminol can act directly on these receptors but typically are first absorbed by the adrenergic nerve endings and subsequently released upon the arrival of impulses at the presynaptic terminal. Metaraminol is an alpha agonist both directly and indirectly, while ephedrine is a beta agonist directly but stimulates alpha receptors when released by adrenergic nerve endings. On the other hand, phentolamine and phenoxybenzamine are effective alpha antagonists and thus effectively block alpha receptors. Propranolol is a beta blocker.

Drugs Acting on Autonomic Nerve Endings

There are no known drugs to stimulate the release of ACh from the presynaptic terminals of cholinergic nerve endings. However, botulinum toxin is a potent inhibitor of ACh release. Adrenergic nerve endings are more commonly manipulated by drug action. Both tyramine and amphetamine promote the release of endogenous norepinephrine from these nerve endings. Ephedrine and metaraminol are also potentiators at these sites by the indirect action of being absorbed into the terminals and subsequently being released as false transmitters. Reserpine and guanethidine are effective inhibitors here by the action of depleting stores of norepinephrine in synaptic vesicles and preventing their further uptake and storage.

Drugs Acting on Autonomic Ganglia

Drugs active at parasympathetic ganglia are equally effective at sympathetic ganglia, and vice versa. Nicotine stimulates postganglionic neuron receptors in the autonomic ganglia. Hexamethonium and mecamylamine effectively block these "nicotinic" receptor sites.

Nonautonomic Drugs

It is worth pointing out that there are several drugs which are active at the skeletal neuromuscular junction which are not active in the autonomic nervous system. For example, curare and succinylcholine effectively block the action of ACh on skeletal muscle receptors but have no similar ACh blocking action on cardiac and smooth muscle receptors.

REVIEW QUESTIONS

1 All of the following statements concerning the autonomic ganglia are true, *except:*
   a The ganglia in the sympathetic chain are paired.
   b Each ganglion in the sympathetic chain has both a gray and a white ramus.
   c The prevertebral autonomic ganglia in the abdomen and pelvis are paired.
   d Each spinal nerve carries some postganglionic sympathetic fibers.
2 The following is (are) true concerning the sympathetic outflow:
   a The cell bodies of preganglionic neurons are located in lamina VII (intermediolateral horn) of the spinal cord between T1 and L2.

    b The cell bodies of the postganglionic sympathetic neurons to the stomach are located in a paravertebral ganglion.

    c Postganglionic sympathetic fibers primarily enter the spinal nerves through the white rami.

    d Preganglionic sympathetic fibers are typically longer than preganglionic parasympathetic fibers.

3 The following is (are) true concerning the parasympathetic outflow:

    a There are always two neurons from the CNS to the effector organ innervated.

    b Cranial nerve V carries some preganglionic parasympathetic fibers.

    c Parasympathetic ganglia are typically quite distant from the effector organs innervated.

    d Some preganglionic parasympathetic fibers originate in the lumbar section of the cord.

4 All of the following statements about autonomic neurotransmitters are true, *except:*

    a Both sympathetic and parasympathetic preganglionic neurons are cholinergic.

    b Postganglionic parasympathetic neurons are cholinergic.

    c Sweat glands are innervated by postganglionic, sympathetic, cholinergic neurons.

    d The adrenal medulla is innervated by adrenergic fibers of the sympathetic nervous system.

5 The following is (are) true concerning metabolism of autonomic neurotransmitters:

    a Most synaptically released ACh is enzymatically degraded in the synaptic cleft.

    b Norepinephrine synthesis typically begins with the amino acid tyrosine.

    c Most of the synaptically released norepinephrine is enzymatically degraded in the synaptic cleft.

    d Choline acetyltransferase is the enzyme responsible for hydrolyzing ACh.

6 All of the following are true concerning the effects of autonomic stimulation on various effector organs of the body, *except:*

    a Sympathetic stimulation promotes contraction of the gall bladder and ducts.

    b Sympathetic stimulation decreases motility and tone in the. intestine.

    c Parasympathetic stimulation promotes decreased conduction velocity in the Purkinje system of the heart.

    d Parasympathetic stimulation causes profuse, watery secretion in the salivary glands.

    e Sympathetic stimulation causes lipolysis of adipose tissue.

7 All of the following responses are associated with beta receptors, *except*

    a vasodilation

    b glycogenolysis

    c bronchial relaxation

    d mydriasis (pupil dilation)

    e vasoconstriction

8 An inhibitory drug at autonomic ganglia is

    a pilocarpine

    b isoproterenol

    c reserpine

    d botulinum toxin

    e hexamethonium

    f guanethidine

9 All of the following drugs stimulate adrenergic receptors on autonomic effector organs, *except*
   a norepinephrine
   b epinephrine
   c phentolamine
   d isoproterenol
   e phenylephrine

10 Beta$_2$ receptors are particularly responsible for mediating
   a vasodilation
   b bronchial relaxation
   c increased cardiac strength
   d increased cardiac rate

The Hypothalamus and Thalamus

The diencephalon (throughbrain or betweenbrain) includes the thalamus, hypothalamus, epithalamus, and subthalamus. It represents the highest part of the brainstem and is capped by the telencephalon (cerebral hemispheres). Except for the interthalamic adhesion, the diencephalon is divided by the cerebrospinal-fluid-filled third ventricle. It is bounded caudally by the midbrain and rostrally by the frontal lobes of the cerebrum. In this chapter we will examine both the hypothalamus and thalamus.

THE HYPOTHALAMUS

The hypothalamus forms the floor of the third ventricle and is separated from the thalamus above by the hypothalamic sulcus in the ventricle's lateral walls. It is composed of a discrete set of nuclei (Fig. 15-1) which are involved in the following functions:

1 Autonomic control
2 Temperature regulation
3 Thirst and control of body water
4 Appetite control

5 Endocrine control
6 Emotional reactions
7 Sleep and wakefulness
8 Stress response

Hypothalamic Nuclei

Several nuclei have been identified in the hypothalamus. Some have become associated with specific physiological activities, while the functions of others are less clear and in some cases unknown. Their relative locations are illustrated in midsagittal section in Fig. 15-1. Therefore it is important to recognize that you are seeing the nuclei on the right side of the third ventricle only. In other words, each of the nuclei is paired.

The nuclei are often grouped in four general areas. The *preoptic area* includes the medial and lateral preoptic nuclei, which extend through the lamina terminalis. The *supraoptic area* includes the supraoptic, anterior hypothalamic, and paraventricular nuclei. The *tuberal area* includs the lateral hypothalamic, posterior hypothalamic, dorsomedial, and ventromedial nuclei. Finally, the *mammillary area* is composed of the medial and lateral mammillary nuclei.

Hypothalamic Connections

For the hypothalamus to play an effective role in the functions listed above, it is necessary that it be in neural contact with many areas of the brain and spinal

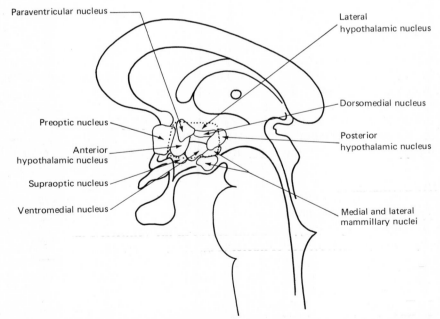

Figure 15-1 Principal nuclei of the hypothalamus. Each of the nuclei shown is paired, with only half of each pair shown in this saggital section.

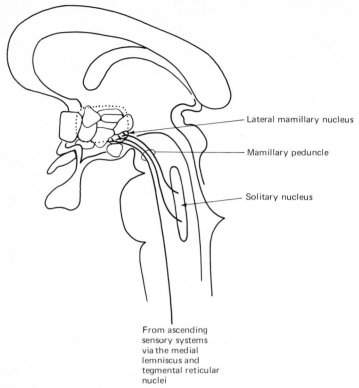

Lateral mamillary nucleus

Mamillary peduncle

Solitary nucleus

From ascending
sensory systems
via the medial
lemniscus and
tegmental reticular
nuclei

Figure 15-2 Afferent input to the hypothalamus via the mammillary peduncle.

cord. The fiber systems involved can be described as either afferent or efferent
to the hypothalamus. Some of the principal systems are presented below.

Hypothalamic Afferent Input Fibers in the _mammillary peduncle_ represent a major ascending input to the hypothalamus (Fig. 15-2). It arises in the
tegmentum of the midbrain and is formed by fibers carrying information from
SVA and GVA fibers which terminate in the solitary nucleus. Similarly, ascending information from the spinal cord relayed through the medial lemniscus
also contributes fibers to this system. The hypothalamic termination is chiefly
in the lateral mammillary nuclei.

The _corticohypothalamic fibers_ project to a number of hypothalamic
nuclei. It is no doubt through such connections that conscious thought is often
able to give rise to autonomic and visceral responses such as, for example, in-
digestion from worry, sweating from fear, and sexual arousal from certain
kinds of thoughts. Nevertheless, the hypothalamus is not ordinarily under cortical control as evidenced, for example, by our inability to raise or lower the
blood pressure at will.

Several corticohypothalamic routes are illustrated in Fig. 15-3. Fibers

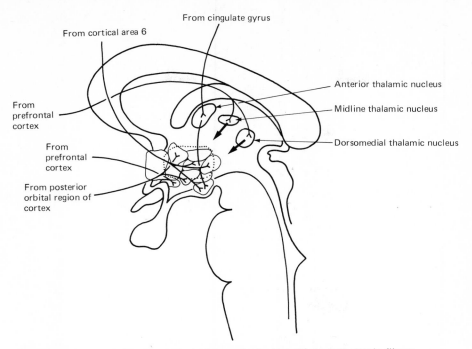

Figure 15-3   Schematic illustration of the principal corticohypothalamic fibers.

from cortical area 6 pass through the septal region to terminate chiefly in the posterior hypothalamic and lateral hypothalamic nuclei as well as the mammillary nuclei. Fibers from the prefrontal cortex project to the supraoptic nucleus as well as indirectly to the hypothalamus through synapses in the anterior, midline, and dorsomedial thalamic nuclei. Projections from the olfactory posterior orbital region of the cortex project to the paraventricular and ventromedial nuclei. The cingulate cyrus also indirectly influences the hypothalamus via an intermediate synapse in the anterior thalamic nucleus. Thalamomammillary fibers are also present.

The *thalamohypothalamic fibers* fall into two general groups; the thalamomammillary fibers which project from the anterior thalamic nucleus to the medial mammillary nucleus, and a group which passes from the midline and dorsomedial thalamic nuclei principally to the anterior hypothalamic nucleus. There are probably other connections as well between the thalamus and hypothalamus (Fig.15-4).

The *corticomammillary fibers* (fornix) project from the hippocampus of the temporal lobe to the mammillary nuclei via a long loop (Fig.15-5). The *stria terminalis* is composed of fibers which originate in the amygdala of the temporal lobe and pass caudally along the tail of the caudate nucleus and arch over the dorsal aspect of the thalamus to terminate in the septal nuclei as well as the preoptic, anterior hypothalamic, and ventromedial nuclei.

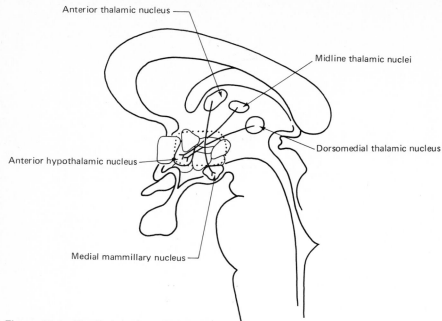

Figure 15-4 The thalamohypothalamic fibers.

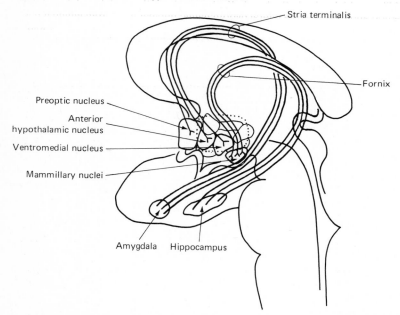

Figure 15-5 Schematic illustration of the corticomammillary fibers (fornix) from the hippocampal nucleus to the lateral mammillary body. Also pictured are the fibers of the stria terminalis from the amygdala to the preoptic, anterior, and ventromedial nuclei of the hypothalamus. Both the amygdala and hippocampus are located in the temporal lobe of the brain.

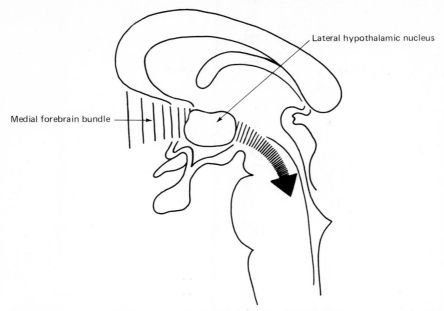

Figure 15-6 Loosely structured schematic illustration of the medial forebrain bundle. It is a complex group of fibers which arise in the basal olfactory regions, the septal nuclei, and the periamygdaloid region and pass into the lateral hypothalamic nuclear area, from which it has numerous connections with other hypothalamic nuclei. Many fibers continue into the midbrain tegmentum, from which signals are relayed to the autonomic- and visceral-controlling nuclei of the brainstem.

The *medial forebrain bundle* is a complex group of fibers which arise in the basal olfactory region, the septal nuclei, and periamygdaloid region and pass to the lateral hypothalamic nuclear area (Fig. 15-6). Many medial forebrain bundle fibers continue into the midbrain tegmentum while others project to additional hypothalamic nuclei. Those reaching the midbrain tegmentum relay signals to the autonomic and visceral controlling nuclei of the brainstem. Hence the bundle is both an afferent and efferent system with respect to hypothalamic nuclei.

Hypothalamic Efferent Output The anterior thalamic and mammillary nuclei are reciprocally related and therefore a *mammillothalamic tract* exists. Through projection fibers from the anterior thalamic nucleus to the cingulate gyrus, the hypothalamus is able to influence activity in this region of the cerebral cortex. This system and the mammillotegmental fibers which project to the reticular nuclei of the brainstem tegmentum are illustrated in Figure 15-7.

The *periventricular fibers* represent a large descending fiber system originating in the supraoptic, posterior hypothalamic, and tuberal nuclei. While there is a small ascending component to thalamic nuclei, most of the fibers descend to synapse in various parasympathetic brainstem nuclei as well as the

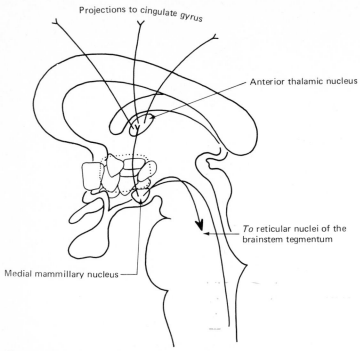

Projections to cingulate gyrus

Anterior thalamic nucleus

To reticular nuclei of the brainstem tegmentum

Medial mammillary nucleus

Figure 15-7   Schematic illustration of the mammillothalamic and mammillotegmental fibers.

respiratory and vasomotor centers. Some also terminate in the reticular nuclei of the brainstem tegmentum. Reticulospinal fibers as well as some periventricular fibers which don't synapse in the brainstem, descend into the spinal cord to influence preganglionic sympathetic and parasympathetic neurons in the intermediolateral region (Fig. 15-8).

The *hypothalamohypophyseal* tract is a group of fibers which run from the paraventricular and supraoptic nuclei to the posterior lobe of the pituitary gland. This tract mediates release of the posterior pituitary hormones, oxytocin, and antidiuretic hormone (ADH). Oxytocin is synthesized in the paraventricular nucleus and transported through the axons of fibers projecting to the posterior lobe. ADH is synthesized in the supraoptic nucleus and similarly transported through the hypothalamohypophyseal tract to the posterior lobe (Fig. 15-9). The hormones are stored in the terminal endings of these fibers until they are released into the circulation.

The Hypothalamus and the Autonomic Nervous System

The hypothalamus has long been suspected of playing a role in autonomic nervous system regulation. Most of the evidence for this is based on the observation that electrical stimulation of various areas of the hypothalamus produce autonomic effects. While there is no clear-cut demarcation line, stimulation of

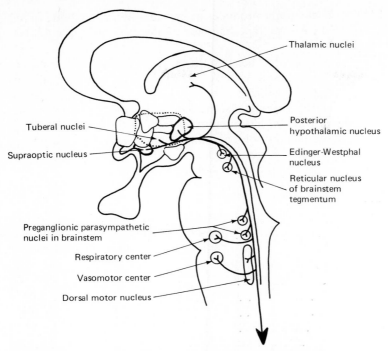

Thalamic nuclei

Tuberal nuclei

Supraoptic nucleus

Posterior hypothalamic nucleus

Edinger-Westphal nucleus

Reticular nucleus of brainstem tegmentum

Preganglionic parasympathetic nuclei in brainstem

Respiratory center

Vasomotor center

Dorsal motor nucleus

Figure 15-8 The periventricular fibers. See text for explanation.

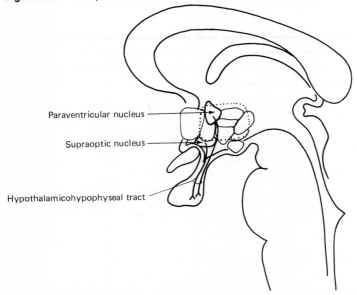

Paraventricular nucleus

Supraoptic nucleus

Hypothalamicohypophyseal tract

Figure 15-9 Schematic illustration of the fibers of the hypothalamohypophyseal tract. The paraventricular nucleus (PVN) is the origin of the posterior pituitary hormone, oxytocin, while the supraoptic nucleus (SON) is the source of synthesis for antidiuretic hormone (ADH).

the caudal hypothalamus generally produces an increase in sympathetic activity, while stimulation of the rostral hypothalamus produces parasympathetic effects.

It is reasonable to assume that the hypothalamus is not the sole, or even the principal, regulator of autonomic activity. While it can certainly modify autonomic activity via direct and indirect pathways to preganglionic neurons in the brainstem and spinal cord, we must also recognize that the hypothalamus itself receives input from a wide variety of sources in both the brain and spinal cord. Thus, while the hypothalamus can certainly modify autonomic response, the question of ultimate control is certainly larger and more complex than can be explained by a model based on hypothalamic control alone.

The Hypothalamus and Temperature Regulation

Temperature regulation is an important homeostatic activity which is primarily controlled by the hypothalamus. If we consider the dangerous effects of temperature extremes on the body, a center designed for regulating this variable is of obvious importance.

Electrical stimulation of the anterior hypothalamus, particularly the supraoptic area, triggers a thermolytic response. That is, those activities which cause the body temperature to drop are set into operation. Conversely, stimulation of the posterior hypothalamus, particularly the tuberal area, triggers a thermogenic response, reflected both in increased heat conservation and production. Thermolytic responses include cutaneous vasodilation in order to increase heat loss by radiation, sweating to increase heat loss by evaporation, and panting in animals like the dog. Thermogenic responses include cutaneous vasoconstriction to prevent heat loss by radiation, shivering to produce heat by increased muscular activity, cessation of sweating to reduce heat loss by evaporation, and an increase in the production and release of thyroxine in order to increase the metabolic rate.

Thermoreceptors in the hypothalamus are sensitive to very small changes in the temperature of circulating blood. Because blood temperature varies closely with changes in core temperature, the hypothalamus is continually kept informed of changes in the overall temperature of the body. Subsequently it can activate appropriate thermolytic or thermogenic activities in order to restore body temperature to normal. The hypothalamus also receives input from cutaneous thermoreceptors which keep it informed of changes in the environmental temperature. Consequently the hypothalamus is continually informed of both external and internal temperature changes and is well equipped through neural activation of appropriate effectors to prevent temperature fluctuations by regulating body temperature within very narrow limits.

The Hypothalamus, Thirst, and Control of Body Water

The hypothalamus is well equipped to respond to changes in the total amount of body water. A poorly localized area of the hypothalamus called the *"thirst center"* is stimulated by a dry mouth as well as body dehydration. Projections from the thirst center to the thalamus and then to the conscious cortex inform us of the need for water. This triggers the sensation of thirst and initiates the conscious desire for water.

The hypothalamus also takes subconscious steps to correct dehydration. Osmoreceptors in the supraoptic nuclei respond to dehydration (typically associated with increased osmolality in the circulating blood) by increasing the production and release of antidiuretic hormone (ADH). This hormone is produced in the supraoptic nucleus (SON) and transported via the axons of the hypothalamohypophyseal tract to the posterior pituitary lobe for temporary storage and ultimate release into the circulation. Once released, ADH promotes an increase in total body water by facilitating water reabsorption in the kidneys so that more is returned to the blood and less is lost in the urine. ADH operates by increasing the water permeability of the distal tubules and collecting ducts of the nephrons. This causes water to be osmotically reabsorbed from the less osmotic glomerular filtrate to the more osmotic extracellular fluid of the kidney medulla and renal blood supply.

The Hypothalamus and Appetite

Studies on animals have confirmed the relationship between the hypothalamus and appetite. The lateral hypothalamic nuclei function in part as a "feeding center." This is based primarily on the observation that electrical stimulation of this region in the rat triggers a strong feeding response which is observed even if the animal has just eaten his fill. Conversely, the ventromedial nucleus is described as the "satiety center" because stimulation of this region stops all feeding activity on the part of the animal. It is certainly possible that these two nuclei are neurally related in such a way that each inhibits the other. In this way, when the lateral hypothalamic nucleus is directing feeding, it can also simultaneously inhibit the satiety center, and vice versa. At present, the system is poorly understood in humans. If such a mutually exclusive system exists, however, it is obviously capable of conscious modification, as we can eat when full and refrain from eating even when hungry.

The Hypothalamus and the Endocrine System

If, as it is often said, the pituitary is the master gland of the endocrine system, it can equally be said that the hypothalamus is master of the pituitary. It influences the production and release of hormones from both the posterior lobe (pars nervosa or neurohypophysis) as well as from the anterior lobe (pars distalis or adenohypophysis). Unlike the anterior lobe, which is not derived from neural tissue, the posterior lobe has an intimate embryological relationship with the hypothalamus. Because of this difference, the hypothalamus exerts its influence in a different manner on each lobe.

Control of the Posterior Lobe The two known posterior pituitary hormones are oxytocin and antidiuretic hormone, also called vasopressin. Each is an octapeptide whose amino acid sequence is well known. There are no secretory cells in the posterior pituitary, however, and both hormones are produced in the hypothalamic nuclei and subsequently transported to the posterior lobe.

Oxytocin is probably produced in the paraventricular nucleus (PVN). Its target tissues include the breast, where it promotes the letdown of milk, and the uterine musculature, where it promotes smooth muscle contractions. It's released in response to several stimuli. These include mechanical stimulation of the nipple area by the suckling infant, uterine and cervical contractions associated with birth, and psychic factors via poorly understood circuits from the conscious cortex. The latter is apparent when the cry of a hungry infant is often a sufficient stimulus for milk letdown in the lactating mother, requiring no mechanical stimulation at all.

Antidiuretic hormone is produced in the supraoptic nucleus and similarly transported to the posterior lobe. The stimulus for its release (stimulation of the thirst center, dehydration, and increased body fluid osmolality) have previously been discussed. ADH is also called vasopressin because of its ability to vasoconstrict blood vessels. Once synthesized, the hormones are transported to the posterior lobe via axonal transport through fibers of the hypothalamohypophyseal tract. Here they are temporarily stored bound to a protein (neurophysin) until their release is called for.

Control of the Anterior Lobe   There are no direct nerve fiber pathways from the hypothalamus to the anterior lobe. And unlike the posterior lobe, it is rich in secretory cells. Thus, the hormones of the anterior lobe are both produced in and released from the adenohypophysis. The known hormones from the anterior lobe include: growth hormone (GH), adrenocorticotrophic hormone (ACTH), thyroid-stimulating hormone (TSH), follicle-stimulating hormone (FSH), luteinizing hormone (LH), luteotropic hormone (LTH), and melanocyte-stimulating hormone (MSH). Luteinizing hormone is called *interstitial cell–stimulating hormone* (ICSH) in the male.

While these hormones are actually synthesized in the anterior lobe of the pituitary, the signal for their release comes from the hypothalamus in the form of small polypeptides called *releasing factors*. At the appropriate time a particular releasing factor is secreted near the capillary network in the median eminence (Fig. 15-10) by fibers from one or more of the hypothalamic nuclei. It then diffuses into the capillaries and travels into the adenohypophysis via the *hypothalamohypophyseal portal system*. Once in the anterior lobe, the portal system again gives rise to a capillary network. The releasing factor then diffuses out of the capillaries and causes specific groups of secretory cells to release their hormone into the capillaries for distribution to the main circulation. Figure 15-10 illustrates the various known releasing factors as well as their hormones and target tissues.

The Hypothalamus and Emotion: The Limbic System

In addition to its other functions, the hypothalamus also plays a role in the physical expression of emotion. Parts of the hypothalamus are closely integrated with the *limbic lobe* of the brain. This lobe, illustrated in Fig. 15-11,

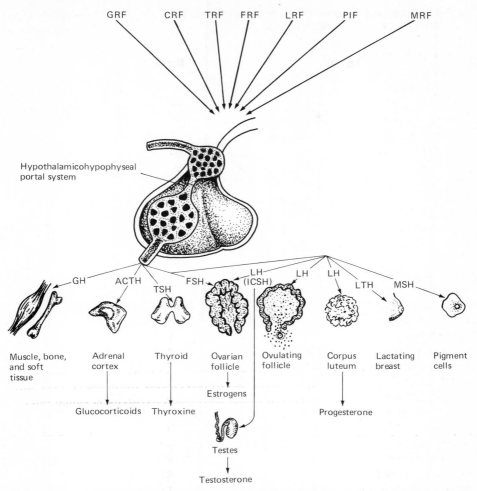

Figure 15-10 The hypothalamus and hormones of the anterior piruitary gland. See text for explanation. GRF, growth hormone–releasing factor; CRF, corticotropin-releasing factor; TRF, thyrotropin-releasing factor; FRF, follicle-stimulating hormone–releasing factor; LRF, luteinizing-hormone–releasing factor, PIF, prolactin inhibitory factor; MRF, melanocyte-stimulating hormone–releasing factor; GH, growth hormone; ACTH, adrenocorticotrophic hormone; TSH, thyroid-stimulating hormone; FSH, follicle-stimulating hormone; LH, luteinizing hormone; also called interstitial cell–stimulating hormone (ICSH); LTH, luteotropic hormone; MSH, melanocyte-stimulating hormone.

includes the cingulate gyrus, isthmus, and parahippocampal gyrus and uncus. The limbic lobe together with the amygdala, hippocampus, olfactory bulbs and trigone, fornix, and mammillary bodies comprise the *limbic system*. In lower vertebrates this system is primarily involved with smell. However in humans, its principal role appears to be in the arousal of emotion.

The cerebral cortex is associated with the subjective aspects of "feelings"

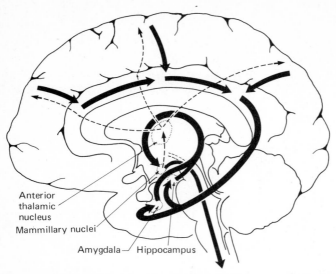

Anterior
thalamic
nucleus
Mammillary nuclei
Amygdala — Hippocampus

Figure 15-11 Diagrammatic illustration of the limbic system. It is composed of the limbic lobe together with the amygdala, hippocampus, olfactory bulbs and trigone, fornix, and mammillary bodies. In lower vertebrates this system is primarily involved with smell. However, in humans its principal function appears to be associated with the arousal of emotion. See text for explanation.

and emotions while the autonomic nervous system promotes many of the physical expressions associated with them. It does this through changes in such activities as heart rate, blood pressure, sweating, salivation, and gastrointestinal activity. One theory is that the limbic system ties the cerebral and autonomic components of emotion together. We all know that it is possible to worry enough about something to the point where it brings on physical symptoms such as stomach upset, sweating, etc.

Figure 15-11 illustrates a model for this phenomenon. The conscious neocortex is reciprocally connected to the cingulate gyrus, which in turn transmits to the parahippocampal gyrus and uncus of the temporal lobe via the isthmus. These cortical areas project to the subcortical hippocampal and amygdaloid nuclei. Fibers projecting from these nuclei pass through the looping arch of the fornix to the mammillary nuclei. These, together with other hypothalamic nuclei, promote autonomic responses through descending fibers to autonomic nuclei within the brainstem and spinal cord.

The system probably works in reverse also. If strong autonomic activity is going on at a subconscious level, the conscious cortex often becomes aware of it. This awareness is probably mediated over mammillothalamic fibers which project to the anterior nucleus of the thalamus, which then project to the cingulate gyrus and the conscious cortex. It must be understood that the pathways described here certainly do not represent the complete network between the cerebral and autonomic components of emotion. This is clearly an area about which we know very little.

THE THALAMUS

The thalamus represents the most rostral part of the diencephalon. It is composed of two large ovoid gray masses separated by the third ventricle but generally connected by a narrow commissural structure, the interthalamic adhesion (Figs. 15-12 and 15-13). The thalamus is separated from the hypothalamus

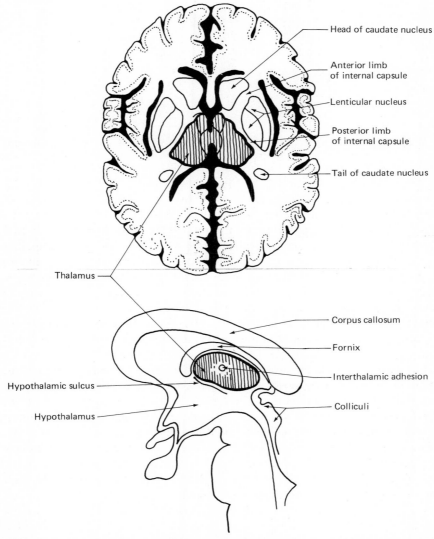

Head of caudate nucleus

Anterior limb
of internal capsule

Lenticular nucleus

Posterior limb
of internal capsule

Tail of caudate nucleus

Thalamus

Corpus callosum

Fornix

Interthalamic adhesion

Hypothalamic sulcus

Colliculi

Hypothalamus

Figure 15-12   The location of the thalamus. Horizontal section (above) and midsagittal section (below).

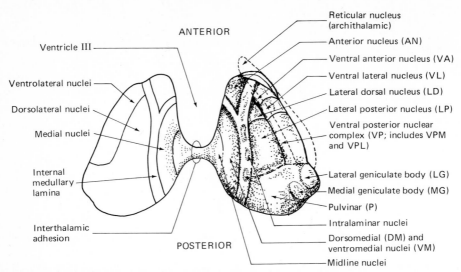

Figure 15-13 Superior view of the thalamus. General divisions to the left and specific thalamic nuclei to the right.

below by a narrow depression in the lateral wall of the third ventricle, the hypothalamic sulcus. It is bounded laterally by the internal capsule and anteriorly by the head of the caudate nucleus (Fig. 15-12).

The thalamus is certainly a very important relay station in the brain and undoubtedly an important subcortical integrator as well. All of the principal sensory paths (except the olfactory system) send fibers to the thalamic nuclei. In addition, it receives input from the basal nuclei, the hypothalamus, the cerebellum, the visual and auditory systems, and most areas of the cerebral cortex.

The gray matter of the thalamus is divided internally by a somewhat myelinated band, the *internal medullary lamina,* which opens into a Y at the anterior pole of the thalamus to effectively demarcate the *anterior nucleus* (AN) (Fig. 15-13).

Except for the intralaminar nuclei, the remaining nuclei of the thalamus are located in three anterior-posterior bands: the *ventrolateral nuclei,* the *dorsolateral nuclei,* and the *medial nuclei.* The latter two groups are separated by the internal medullary lamina. These groups, and the specific nuclei which compose them, are illustrated in Fig. 15-13. The various afferent and efferent connections these nuclei make with the rest of the nervous system are schematically illustrated in Fig. 15-14.

A summary of the various thalamic nuclei and their connections with other components of the nervous system is presented here.

The Anterior Nuclei

These are located in the most anterior and superior part of the thalamus bounded by the Y of the internal medullary lamina. While we of speak of the anterior nucleus (AN) in the singular, it is actually composed of several nuclei.

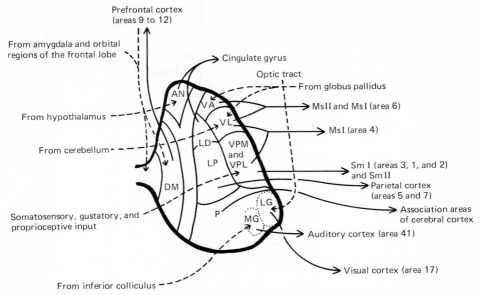

Figure 15-14 Schematic illustration of a superior view of the right thalamus showing principal afferent (dashed lines) and efferent (solid lines) connections with other parts of the nervous system. AN, anterior nucleus; VA, ventral anterior nucleus; VL, ventral lateral nucleus; LD, lateral dorsal nucleus; VPM, ventral posterior medial nucleus; VPL, ventral posterior lateral nucleus; DM, dorsomedial nucleus; LG, lateral geniculate body; MG, medial geniculate body; LP, lateral posterior nucleus; P, pulvimar.

They have reciprocal connections with the hypothalamus via the mammillothalamic fibers as well as with the limbic lobe of the cortex, particularly the cingulate gyrus.

The Medial Nuclei

The principal nuclei here are the large *dorsomedial nucleus* (DM) and the *ventromedial nucleus* (VM). The dorsomedial nucleus has reciprocal connections with the frontal lobe of the cortex, areas 9, 10, 11, and 12. It also receives input from the amygdala and orbital regions of the frontal lobe. It is reciprocally connected with most of the other thalamic nuclei as well.

The Midline Nuclei

The midline nuclei receive input from the brainstem reticular formation. They are also connected with the hypothalamus as well as the dorsomedial nuclei on both sides via the interthalamic adhesion. The prefrontal cortex, amygdala, and orbital region of the frontal lobe also project into these nuclei.

The Dorsolateral Nuclei

This group includes the *lateral dorsal nucleus* (LD), the *lateral posterior nucleus* (LP), and the *pulvinar* (P). The lateral dorsal nucleus is reciprocally related to the posterior cingulate gyrus, the precuneate region of the inferior parietal lobe, and the mammillary nuclei. The lateral posterior nucleus receives input from the medial and lateral geniculate bodies and the ventral posterior nucleus (VP). It also has extensive interconnections with the postcentral gyrus of the parietal lobe, specifically areas 5 and 7 and the precuneus. Likewise, the pulvinar also receives input from the medial and lateral geniculate bodies and the ventral posterior nucleus (VP). In addition, it may also receive direct input from the optic tract. It has reciprocal connections with the association areas of the parietal, occipital, and temporal cortexes.

The Ventrolateral Nuclei

This group includes the *ventral anterior nucleus* (VA), the *ventral lateral nucleus* (VL), and the *ventral posterior nuclear complex* (VP). The latter includes the *ventral posteriomedial nucleus* (VPM) and the *ventral posteriolateral nucleus* (VPL). Both the ventral anterior and ventral lateral nuclei receive input from the globus pallidus, while the ventral lateral nucleus also receives input from the cerebellum and the red nucleus. Both nuclei project to area 6 of the primary motor area (MsI) and to the secondary motor area (MsII) as well. The ventral lateral nucleus also projects to area 4 of MsI. The ventral anterior nucleus is reciprocally related to the caudate nucleus.

The ventral posterior nuclear complex is the principal thalamic receiving area of the large ascending sensory systems. The VPL receives somatosensory and proprioceptive input from the medial lemniscus and the spinothalamic tracts. The VPM receives input from the trigeminal and gustatory pathways. The principal cortical projections from the VPM and VPL pass through the posterior limb of the internal capsule to the primary and secondary somatosensory areas (SmI and SmII) of the cerebral cortex. SmI and SmII also project to these nuclei.

The Intralaminar Nuclei

This group includes the *centromedian nucleus* (CM) and *parafascicular nucleus* (PF). Both are reciprocally related to the entire neocortex as well as other thalamic nuclei. Both also receive input from the spinothalamic tracts and the brainstem reticular formation. In addition, the globus pallidus and cortical area 4 project to the centromedian nucleus, while the parafascicular nucleus receives input from area 6.

The Reticular Nucleus of the Thalamus

This is a long curved nucleus which separates the lateral thalamus from the fibers of the posterior limb of the internal capsule. It receives input from the entire neocortex, the brainstem reticular formation, and the globus pallidus. Its output is primarily directed to other thalamic nuclei, and it is thought to play an important part in the reticular activating system associated with wakefulness.

The Medial and Lateral Geniculate Bodies

The caudal region of the ventral thalamus contains two round swellings, the *medial geniculate body* (MG) and the *lateral geniculate body* (LG). The former is an important relay center in the conscious auditory pathway. Fibers project from here to the auditory cortex of the temporal lobe. The latter is an important relay and integration center in the conscious visual pathway. It receives input from optic nerve fibers and projects output fibers to the visual cortex over the optic radiation. The pulvinar has also been shown to be neurally connected with the lateral geniculate body.

In summary, it must be recognized that the list of thalamic connections is incomplete, as new studies are constantly showing additional pathways. We can also assume that the thalamic nuclei are intricately connected to each other, further clouding our understanding of any clear mechanisms which the thalamus employs in integrating the information it receives.

REVIEW QUESTIONS

1 The tuberal area of the hypothalamus includes
   a the medial and lateral preoptic nuclei
   b the lateral hypothalamic, posterior hypothalamic, dorsomedial, and ventro-
        medial nuclei
   c the medial and lateral mammillary nuclei
   d the supraoptic, anterior hypothalamic, and paraventricular nuclei
2 A major route of ascending input to the hypothalamus is
   a the mammillary peduncle
   b the corticohypothalamic tract
   c the medial forebrain bundle
   d the periventricular tract
   e none of the above
3 A pathway of afferent fibers from the hippocampus to the mammillary nuclei is the
   a fornix
   b stria terminalis
   c medial forebrain bundle
   d mammillohippocampal tract
4 All of the following statements about the hypothalamus and temperature regulation
   are true, *except*:
   a Electrical stimulation of the anterior hypothalamus, particularly the supraoptic
        area, triggers a thermolytic response.
   b Hypothalamic thermoreceptors are sensitive to changes in the temperature of
        circulating blood.
   c Cutaneous thermoreceptors signal changes in body surface temperature to the
        hypothalamus.
   d The hypothalamus directs the release of thyroxine as a thermolytic activity.
5 All of the following statements concerning the hypothalamus and the endocrine
   system are true, *except*:
   a The hypothalamus influences the release of anterior pituitary hormones via the
        hypothalamohypophyseal tract.
   b Neurohypophyseal hormone release is mediated through releasing factors.
   c Growth hormone–releasing factor (GRF) travels to the adenohypophysis via
        the hypothalamohypophyseal portal system.
   d The posterior pituitary hormone oxytocin is probably produced in the paraven-
        tricular nucleus (PVN) of the hypothalamus.

6 The ventral posteriolateral nucleus (VPL) of the thalamus is part of
   a the anterior nuclei
   b the medial nuclei
   c the midline nuclei
   d the dorsolateral nuclei
   e the ventrolateral nuclei

7 The anterior nucleus of the thalamus
   a is a relay station in the limbic system
   b receives substantial input from the cerebellum
   c is a principal part of the reticular activating system
   d is an inportant relay station in the cortically originating extrapyramidal system (COEPS)

8 All of the following statements about the thalamus are true, *except*:
   a It is bounded laterally by the posterior limb of the internal capsule.
   b It is bounded anteriorly by the head of the caudate nucleus.
   c Its two lobes are typically connected by the interthalamic adhesion.
   d Its medial walls are bathed by the CSF of the fourth ventricle.

9 A major portion of the hypothalamic output to the thalamus is received by the
   a lateral posterior nucleus
   b anterior nucleus
   c dorsomedial nucleus
   d medial geniculate body
   e ventrolateral nucleus

10 The principal hypothalamic route to autonomic nuclei is via the
   a periventricular fibers
   b mammillothalamic tract
   c mammillary peduncle
   d stria terminalis

Chapter 16

The Cerebral Cortex, Basal Nuclei, and Motor Control

The cerebral cortex is a thin layer of gray matter which completely covers the telencephalon and is responsible for directing skeletal muscle movement, receiving sensory information from both inside and outside the body, and integrating sensorimotor activity. It also stores and processes memory, initiates and coordinates learning and all higher cognitive functions, and mediates such phenomena as love, hate, joy, appreciation, etc. In this chapter we will examine only the sensory and motor roles of the cortex.

Subcortical clusters of gray matter called *basal nuclei* are also important in coordinating muscle movement and motor control. In this respect, they cooperate with the cerebral cortex, the cerebellum, and the brainstem in bringing about coordinated and perfectly timed movements when a purposeful motor act is required. In the present chapter we will examine these nuclei and the manner in which they are incorporated into the motor control system.

THE CEREBRAL CORTEX

Phylogenetically, the human cerebral cortex is composed of a relatively recent and extensive portion, the neocortex, and an older relatively small region, the allocortex. The *allocortex* comprises only about 10 percent of the total cortical area and is limited to the olfactory cortex and the cingulate, parahippocampal,

Tabe 16-1   Neocortical Laminae

Lamina	Layer	Description
I	Molecular	Primarily composed of the sparsely scattered horizontal cells of Cajal and the horizontal fibers of pyramidal cells, stellate cells, and cells of Martinotti.
II	External granular	Composed of densely packed stellate and small pyramidal cells. This area is traversed by vertical fibers from both ascending axons and apical dendrites of large pyramidal cells in lamina V. The ascending axons often synapse with the apical dendrites in this layer.
III	External pyramidal	Medium-sized pyramidal cells are located here. Stellate and basket cells are also present.
IV	Internal granular	This layer is characterized by stellate cells and small pyramidal cells. The *external band of Baillarger,* a concentrated band of horizontal fibers, also runs through this layer.
V	Internal pyramidal	This is a dense layer composed of large pyramidal cells. It is also characterized by many ascending and descending fibers. A horizontal band of concentrated fibers, the *internal band of Baillarger,* traverses this layer.
VI	Multiform	Most of the cells in this layer are small and represent a variety of morphological types.

and dentate gyri. It is functionally subordinate to the much larger *neocortex,* which comprises almost 90 percent of the cortex and represents almost all of the highly convoluted hemispheres seen in the exposed brain. The neocortex is composed of six distinguishable layers (*laminae*) which vary in thickness and density from one cortical region to another. The laminae are distinguishable from each other by the cell types found in each and by the type and direction of fibers which pass through them. The laminae are numbered from I to VI, with I being at the cortical surface and the others lying progressively deeper. The six laminae are described in Table 16-1.

Physiologists often subdivide the cerebral cortex into regions based on the functional characteristics of cortical layers in that region. Typically included are the sensory cortex (koniocortex), association cortex (homotypical cortex), and the motor cortex (heterotypical cortex). The *sensory cortex* includes the principal sensory receiving areas, while the *association cortex* covers major portions of the brain including the frontal, parietal, and temporal lobe. The *motor cortex* includes the principal motor areas. The relative thickness of cortical laminae IV and V is the noticeably variable feature between the three regions. The internal granular layer (IV) is the main receiving area for the sensory projection fibers from the thalamus. Consequently lamina IV is thickest in the sensory cortex. The internal pyramidal layer (V) is characterized by large pyramidal cells whose descending axons represent the motor fibers of the corticospinal system. Not surprisingly lamina V is largest in the motor regions of the cortex. Both laminae appear to be equally important in the association cortex as it receives some sensory input and gives rise to some motor output. It is also inportant to note that while the sensory cortex is primarily concerned with sensory input, it does give rise to a small motor component. Likewise the motor cortex receives a small degree of sensory input.

The circuitry of the cerebral cortex has been much more difficult to evaluate than that of the cerebellar cortex. Because of the dense nature of neuronal elements, the extensive nature of dendritic processes called *neutropil,* and lack of repetitious patterns of neuronal contacts, meaningful evaluation of cortical neuronal circuitry has been difficult and not very fruitful. Recall that the neuronal makeup of the cerebellar cortex is everywhere identical and shows very symmetrical and repeated patterns. This, coupled with low neuronal density in the cerebellar cortex, has made experimentation and evaluation of cerebellar circuitry much easier than is true for the cerebral cortex. Another factor related to the difficulty of examining cerebral cortical circuitry is that fibers afferent to the cortex do not show the same consistency in their terminations as seen in the cerebellar cortex. Recall the climbing fiber–Purkinje cell and mossy fiber–granular cell synapses observed in the latter. Nevertheless, the efferent output from the cerebral cortex is primarily through axons of pyramidal cells in laminae II to V with the largest cells in lamina V. Cortical afferents project to all six laminae, with lamina IV of the sensory cortex receiving the largest number of collateral synapses.

Brodmann's Areas

Brodmann, an early twentieth-century German neurologist, described the six-layered cortex just discussed. Using Nissl stain, which clearly shows cell bodies but not neurites, he identified six distinct layers. Later work utilizing Golgi and Weigert stains brought out additional detail not previously seen. Brodmann mapped the cerebral cortex into many areas based on variations in the six layers. Many attempts have been made by physiologists to ascribe specific functional importance to these areas. In some cases this has been possible (e.g., Brodmann's area 17 and the primary visual cortex), but in many cases no distinct relationship exists. More often than not, specific functional regions seem to overlap several areas. Nevertheless, Brodmann's areas are quite useful as landmark indicators because of their worldwide recognition. The cortical areas of Brodmann are illustrated in the lateral and median sagittal views of Fig. 16-1.

Electrophysiological Studies of the Cortex

Most of what we know concerning the functional role of the cortex is based on electrophysiological studies. Carefully probing the cortex with a stimulating electrode and observing the muscular responses produced has been the most

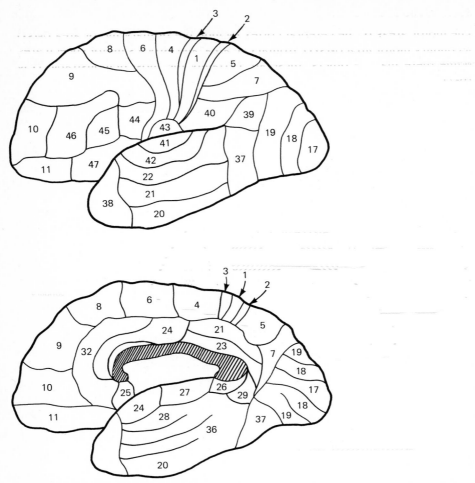

Figure 16-1 The cerebral cortical areas of Brodmann. Lateral surface in the upper view and medial surface in the lower view.

useful technique to uncover those cortical areas capable of initiating movement. Similarly, stimulating peripheral receptors and recording their "evoked responses" with cortical recording electrodes has enabled researchers to determine those cortical areas which receive sensory input. Not surprisingly there is considerable overlap of the "motor" and "sensory" cortical areas. Those areas adjudged to be motor because they produce muscular movement when electrically stimulated are also capable of generating evoked responses when peripheral receptors are stimulated. Likewise, the "sensory" areas show a small motor component as well. Nevertheless, one function seems to predominate, and this has led to the establishment of a commonly used classification scheme which we will examine now.

Motor Areas of the Cortex

The motor areas of the cerebral cortex include the primary motor area (MsI), secondary motor area (MsII), frontal eye area, and Broca's motor speech area. While there may be others, these are certainly the most demonstrable (Fig. 16-2).

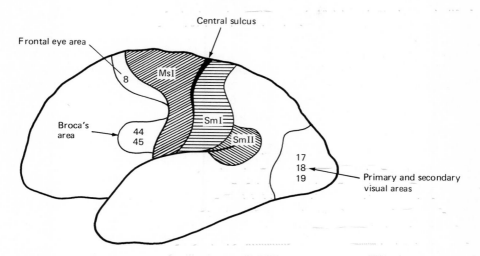

LATERAL VIEW OF CEREBRAL CORTEX

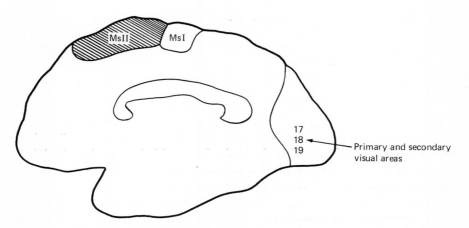

MEDIAL VIEW OF CEREBRAL CORTEX

Figure 16-2 Significant functional areas of the lateral and medial cerebral cortex: primary motor area (MsI), supplementary motor area (MsII), primary somatic sensorimotor area (SmI), secondary somatic sensorimotor area (SmII).

The Primary Motor Area (MsI)   This area is located immediately anterior to the central sulcus. Electrical stimulation of the cortex in this region produces movements in the appropriate part of the body on the contralateral side. It is important to note that movements initiated in this way are not single uncoordinated contractions of given muscles, but rather movements accompanied by contraction of agonists and relaxation of antagonists. Nevertheless, these movements are very simple, and are similar to those which might be produced by an infant. Obviously more advanced movements must require the incorporation of additional systems.

The primary motor area (equivalent to Brodmann's area 4 and an adjacent strip of area 6) extends over the superior medial border of the hemisphere onto the medial surface. The body is represented as a homunculus with the head and face regions located near the lateral fissure and the leg and foot areas extending onto the medial surface. The back extends anteriorly over area 4 onto the adjacent strip of area 6. The fingers and toes extend over the cortical surface in the central sulcus.

Area MsI also has a small sensory component which receives input from a number of sources. The lemniscal system to the VPL nucleus of the thalamus ultimately projects from this nucleus to area 4 of MsI. The cerebellum projects to the VL nucleus of the thalamus, which in turn projects to areas 4 and 6 of MsI. Finally, the globus pallidus sends fibers to both the VA and VL nuclei of the thalamus which then project to area 6 of MsI. Much of the input to MsI is proprioceptive, but sensory input from other sources is also noted.

The Supplementary Motor Area (MsII)   The extension of area 6 onto the medial surface of the cortex represents the supplementary motor area (MsII). The body is represented horizontally here with the head forward, the back region lying adjacent to the cingulate gyrus, and the fingers just reaching the upper surface of the hemisphere. Electrical stimulation of this area produces somewhat complex bilateral avoidance movements. They are not as specifically distinct as those produced by MsI stimulation. The VA and VL nuclei of the thalamus both project sensory input to MsII. Both nuclei receive input from the globus pallidus, while the cerebellum projects only to the VL nucleus.

The Frontal Eye Area   This region coincides with area 8. Electrical stimulation here produces deviation of the eyes, head, and neck to the opposite side.

Broca's Motor Speech Area   This area corresponds roughly to areas 44 and 45 of the frontal lobe. Most of our information concerning its role comes from ablation studies and stimulation. Curiously, the left hemisphere appears to be dominant as ablation here usually abolishes sound production and often produces a motor aphasia or speech paralysis in humans. The effects typically aren't observed with ablation of the same area in the right hemisphere. It is estimated that 90 percent of us are left hemisphere dominant in this respect, regardless of right- or left-handedness.

Sensory Areas of the Cortex

The Primary Somatic Sensorimotor Area (SmI)   Areas 3, 1, and 2 produce the largest evoked responses when somatic sensory receptors are stimulated. Smaller responses are recorded in the primary motor area (MsI) of the precentral gyrus. Input from touch, pressure, pain, temperature, and proprioceptors projects to the VPL nucleus of the thalamus, which then projects heavily to SmI, truly the principal receiving area for somatic sensation.

The body homunculus represented in SmI is essentially a mirror image of that found in the primary motor area (MsI) anterior to the central sulcus. Studies with monkeys have indicated that the topographic organization of SmI consists of a series of overlapping bands at right angles to the central sulcus. Each of these bands is the cortical area for the representation of a single dermatome

It is also now well established that electrical stimulation of the postcentral gyrus (SmI) produces motor responses as well. It was originally thought that such movements were the result of current spread from the stimulating electrodes to the precentral gyrus. However, it is now quite clear that this is not the case and that SmI is capable of producing motor responses on its own, although requiring higher stimulation intensities than MsI.

The Secondary Somatic Sensorimotor Area (SmII)   This area, located immediately posterior to the face region of SmI, is characterized by a homunculus with the head represented anteriorly, the leg muscles posteriorly, the back inferiorly, and the hands and feet superiorly. Stimulation here causes gross movements of postural adjustments which are diffuse and widespread.

The Visual Cortex   A large area over the occipital pole of the occipital lobe (areas 17, 18, and 19) represents the visual cortex. Included are two functionally different areas: the primary visual area and the visual association area. The *primary visual area* (area 17) is the principal receiving area for visual signals projected along the optic radiation from the lateral geniculate body (LG). Recall that viewed objects in the left visual field of both eyes project to the right hemisphere while those in the right visual field project to the left hemisphere. Further, objects viewed in the lower quadrants of each visual field give rise to images in the cuneal regions of area 17 while those in the upper quadrants project images to the lingular regions.

Total ablation of area 17 renders a person blind. Nevertheless, more than area 17 is required in order to comprehend the image in the visual field which is projected on the visual cortex. Areas 18 and 19 immediately surround the primary visual area and comprise the *visual association area*. This area applies cognition to the visual signal and helps to "make sense" out of the projected image.

The Auditory Cortex   This region includes the middle portion of the superior temporal gyrus of the temporal lobe and a good portion of the insular cortex. Like the visual cortex, it is composed of two functionally different areas: the primary auditory area and auditory association area. The *primary auditory* *area* is a relatively small region in the middle of the superior temporal convolution, extending over the superior surface to part of the lateral and medial lip. This is roughly equivalent to area 41. The medial geniculate body relays signals to this area in response to input over the conscious auditory pathway. When auditory impulses reach this area, the sound is heard but not fully comprehended. Comprehension requires the participation of the *auditory association area*. This area, covering the insular cortex and a region surrounding the primary area on the lateral surface of the temporal lobe (areas 42 and 22), has extensive interconnections with area 41.

The Gustatory Cortex   This area is located near the most inferior lateral extension of the primary sensorimotor area (SmI) and may include area 43. Taste signals relayed through the VPM nucleus of the thalamus project to this area.

The Olfactory Cortex   You will recall that the olfactory tracts divide into a medial and lateral stria as they approach the anterior perforated substance. The lateral olfactory tract terminates in the prepyriform cortex and parts of the amygdala of the temporal lobe. These areas represent the *primary olfactory cortex*. Fibers then project from here to area 28, the *secondary olfactory area*, for sensory evaluation. The medial olfactory tract projects to the anterior perforated substance, the septum pellucidum, the subcallosal area, and even the contralateral olfactory tract. Both the medial and lateral olfactory tracts contribute to the visceral reflex pathways causing the viscerosomatic and viscerovisceral responses described in Chap. 7. It is worth pointing out that unlike other sensory systems, no relay through a thalamic nucleus occurs in the olfactory system.

Cerebral Dominance

Certain behavioral patterns appear to be associated with one or the other hemisphere. These include handedness, the performance of speech, understanding the spoken and written word, and spatial appreciation. Approximately 90 percent of adults are right-handed (controlled by the left cerebral hemisphere) and over 96 percent of adults have their speech centers (Broca's motor speech area) located in the left hemisphere. This is evidenced by the fact that almost all aphasic patients with speech disorders have left-hemisphere lesions in Broca's area. Additional studies with humans have clearly established that the left hemisphere is best suited for written and oral language expression as well as analytic calculation, while the right hemisphere is particularly suited for appreciation of spatial relationships and aesthetic and nonverbal expression. Thus, the left hemisphere is often called the *major or dominant hemisphere*, while the right is the *minor hemisphere*. It should be noted that in those individuals who are left-handed, there is no similar shift in control from left to right hemisphere of the other behavioral observations listed above.

Split-Brain Studies   The commissural fibers (corpus callosum and anterior, posterior, and hippocampal commissures) serve to connect the two hemispheres. We have learned a great deal about the different functions of the two hemispheres from individuals who have had a complete sectioning of the corpus callosum in order to prevent the spread of epileptic seizures from one hemisphere to the other. These "split-brain" individuals retain normal behavioral patterns and can perform and learn as well as normal people. However, cerebral dominance shows up in carefully planned experiments.

Much of this work has been performed by R. W. Sperry. If an unfamiliar object is placed in the left hand of blindfolded split-brain individuals, they will be able to fully appreciate its shape and touch by feeling it but will be unable to orally describe it or accurately draw a picture of it with their right hand. They cannot describe it orally because the right hemisphere, which received the sensory input from the object, is unable to communicate with the speech area of the dominant left hemisphere. Similarly, they will be unable to accurately draw it with the right hand because the important spatial information received by the right hemisphere cannot be transmitted to the dominant hemisphere. Thus, the apparent role of the cerebral commissures is the bilateral hemispheric integration of written and oral expression.

Visual input to the split-brain individual likewise demonstrates cerebral dominance if carefully designed tests are performed. As the reader will recall, objects viewed in the left visual fields of both eyes are transmitted to the right occipital lobe. One such test involves having the individual look straight ahead at a table upon which are laid a variety of common objects such as a paper clip, screwdriver, bottle, key, etc. If a card bearing the printed name of one of these objects is flashed for 0.1 s in the left visual field, the individual is quite successful when asked to reach out and take the item named on the card with the left hand. This is so because the right hemisphere received the visual signal, and this same right hemisphere directs the movement of the left hand to the appropriate item. The subject could even crudely write the name of the retrieved item by writing with the left hand, since the right hemisphere, which received the signal, directs the activity of the left hand. However, because of the failure of the right (minor) hemisphere to communicate its information to the left (major) hemisphere because of the severed commissure, the individual cannot verbally say what name was seen on the card or what item was retrieved by the left hand. The left "speaking" hemisphere has not been informed of the actions of the right hemisphere. Indeed, the individual verbally denies even seeing such a card. Similarly, if asked to use the right hand to write the name of the item retrieved with the left hand, the subject would be unable to do so because the left "writing" hemisphere received none of relevant information.

Identical results have now been observed in individuals who have their brains essentially "chemically split" by the injection of short-acting anesthetics into the left carotid artery, which anesthetizes the left hemisphere.

Evaluation of Cortical Areas by Lesion Studies

Much of our knowledge of the behavioral role of the various cortical areas has been obtained by accidental or disease-produced lesions in the human cerebral cortex. For example, lesions in areas 18 and 19 don't produce blindness, as visual signals still reach area 17 and objects can be clearly seen, but they are neither recognized identified, nor understood. This condition is known as *visual agnosia*, meaning that the viewed object is "not known." Lesions limited to area 17, however, produce outright blindness.

Lesions to Broca's motor speech area (44 and 45) in the major hemisphere cause an *expressive* or *motor aphasia*. The patient can't speak intelligibly. He or she knows what to say but can't do it. There is no paralysis of the muscles themselves, but the patient speaks very slowly often leaving out nouns and verbs and has considerable difficulty with phrases.

The caudal aspect of the superior temporal gyrus, known as *Wernicke's area* (area 22), is important for understanding the spoken word. Lesions to this area, typically in the major hemisphere, leave individuals able to hear normally, but spoken words appear to be meaningless. Such people can speak but make grammatical errors because of their failure to understand their own spoken words. This region receives many fibers from other association areas, including visual (18 and19), auditory (41 and 42), and somesthetic (5 and 7). The condition, *auditory aphasia*, is most severe if the lesion involves both hemispheres, leaving these individuals unable to communicate orally in any intelligible fashion.

The *angular gyrus* (area 39) is located at the caudal end of the lateral fissure between the supramarginal gyrus and Wernicke's area. Like Wernicke's area it has extensive connections with visual, auditory, and somesthetic association areas. A lesion of area 39 in the major hemisphere leaves the individual unable to comprehend written language. He or she can see words, but cannot understand them. This inability to read (*alexia*) does not prevent the individual from speaking normally but is usually accompanied by the inability to write (*agraphia*).

Lesions to area 40, the *supramarginal gyrus,* inflicts a person with tactile and proprioceptive losses. This individual demonstrates *astereognosis* (the inability to identify familiar objects by touch) amd makes errors in judgment concerning body position.

While we can learn much about the contribution made by particular areas of the cerebral cortex from such lesion studies, it is important to recognize that the areas involved may simply be "links" in a chain as far as their affected sensorimotor observations are concerned. Other cortical areas may also be heavily involved. Further, eventually unraveling the sequences of cortical area involvement in a given behavioral pattern will still leave this greater mystery unsolved: What is the pattern of neuronal sequencing and synaptic integration?

The Corticomotor Reflex

Current research supports a theory that the motor cortex is composed of narrow, deep columns which represent the functional units around which sensorimotor activity is organized. These columns extend vertically through the entire seven-layered cortex. Each may be as narrow as a single millimeter. Part of the basis for the columnar idea is based on observations that the cutaneous receptive field of a given column of cortical neurons lies in the path of movement produced by electrical stimulation of this same column. Thus as the muscles of a limb contract, objects encountered by the leading edge of the moving limb may possibly stimulate cutaneous receptors which reflexly reinforce the movement by projecting back to the same cortical column. Therefore, cutaneous inputs may be constantly providing feedback to guide limb movements via this *corticomotor reflex*. It is possible that this feedback may also involve muscle and joint receptors, causing the reflex to behave somewhat like a tracking system by directing the limb to follow the path of tactile and proprioceptive stimulation.

The corticomotor reflex may also behave much like the stretch reflex in providing background muscle tone upon which the cortically originating voluntary motor command is superimposed. Each cortical column in the motor cortex is thought to have a facilitatory or inhibitory effect. Activity in horizontal association fibers from one cortical column to adjacent columns may provide the integration necessary for appropriate coordination of agonists and antagonists.

THE BASAL NUCLEI AND MOTOR CONTROL

The white matter of the cerebrum is composed for the most part of the myelinated axons of neurons with cell bodies located in gray areas of the CNS. These gray areas include the cerebral cortex, thalamus, and basal nuclei (Figs. 16-3 and 16-4). The basal nuclei along with the cerebellum play an important role in muscle coordination. They include the caudate nucleus, putamen, globus pallidus, and claustrum. However, the claustrum is often excluded when describing the functional role of the basal nuclei in motor control.

The *putamen* is continuous anteriorly with the head of the *caudate nucleus*, which arches upward and backward and finally curves around anteriorly and laterally to enter the temporal lobe ending in the amygdala (Fig. 16-3). The caudate nucleus and putamen are collectively called the *corpus striatum*, while the putamen and globus pallidus represent the *lenticular nucleus*. Taken together, the caudate nucleus, putamen, and globus pallidus make up the *basal nuclei*.

The Internal Capsule

The oval thalamic mass lies just medial and posterior to the lenticular nucleus on either side of the brain. With the exception of the auditory radiation from the medial geniculate body and the optic rediation from the lateral geniculate body, all ascending and descending pathways between the cerebral cortex and the brainstem pass through the *internal capsule*. This vertical group of fibers is bounded laterally by the lenticular nucleus, anteriomedially by the head of the caudate nucleus, and posteriomedially by the thalamus (Fig. 16-4). The *corona radiata* is a fanlike radiation of ascending and descending fibers between the internal capsule and cerebral cortex.

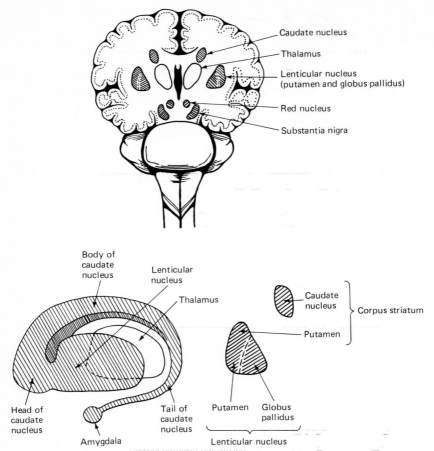

Figure 16-3 Illustration of the basal nuclei. The upper coronal section shows the basal nuclei in relation to the thalamus. The lower left illustration shows the caudate nucleus in relation to the lenticular nucleus, amygdala, and thalamus. The basal nuclei are grouped by commonly used terms in the lower-right illustration.

In cross section, the internal capsule forms a V-shaped region in each hemisphere (Fig. 16-4). The principal ascending and descending fibers of the internal capsule are also illustrated in this figure. The *anterior limb* of the capsule is partly formed by the frontopontine fibers which arise in the cortex of the frontal lobe and descend to the pontine nuclei, where most of them synapse. The anterior limb also carries ascending fibers of the thalamocortical tract from the thalamus to the frontal cortex.

Corticobulbar fibers from the motor cortex to cranial nerve nuclei controlling head and neck movements pass through the *genu* and anterior part of the *posterior limb*. Also located in the posterior limb, in increasingly posterior order, are corticospinal fibers to the limb and trunk muscles and the parietopontine and occipitopontine fibers connecting the parietal and occipital cortex with

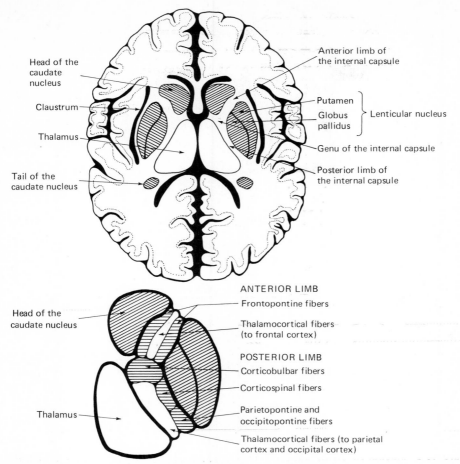

Figure 16-4   The upper illustration shows a cross section through the brain indicating the relationship between the basal nuclei and the thalamus. Notice how the internal capsule is formed between them. The bottom illustration shows the relative positions of the various ascending and descending tracts through the anterior and posterior limbs of the internal capsule. The ascending tracts are white and the descending tracts are cross-hatched.

pontine nuclei. Most of the medial portion of the posterior limb is taken up by the thalamocortical fibers, which project to the parietal and occipital cortex.

MOTOR CONTROL AND CENTRAL NERVOUS SYSTEM INTERACTION

Coordinated muscle activity is controlled by the close and harmonious interaction of the cerebral cortex, cerebellum, and basal nuclei. Through their output to the pyramidal and extrapyramidal systems, they are able to initiate and modify the timing and sequencing of motor acts.

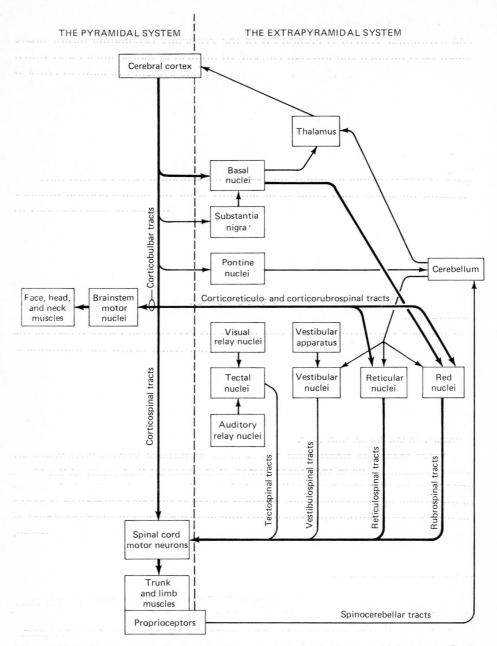

Figure 16-5 Diagrammatic illustration of the pyramidal and extrapyramidal systems. Explanation in text.

The Pyramidal System

The *pyramidal system* is composed of the cortically originating motor fibers which pass through the internal capsule to brainstem motor nuclei and spinal cord motor neurons (Fig. 16-5). The fibers of this system originate in cortical lamina V, primarily as the axons of pyramidal cells in the motor cortex of the precentral gyrus. Some fibers originate in the postcentral gyrus as well. After leaving the cortex, the descending fibers converge in the corona radiata and pass through the genu and posterior limb of the internal capsule. The body musculature innervated is represented with the head near the genu, while lower parts of the body lie more posteriorly. The fibers then pass into the middle third of the cerebral peduncle, where the body representation twists so that those innervating the lower body come to lie laterally while the medial portion supplies the upper body and head. The fibers then continue through the anterior pons to appear as the rounded medullary pyramids, which give the system its name.

Corticobulbar fibers of the pyramidal system terminate in brainstem motor nuclei, while the *corticospinal fibers* continue on into the spinal cord as the anterior and lateral corticospinal tracts. The *lateral corticospinal tract* (crossed portion) descends all the way to sacral levels with fibers continually leaving to synapse on interneurons in laminae IV, V, VI, VII, and VIII. Some even synapse directly on alpha and gamma motor neurons in lamina IX (Fig. 6-3). The *anterior corticospinal tract* (uncrossed fibers) continues to descend on the same (ipsilateral) side of the cord but does not reach below the midthoracic level. At various levels, fibers leave the tract and cross over in the anterior white commissure to synapse on interneurons in lamina VIII. The corticospinal tracts appear to be directed most effectively to facilitating movements requiring skill and dexterity of the distal musculature (Chap. 6), while the corticobulbar tracts mediate movements of the facial muscles and other muscles of the head and neck.

Since there are many more fibers in the pyramidal system than there are giant pyramidal cells in the motor cortex, it is apparent that many of the fibers arise from smaller pyramidal cells located over the pre- and postcentral regions of the frontal and parietal cortex. Further evidence for this assumption is based on the fact that retrograde (backward) impulse transmission over the fibers of the pyramidal system, when the medullary pyramids are electrically stimulated, produces evoked responses in both pre- and postcentral areas.

The Extrapyramidal System

The *extrapyramidal system* is composed of motor fibers which do not pass through the medullary pyramids but which nevertheless exert a measure of control over bodily movements. The system is difficult to describe, partly because of the complexity of pathways and feedback loops which compose it. Nevertheless, the extrapyramidal system can be divided into three controlling systems: the cortically originating indirect pathways, the feedback loops, and the auditory-visual-vestibular descending pathways.

Cortically Originating Indirect Descending Pathways   At the same time signals are being transmitted over the pyramidal system to produce a specific movement, additional signals relative to the movement are also relayed to the basal nuclei, red nucleus, and brainstem reticular formation. The basal nuclei evaluate the command signal sent down the pyramidal pathways and may contribute to the establishment of needed background muscle tone for the movement. The nuclei are able to do this in part by projecting to the red nuclei, which influence spinal cord alpha and gamma motor neurons via rubrospinal tracts. Similar indirect routing to the spinal cord is achieved through corticoreticulospinal and corticorubrospinal pathways (Fig. 16-5).

The function of these indirect pathways to the spinal cord motor neurons may include more than providing background muscle tone for movements directed by the motor cortex. Recall from Chap. 6 that ablation studies in which the rubrospinal tracts are experimentally cut have shown that the corticospinal and rubrospinal tracts have somewhat similar effects on spinal motor neurons. When the rubrospinal tracts of monkeys were damaged along with earlier pyramidal tract sections, the loss of skilled control in distal muscles became even more severe and yet there was little or no loss of proximal muscle control. Even so, because the red nucleus receives input from the basal and cerebellar nuclei as well as direct input from the cerebral cortex, its function may include modifying or "fine tuning" the motor neurons which innervate the muscles involved in a given movement.

Feedback Loops   The feedback loops described here include neural circuits in which a signal sample is fed back to a "comparator," which is in a position to compare the signal with some desired condition and subsequently take steps to "adjust" or "modify" it. The extrapyramidal system includes two such feedback systems: the cortically originating extrapyramidal system feedback loops (*COEPS feedback loops*) and the proprioceptor originating extrapyramidal system feedback loops (*POEPS feedback loops*).

The COEPS feedback loops are composed of fibers originating in the motor cortex which synapse in subcortical centers. After integrating and evaluating the signals, the centers project fibers back to the cortical source for modification. Three such loops are illustrated in Fig. 16-6. In loop A the signal is "tapped off" to the corpus striatum (caudate and putamen), which in turn project to the globus pallidus. Pallidothalamic fibers then project to the thalamus, which completes the loop by projecting back to the cortical source. Somewhere in this loop the original signal sent down the pyramidal tracts is compared and evaluated with other input relative to the movement. After appropriate integration, modifying feedback signals are returned to the cortex via the thalamocortical fibers. In loop B the sample signal is sent to pontine nuclei for subsequent referral to the cerebellum, where it is probably compared to proprioceptive input coming from muscles, tendons, and joints involved in the movement. This input probably includes such things as the current state of muscle tone and the relative position and movement of the limb involved. Following integration of

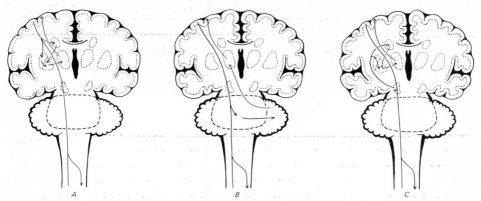

Figure 16-6 Schematic illustration of three cortically originating extrapyramidal system feedback loops (COEPS feedback loops). *A.* Corticostriatopallidothalamocortical feedback loop. *B.* Corticopontocerebellothalamocortical feedback loop. *C.* Corticonigrostriatopallido-thalamocortical feedback loop. These are three of many such loops in the brain.

this input, the cerebellum then projects its output to the thalamus (via dentatothalamic tracts) which then completes the loop by sending fibers back to the cortical source through thalamocortical projections. In loop C, the sample signal is sent to the substantia nigra, which projects in turn to the corpus striatum. From here the feedback circuit is identical to that illustrated in loop A. The importance of these feedback loops to normal motor control can be most clearly seen by an examination of the clinical signs associated with dysfunction of the basal nuclei and their related brainstem areas, which we will examine later.

The other feedback loop system which is included in the extrapyramidal system is composed of the POEPS feedback loops. In this system the modification is not directed back toward the cortical source (as are the COEPS loops), but to the spinal cord motor neurons instead. The principal loop involves the relay of muscle, tendon, and joint proprioceptive information to the cerebellum via the spinocerebellar tracts. The signals are integrated in the cerebellum and probably compared with the intended signals sampled by corticopontocerebellar pathways. In this way the cerebellum might compare the intended movement with the instantaneous performance of that movement as sampled by the proprioceptors of the spinocerebellar tracts. It could then direct modification through its projections to the vestibular, reticular, and rubral nuclei and their respective descending tracts to the appropriate motor neurons of the spinal cord.

Auditory Visual Vestibular Descending Pathways   Postural adjustments in response to auditory, visual, and vestibular signals is an additional way to regulate the activity of spinal motor neurons. Auditory and visual input to the tectal nuclei of the midbrain may be responsible for producing reflex movements of the body in response to a sudden sound or bright light. Similarly, input from the vestibular apparatus to the vestibular nuclei and cerebellum no doubt plays a role in reflex postural adjustments through the vestibulospinal and other tracts.

It should be pointed out here that because of the complex nature of the neural circuits which effect motor control through routes other than the pyramidal system, a precise and universally agreed upon definition of the extrapyramidal pathways has never been achieved.

Clinical Signs of Basal Nuclei and Related Brainstem Dysfunction

Certain disease conditions relating to motor control appear to be positively linked to dysfunction of the basal nuclei and those structures functionally related to them including the thalamus, subthalamus, and substantia nigra.

Chorea is a condition characterized by uncontrolled random movements of the body often accompanied by facial grimaces. Evidence indicates that the condition is often associated with dysfunction of the corpus striatum. It is often seen as a complication of rheumatic fever in children. Recovery from this childhood form of the disease, *Sydenham's chorea*, is usually complete with no subsequent lingering effects. A more severe form, *Huntington's chorea*, is a hereditary disease which becomes progressively worse and often leads to severe mental debilitation. *Athetosis* is a condition characterized by slow wormlike movements of the peripheral appendages, and is also associated with damage to the corpus striatum and lateral parts of the globus pallidus. Voluntary movements in the affected appendages are often impaired. Violent flinging of a limb or limbs is a rare condition called *ballismus*. If one limb is involved the condition is called *monoballismus*, and if both limbs on a single side are affected the term is *hemiballismus*. It is generally associated with damage to the subthalamus and can occur spontaneously or be brought on by the initiation of a voluntary movement involving the affected limb.

Perhaps the most familiar disease condition in this group is *Parkinson's disease* (paralysis agitans). It is characterized by an increasing tremor during rest. Also observed are a "pill-rolling" action of the fingers, a poverty of movement expressed by difficulty in initiating voluntary movements such as getting up from a chair and walking, a plastic or deathlike rigidity often demonstrated by a "cog-wheeling" phenomenon when a limb is passively moved, and an increasing masklike fixed expression to the face.

The cog-wheeling phenomenon that occurs as a limb is passively moved is tentatively explained by the following mechanism. Initial resistance is due to muscle tone as the limb is moved. Release comes when group Ib afferents from Golgi tendon organs inhibit homonymous alpha motor neurons. Then as the passive movement of the limb continues, tension again develops until the threshold of the Golgi tendon organs is once again reached, causing a second release. This rachetlike movement continues as the limb is passively moved. Parkinson's disease is usually associated with dysfunction of the basal nuclei and the substantia nigra.

Feedback loops in electronic systems must be finely tuned in order to prevent oscillations. In physiological systems the feedback loops must also be working properly in order to prevent oscillations in muscle systems. In Parkinson's disease, the fine tuning is lost and oscillating signals to motor neurons produce tremors. It appears that the principal site of malfunction lies in the dopamine-releasing fibers of the nigrostriatal pathway. There are both excitatory cholinergic nigrostriatal fibers and inhibitory dopaminergic nigrostriatal fibers. Fine tuning seems to require the complete integrity of both types. In Parkinson's disease, the feedback system becomes "untuned" by the inability of the inhibitory dopaminergic neurons to produce and release dopamine. Some success has been achieved in the treatment of this condition by the adminstration of L-dopa, a dopamine precursor which is taken up by dopaminergic nigrostriatal fibers and converted to dopamine. With this subsequent "replacement" of the missing transmitter, some degree of fine tuning is restored and the severity of symptoms is often reduced.

REVIEW QUESTIONS

1 Cerebrocortical lamina IV (internal granular) is relatively largest in
   a   the sensory cortex
   b   the association cortex
   c   the motor cortex
   d   the heterotypical cortex
2 Input to the cerebral cortex from touch, pressure, pain, temperature, and proprioceptors is primarily directed to
   a   MsI
   b   MsII
   c   SmI
   d   SmII
   e   none of the above
3 A relatively small region in the middle of the superior temporal convolution, extending over the superior surface to the lateral and medial lip, is
   a   the gustatory area
   b   Broca's motor speech area
   c   the primary auditory area
   d   the olfactory area
4 All of the following statements about cerebral dominance are true, *except:*
   a   The left hemisphere is best suited for aesthetic and nonverbal expression.
   b   The right hemisphere is best suited for appreciation of spatial relationships.
   c   The left hemisphere is best suited for written language expression.
   d   The left hemisphere is best suited for oral language expression.
5 Wernicke's area (area 22) is important for
   a   the comprehension of written language
   b   the comprehension of spoken language
   c   the ability to identify familiar objects by touch
   d   the ability to write

6 Alexia and agraphia are usually associated with destruction of
   a the angular gyrus
   b the supramarginal gyrus
   c Broca's area
   d areas 5 and 7

7 The corpus striatum includes
   a the putamen and globus pallidus
   b the amygdala and hippocampus
   c the caudate nucleus and putamen
   d the caudate nucleus and globus pallidus
   e none of the above

8 Passing through the anterior limb of the internal capsule are
   a the parietopontine fibers
   b the thalamocortical fibers to the frontal cortex
   c the occipitopontine fibers
   d the frontopontine fibers

9 All of the following statements about the pyramidal and extrapyramidal systems are
   true, *except*:
   a The anterior corticospinal tract is part of the pyramidal system.
   b The COEPS feedback loops are part of the pyramidal system.
   c The pyramidal system is so named because its fibers originate in pyramidal cells
       of the cerebral cortex.
   d The rubrospinal tract is considered part of the extrapyramidal system.

10 All of the following are associated with damage to the basal nuclei and related
   brainstem nuclei, *except*
   a paralysis agitans
   b athetosis
   c chorea
   d achalasia
   e ballismus

Chapter 17

Neurochemistry

Several aspects of neurochemistry have been previously examined in this text, including the synthesis and degradation of several neurotransmitters and the role of various ions in impulse conduction and muscle contraction. Still, we have not looked at all into the chemical activity within the brain and spinal cord. In this chapter we will examine the activity of various neuroactive chemicals in the brain, including the catecholamines, indoleamines, amino acids, neuropeptides, prostaglandins, and others as well as energy metabolism within the brain itself.

The brain, like other organs of the body, requires an adequate vascular system in order to supply it with nutrients and oxygen and to remove metabolic wastes and carbon dioxide. Unlike most other organs, however, capillary exchange of these and other materials in the brain is complicated by the presence of a transport-limiting system, the *blood-brain barrier*.

BLOOD-BRAIN BARRIER

Electron miscroscope studies have shown that capillaries in the brain have a continuous capillary endothelium with tight junctions and are therefore unlike the more permeable capillaries found elsewhere in the body. This effectively

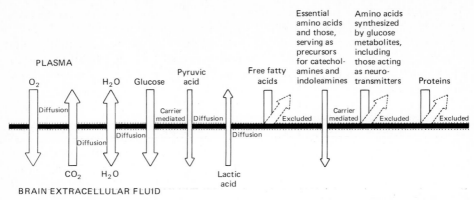

Figure 17-1 The permeability of the blood-brain barrier to several different metabolic substances.

excludes the passage of many materials including proteins and molecules with molecular weights as low as 2000. The existence of the barrier was first demonstrated by Paul Ehrlich and later by Goldman, who in 1909 injected large amounts of the dye trypan blue into the vascular circulation and observed that all tissues became intensely stained while the brain remained "snow white." We now know that trypan blue was excluded from the brain because it rapidly complexed with albumen in the plasma and could not cross cerebral capillaries in this form.

Many materials do, however, cross the barrier from plasma to brain. Nevertheless, it's a "selective" barrier where some materials are excluded or cross with difficulty and others pass quite freely. Because of the heavy dependence of the brain on a steady supply of oxygen for cellular respiration and glucose for energy metabolism, it is not surprising to find that they pass freely into the brain with little hindrance. Similarly, metabolic wastes and carbon dioxide readily pass across the barrier from brain to plasma. On the other hand, free fatty acids, an easily accessible alternate energy source for most other cells of the body including muscle, are virtually excluded from the brain. A summary of the permeability of the blood-brain barrier to several different metabolic substances is illustrated in Fig. 17-1.

Diffusion Across the Barrier

O_2, CO_2, N_2O, Kr, and Xe are gases which readily diffuse across the barrier. The latter three have been used to calculate cerebral blood flow. Water also readily diffuses into and out of the brain. Its net movement is dictated solely by the osmolality of the plasma. Thus an increase in the plasma osmolality from its normal value of 290 mosmol/L can draw water from the brain by osmosis, and actually shrink its volume. This phenomenon has been employed clinically to reduce intracranial pressure by using plasma expanders such as mannitol to increase plasma osmolality. Mannitol does not cross the blood-brain barrier.

Lipid solubility is an important factor in diffusion across the barrier. Generally the higher the lipid solubility of a substance, the more readily it diffuses. Thus alcohols like ethanol move freely into the brain. Lipid-soluble thiobarbital equilibrates more rapidly between plasma and brain than the slightly less soluble barbital does. Salicylic acid is less soluble yet and thus requires even more time to equilibrate.

Facilitated Transport across the Barrier

Carrier systems appear to be involved in the transport of several materials across the barrier. Glucose, ions, and certain amino acids utilize this type of system. The carrier system for glucose is stereospecific as D-glucose, but not L-glucose, is readily transported into the brain. Lactic, pyruvic, and acetic acids also utilize such carriers.

While proteins are virtually excluded from the brain, certain amino acids pass readily into it. Included are the essential amino acids and those which are precursors for the production of neurotransmitters. The latter include tyrosine (required for norepinephrine and dopamine synthesis) and tryptophan (for serotonin synthesis). Similarly, neuroactive peptides whose amino acid sequences have been clearly identified such as substance P, methionine enkephalin and leucine enkephalin, β-endorphin, ACTH, angiotensin II, oxytocin, vasopressin, somatostatin, thyrotropin-releasing factor, and luteinizing hormone–releasing factor rely on a steady transport of these amino acids from plasma to brain for their continued synthesis.

Ions cross the barrier into brain but do so much more slowly than into other body tissues. An intravenous K^+ administration exchanges much more quickly with muscle tissue that it does with brain. Ca^{2+} and Mg^{2+} transport is equally slow, while Na^+ is somewhat faster. H^+ ion transport into the brain is very slow.

Certain areas of the brain apparently contain no blood-brain barrier. These include the neurohypophysis, median eminence of the hypothalamus, the area postrema, and the pineal gland. Because many circulating hormones control their own release through negative feedback to the hypothalamus, the importance of barrier lack in this area is readily apparent. If such hormones are to influence the hypothalamic output of releasing or inhibiting factors to the anterior pituitary via the hypothalamohypophyseal portal system, they must not be barred from the hypothalamus by a barrier system. Similarly, osmoreceptors of the hypothalamus must be able to constantly and easily detect changes in the osmolality of the plasma if the release of antidiuretic hormone (ADH) is to proceed properly.

CEREBRAL BLOOD FLOW AND OXYGEN CONSUMPTION

The average cerebral blood flow in humans is approximately 55 mL per 100 g of brain tissue per minute. This is a little over 700 mL/min for a 1350-g brain. Thus while the human brain comprises only about 2.5 percent of the body's weight, it receives almost 15 percent of the cardiac output, attesting to the high vascular demands of this organ.

A reliable and frequently used method of determining cerebral blood flow is the method of Kety and Schmidt. It is based on the Fick principle and utilizes the arteriovenous difference of a freely diffusible gas such as N_2O as it passes through the brain. Accordingly, the flow of blood through the brain can be determined by measuring the amount of N_2O removed from the blood by the brain per minute and dividing this by the arteriovenous difference of N_2O as it passes through the brain. The cerebral blood flow is higher in children than in adults, typically exceeding 100 mL per 100 g per minute. However, contrary to popular thinking, the blood flow decreases only slightly with advancing age.

The brain utilizes fully 25 percent of the body's total oxygen consumption. The arteriovenous O_2 difference is relatively high since the brain receives only 15 percent of the cardiac output. The arteriovenous difference is 6.6 mL per 100 mL, falling from 19.6 to 13 mL per 100 mL as blood passes through the brain (Fig. 17-2). Thus we can calculate a cerebral oxygen consumption of approximately 3.5 mL per 100 g per minute. This value is greater in skeletal muscle, skin, and liver, but less in cardiac muscle and kidney.

The utilization of oxygen by the brain is not uniform throughout its mass. The gray matter consumes as much as 94 percent of cerebral oxygen, while the white matter, which makes up fully 60 percent of the brain's mass, consumes only 6 percent. Oxygen consumption, and hence oxygen need, increases as we move up the neuraxis. It is lowest in the spinal cord and increases through the medulla, midbrain, thalamus, cerebellum, and cerebral cortex. Thus it is not surprising to find that the sensorimotor functions of the cerebral cortex are more sensitive to hypoxic damage than are the vegetative functions of the pontomedullary areas.

Progressive decreases in cerebral oxygen consumption are always accompanied by progressive decreases in the level of mental alertness. Compared to the mentally alert young man with an O_2 consumption of 3.5 mL per 100 g per minute, the mentally confused states associated with diabetic acidosis, insulin hypoglycemia, and some forms of cerebral arteriosclerosis might typically show O_2 consumptions rates down to 2.8 mL per 100 g per minute. Finally, the comatose states of diabetic coma, insulin coma, and anesthesia can show consumption rates as low as 2.0 mL per 100 g per minute. On the other hand, O_2 consumption by the brain increases during convulsions.

GLUCOSE METABOLISM

Glucose is virtually the only energy substrate which the brain can use. Free fatty acids, used by most other tissues when glucose is in short supply, are excluded from the brain by the blood-brain barrier. Figure 17-2 shows that the brain extracts 6.6 mL of O_2 from each 100 mL of cerebral blood and returns 6.7 mL of CO_2. Thus the respiratory quotient (RQ) of the brain is approximately

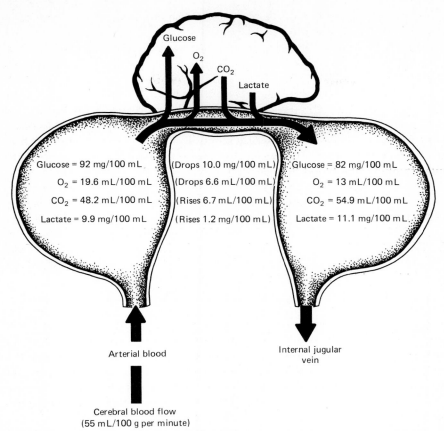

Glucose

O_2

CO_2

Lactate

Glucose = 92 mg/100 mL	(Drops 10.0 mg/100 mL)	Glucose = 82 mg/100 mL
O_2 = 19.6 mL/100 mL	(Drops 6.6 mL/100 mL)	O_2 = 13 mL/100 mL
CO_2 = 48.2 mL/100 mL	(Rises 6.7 mL/100 mL)	CO_2 = 54.9 mL/100 mL
Lactate = 9.9 mg/100 mL	(Rises 1.2 mg/100 mL)	Lactate = 11.1 mg/100 mL

Arterial blood

Internal jugular
vein

Cerebral blood flow
(55 mL/100 g per minute)

Figure 17-2 Arteriovenous differences for glucose, oxygen, carbon dioxide, and lactate. The oxygen and carbon dioxide values indicate that glucose is virtually the only energy source utilized by the brain as the respiratory quotient (RQ) is approximately 1.0. 85 percent of the glucose extracted by the brain is converted to CO_2, while 15 percent is converted to lactic acid.

1.0, indicating carbohydrate utilization only. Brain glucose consumption is normally about 10 mg per 100 mL, accounting for almost 75 percent of the liver's production and further attesting to the brain's heavy dependence on glucose.

Adenosine triphosphate (ATP), produced by the metabolic degradation and oxidative phosphorylation of glucose, is the useful energy currency in brain tissue. About 85 percent of the circulating glucose extracted from the cerebral arterial blood is converted to CO_2 via the tricarboxylic acid (TCA) cycle, while 15 percent is converted to lactic acid. The general scheme for glucose metabolism in the brain is similar to that in other tissues and is illustrated in Fig. 17-3. The enormous ATP requirements of the brain are partly due to neurotransmitter synthesis, release, and reuptake as well as intracellular transport and complex synthetic mechanisms. But undoubtedly the greatest percentage of

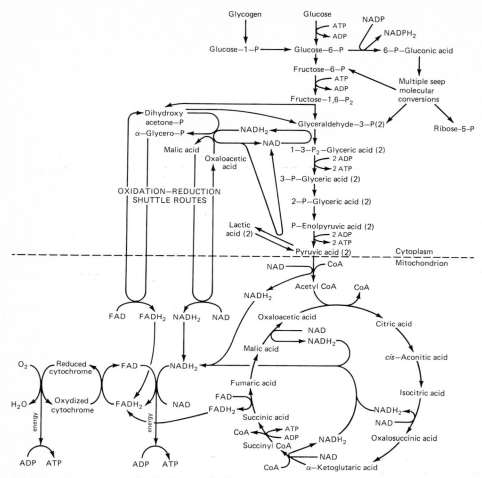

Figure 17-3 Illustration of glucose metabolism in the central nervous system. Because $NADH_2$ does not readily permeate the mitochondrial membrane, alternate "shuttle" molecules mediate the oxidation of cytoplasmic $NADH_2$ and the subsequent reduction of mitochondrial NAD and FAD. The oxaloacetic acid–malic acid system is probably the more important in this respect. Approximately 38 molecules of ATP are formed per molecule of glucose metabolized.

ATP is utilized to power the ion pumps which restore membrane potentials, enabling neurons to maintain their excitability.

REGULATION OF CEREBRAL BLOOD FLOW

Adequate cerebral blood flow (CBF) must be maintained at all times in order to ensure the delivery of sufficient O_2 and glucose to the brain. Fortunately we have automatic regulating systems which ensure adequate flow. The cerebral arterial vasculature is in a normal state of partial constriction and the CBF can be increased by vasodilation, which decreases cerebrovascular resistance. Likewise, increased vasoconstriction causes the cerebrovascular resistance to increase, producing a corresponding decrease in cerebral blood flow. Changes in cerebrovascular resistance and hence cerebral blood flow are caused by (1) fluctuations in perfusion pressure and (2) variations in circulating Po_2 and Pco_2.

Changes in Perfusion Pressure

If we subtract intracranial pressure (ICP) from the mean arterial pressure (MAP), we obtain the effective perfusion pressure (PP) in the brain. Within physiological limits, changes in PP feed back negatively to change cerebrovascular resistance, thus maintaining a constant CBF. If the PP decreases, the expected drop in CBF is not realized because the automatic compensatory decrease in cerebrovascular resistance maintains blood flow near normal limits. Similarly, an increase in PP doesn't produce an increase in CBF because compensatory increases in cerebrovascular resistance again maintain the CBF at normal levels.

This autoregulating compensatory mechanism operates within the PP range of 50 to 180 mmHg. Since the cerebral vessels have presumably dilated maximally when the PP drops to 50 mmHg, further drops in pressure can't be compensated for, and CBF begins to fall accordingly (Fig. 17-4). Likewise, once the PP increases to around 180 mmHg, the vessels are maximally vasoconstricted and cannot compensate for further increases in pressure. Thus beyond 180 mmHg the cerebral blood flow rises directly with the perfusion pressure.

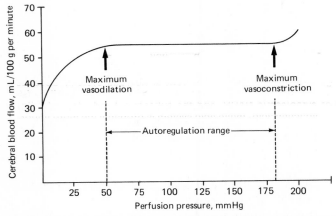

Figure 17-4 Autoregulation of cerebral blood flow as the perfusion pressure changes. The autoregulatory compensating mechanism operates within the range of 50 to 180 mmHg. As the pressure drops within this range, cerebrovascular dilation decreases the cerebrovascular resistance and thus prevents a drop in the cerebral blood flow. Increases in pressure cause an increase in the cerebrovascular resistance, thereby preventing an increase in cerebral blood flow. Outside of this range, the vessels cannot dilate or constrict further, and the cerebral blood flow changes directly with the perfusion pressure.

Changes in Po$_2$ and Pco$_2$

Decreases in arterial Po$_2$ produce no change in cerebrovascular resistance until the level falls to approximately 50 mmHg. Below this level we see vasodilation and an increase in CBF. When the Po$_2$ drops to 30 mmHg, the CBF reaches a level about 50 percent greater than normal. Increases in Po$_2$ above the normal level of 96 mmHg cause a slight increase in cerebrovascular resistance and a subsequent drop in CBF. It is interesting to note that the compensatory rise in CBF caused by falling O$_2$ levels is greater than the drop in CBF caused by higher than normal O$_2$ levels, once again stressing the importance the body puts on supplying adequate O$_2$ to the brain.

Increases in arterial Pco$_2$ profoundly increase the CBF. Blood flow to the brain can be almost doubled by breathing 7 percent CO$_2$. Conversely, hyperventilating can reduce the arterial Pco$_2$ sufficiently to drop the CBF from its normal 55 mL per 100 g per minute to 34 mL per 100 g per minute. It is not surprising to find that dizziness often occurs at this level when you consider that unconsciousness appears at 30 mL per 100 g per minute.

Because pH is profoundly influenced by Pco$_2$, through the reaction of CO$_2$ with H$_2$O to form H$_2$CO$_3$ in the presence of the enzyme carbonic anhydrase, there has been some question as to whether the changes in vasomotor tone are due to CO$_2$ or H$^+$ions. Studies in which carbonic anhydrase has been poisoned by acetazolamide show that the normal effects of altered Pco$_2$ on vasomotor tone are eliminated. This would suggest that CO$_2$ plays only an indirect role while it is actually the change in H$^+$-ion concentration which is the directly acting agent. Further, since the application of acid to the cortex causes no vascular change nor do H$^+$ ions freely enter cells while CO$_2$ does, it is likely that intracellular rather than extracellular H$^+$ ions are involved.

EFFECTS OF OXYGEN DEPRIVATION

Almost all of the oxygen consumed by the brain is utilized for the oxidation of carbohydrate. Sufficient energy is released from this process so that the normal level of oxygen utilization is adequate to replace the 12 mmol or so of ATP which the whole brain uses per minute. However, since the normal brain reserve of ATP and creatine phosphate (CrP) totals only about 8 mmol, less than a minute's reserve of high energy phosphate bonds is actually available if production were to suddenly stop. In the absence of oxygen, the anaerobic glycolysis of glucose and glycogen could supply only another 15 mmol of ATP, as these two energy substrates are stored in such low quantities in brain tissue.

A continuous uninterrupted supply of oxygen to the brain is essential in order to maintain its metabolic functions and to prevent tissue damage. The oxygen-independent glycolytic pathway (anaerobic glycolysis) is insufficient, even at maximum operating levels, to supply the heavy demands of the brain. Thus a loss of consciousness occurs when brain tissue Po$_2$ levels fall to 15 to 20 mmHg. This level is reached in less than 10 s when cerebral blood flow is completely stopped.

Low tissue oxygen levels in the brain (hypoxidosis) can be caused by decreased blood flow (ischemia) or with adequate blood flow accompanied by low levels of blood oxygen (hypoxemia). It is important to recognize that decreased Po_2 caused by ischemia is accompanied by decreased brain glucose and increased brain CO_2 while hypoxemia with normal blood flow is not accompanied by changes in brain glucose or CO_2. With complete cessation of CBF, irreversible damage occurs to brain tissue within a few minutes and the histological effects observed are remarkably similar whether caused by ischemia, hypoxemia, or hypoglycemia.

Experimental studies on rats and mice in which arterial Po_2 is progressively reduced have illustrated some aspects of hypoxemia which are likely to be similar in humans. A drop in arterial Po_2 to 50 mmHg (normal, 96 mmHg) produces no change in CBF, O_2 utilization by the brain, or lactic acid production. However, as Po_2 levels drop to 30 mmHg, a 50 percent increase in CBF is observed along with the onset of coma, decreased oxygen utilization, and increased lactic acid production. When the Po_2 drops further to 15 mmHg, 50 percent of the animals die because of cardiac failure. The remainder show a tremendous increase in lactic acid production, but, suprisingly, levels of ATP, ADP, and AMP remain normal. If cerebral perfusion is artificially maintained while the arterial Po_2 is decreased further, ATP, ADP, and AMP levels still remain normal. The implication is that the coma observed at low oxygen levels may not be due to a decrease in ATP but instead to some still unexplained mechanism. It appears likely that cardiac complications caused by hypoxemia and the subsequent effect on cerebral blood flow may actually be a primary cause of the irreversible pathologic damage to the brain.

Hypoxia, such as that brought on by high altitudes, brings on a number of symptoms, including drowsiness, apathy, and decreases in judgment. Unless oxygen is administered within half a minute or so, coma, convulsions, and depression of the EEG occur.

EFFECTS OF GLUCOSE DEPRIVATION

In the healthy normal functioning brain, glucose is the only substrate utilized for energy metabolism. Thus hypoglycemia presents the brain with a very serious problem. While most other tissues can shift to utilizing free fatty acids (FFA) as an alternative energy source when glucose is lacking, the brain cannot because they are excluded by the blood-brain barrier. While there is some evidence that the brain can utilize β-hydroxybutyric acid for energy metabolism when glucose levels are low or when fats are being mobilized for energy metabolism throughout the rest of the body, the brain could never supply its high energy demands by this method alone in the absence of glucose. Thus the brain is dependent on an uninterrupted supply of blood-borne glucose to energize its cells.

Decreases in blood glucose bring on disturbances in cerebral function. Depending on the level of hypoglycemia, these changes range from mild sensory disturbances to coma. At blood glucose levels of 19 mg per 100 mL or below (normal is 60 to 120 mg per 100 mL), a mentally confused state occurs. Brain O_2 utilization falls to 2.6 mL per 100 g per minute (normal, 3.5 mL per 100 g per minute) and glucose utilization drops as well. Coma commences when glucose levels fall to 8 mg per 100 mL.

Epinephrine can be effective in reversing the effects of hypoglycemia by promoting liver glycogenolysis. However, attempts to solve the problem by substituting other carbohydrate metabolic substrates have been largely unsuccessful, with the single exception of mannose. This is the only monosaccharide other than glucose which the brain appears to utilize directly. It crosses the blood-brain barrier and directly replaces glucose in the glycolytic pathway. However, its normal level in the blood is too low to be of any real help in reversing the cerebral effects of hypoglycemia. Unless reversed quickly, comatose levels of prolonged hypoglycemia will bring on necrosis of cerebrocortical cells and (to a lesser extent) other brain regions as well.

NEUROACTIVE CHEMICALS

Neurons in the CNS produce a large number of special molecules which function as neurotransmitters or are suspected to do so, including acetylcholine (ACh), norepinephrine (NE), dopamine (DA), γ-aminobutyric acid (GABA), aspartic acid, glutamic acid, glycine, and substance P. CNS neurons also synthesize a number of neuropeptides which perform quite specific endocrine roles. We will take a closer look at these neuroactive chemicals now.

Acetylcholine

Acetylcholine has long been recognized as an important neurotransmitter. It's released by preganglionic sympathetic and parasympathetic nerve fiber terminals as well as postganglionic parasympathetic and certain select sympathetic fibers. It is also the only recognized neurotransmitter at the skeletal muscle neuromuscular junction. Unfortunately we don't have nearly as complete a picture of the distribution of cholinergic neurons in the CNS. There appear to be cholinergic fibers associated with the arousal or activating systems of the brain which project from the midbrain reticular formation, hypothalamus striatum, and septum to the neocortex. ACh and the enzymes necessary for its synthesis are also found in the hippocampus, corpus striatum, and retina.

Acetylcholine is formed by the reaction of choline with acetyl coenzyme A (acetyl CoA) in the presence of the enzyme choline acetyltransferase (CAT). Since neurons can't synthesize choline, the ultimate source of choline for ACh synthesis is the choline of the plasma. Acetyl CoA is synthesized within presynaptic cytoplasm by the ATP-energized reaction of acetate with CoA. Once ACH has been synaptically released and has produced its postsynaptic effects on membrane permeability, it is hydrolyzed within microseconds by the enzyme acetylcholinesterase (AChE). Interestingly enough, while negligible amounts of ACh are reabsorbed by presynaptic terminals in the peripheral nervous system (hydrolysis by AChE being overwhelmingly dominant), its reup-

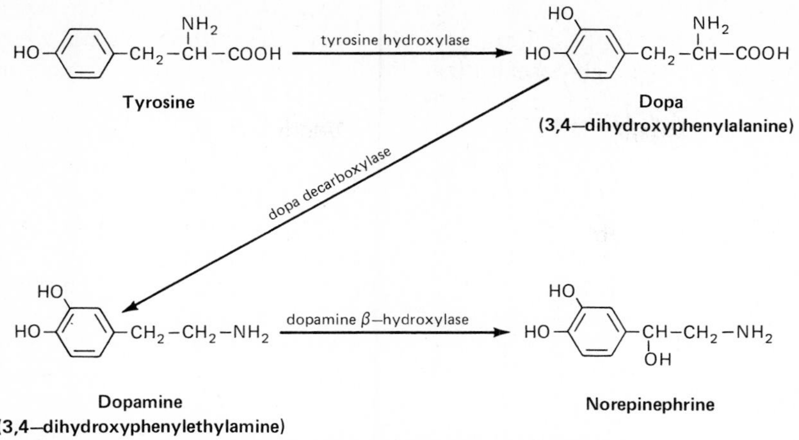

Figure 17-5 Scheme for the synthesis of the catecholamines dopamine (DA) and norepinephrine (NE).

take by the terminals in brain is considerable. Nevertheless, its failure to be resequestered into synaptic vesicles leaves the significance of this process in doubt.

$$\text{Acetate} + \text{CoA} + \text{ATP} \longrightarrow \text{acetyl CoA} + \text{AMP} + 2p_i$$

$$\text{Acetyl CoA} + \text{choline} \xrightarrow{\text{choline acetyltransferase}} \text{acetylcholine} + \text{CoA}$$

$$\text{Acetylcholine} + \text{H}_2\text{O} \xrightarrow{\text{acetylcholinesterase}} \text{choline} + \text{acetate}$$

Catecholamines

The catecholamine neurotransmitters are norepinephrine (NE) and dopamine (DA). The synthesis of both of these amines proceeds from the amino acid tyrosine (Fig. 17-5). Tyrosine is converted to 3,4-dihydroxyphenylalanine (dopa) by the enzyme tyrosine hydroxylase. Subsequent decarboxylation by dopa decarboxylase converts dopa to 3,4-dihydroxyphenylethylamine (dopamine). This is as far as the synthesis proceeds in dopaminergic neurons. In norepinephrinergic neurons, an additional step converts dopamine to norepinephrine by action of the enzyme dopamine β-hydroxylase.

The enzymatic degradation of the two catecholamines is illustrated in Fig. 17-6. Catechol-o-methyltransferase (COMT) and monoamine oxidase (MAO) produce inactive products which have little effect on receptor sites. MAO catalyzes the oxidative deamination of norepinephrine to 3,4-dihydroxymandelic acid and dopamine to 3,4-dihydroxyphenylacetic acid. These products are then methylated by COMT to 3-methoxy-4-hydroxymandelic acid and homovanillic acid, respectively. Alternatively, norepinephrine can first be methylated to normetanephrine and then deaminated to 3-methoxy-4-hydroxymandelic acid.

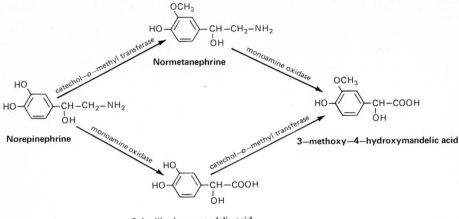

Figure 17-6 Scheme for the degradation, by enzymatic action, of the catecholamines dopamine (DA) and norepinephrine (NE) to physiologically inactive forms.

Distribution of Norepinephrinergic Fibers The distribution of norepinephrinergic fibers in the peripheral nervous system is limited to the majority of postganglionic sympathetic neurons. Norepinephrine-releasing neurons in the central nervous system have their cell bodies located in the midbrain, pons, and medulla, primarily in the reticular formation. Two norepinephrine systems are often described in the mammalian brain: the *locus ceruleus system* and the *lateral tegmental system*. The cell bodies of the former are located in the locus ceruleus, a prominent nucleus in the brainstem reticular formation at the level of the isthmus. This nucleus is composed entirely of norepinephrinergic neurons. Their fibers project to the spinal cord, brainstem, cerebellum, hypothalamus, thalamus, basal telencephalon, and the entire neocortex. The lateral tegmental system includes those norepinephrinergic neurons with cell bodies located in the dorsal motor nucleus of X, the nucleus of the solitary tract, and the adjacent and lateral tegmentum. The fibers of this system project to the spinal cord, brainstem, hypothalamus, thalamus, and basal telencephalon.

Distribution of Dopaminergic Fibers Dopaminergic systems in the CNS are more complex, numerous, and diversely distributed than norepinephrine systems. Seven dopaminergic systems can be identified in the mammalian brain.

Nigrostriatal System   The neurons in this system project from the pars compacta of the substantia nigra and the mediolateral tegmentum to terminate in the caudate nucleus, putamen, and globus pallidus. A marked reduction in dopamine content in the neostriatum (caudate and putamen) is characteristic in patients with Parkinson's disease. There is good evidence that the dopaminergic neurons of the substantia nigra inhibit their target cells in the caudate nucleus.

Mesocortical System   This system is composed of fibers from the substantia nigra and medioventral tegmentum which do not project to the basal nuclei. The fibers terminate in both the neocortex and allocortex. Terminations in the former include the mesial frontal, anterior cingulate, entorhinal, and perirhinal regions. Terminations in the allocortex include the olfactory bulb, anterior olfactory nucleus, olfactory tubercle, piriform cortex, septal area, and amygdaloid complex.

Tuberohypophyseal System   These fibers originate in the arcuate and periventricular hypothalamic nuclei, and project to the neurointermediate lobe of the pituitary gland as well as the median eminence. One function of this system appears to be the inhibition of pituitary prolactin secretion. The pathway to the intermediate lobe may serve to inhibit melanocyte-stimulating hormone (MSH) secretion.

Retinal System   The dopaminergic neurons of this system are the interplexiform cells of the retina which terminate in both the inner and outer plexiform layers of the retina.

Incertohypothalamic System   These fibers project from the zona incerta and the posterior hypothalamus to the dorsal hypothalamic area and the septum. They may play a role in neuroendocrine regulation.

Periventricular System   The cell bodies of these fibers are located in the medulla in the area of the dorsal motor nucleus of X, the nucleus of the solitary tract, and the periaqueductal and periventricular gray matter. They terminate in the periaqueductal and periventricular gray, tegmentum, tectum, thalamus, and hypothalamus. Their function is unknown.

Olfactory Bulb System   This system is composed of the periglomerular cells of the olfactory bulbs which terminate on the mitral cells of the glomeruli. Their function is unknown.

Serotonin and Melatonin

Serotonin and melatonin are neuroactive indolealkylamines. Serotonin functions as a CNS neurotransmitter while melatonin, formed by a two-step process from serotonin, may play a hormonal role in the pineal gland. The highest concentration of serotonin anywhere in the body is in the pineal gland. The next highest concentration is in the raphe nuclei of the lower brainstem. The French neurophysiologist Jouvet demonstrated the role of these sero-

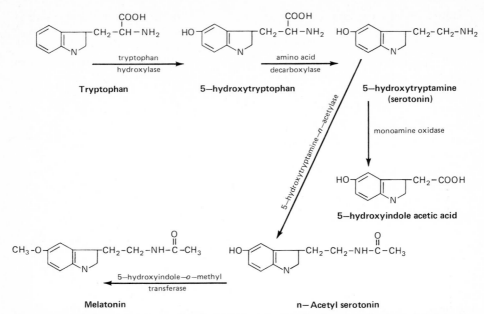

Figure 17-7 Scheme for the synthesis of the indolealkalylamines serotonin and melatonin. The synthesis of melatonin, from serotonin through the intermediary structure *n*-acetyl serotonin, occurs in the pineal gland. Degradation of serotonin, by the enzyme monoamine oxidase (MAO) to 5-hydroxyindole acetic acid, is also shown.

tonergic raphe neurons by performing experiments on cats. He selectively destroyed the raphe neurons, producing a significant reduction in brain serotonin levels, and found that the cats became totally insomniac. He followed this by administering *p*-chlorophenylalanine to another group of cats. This drug, which prevents the conversion of tryptophan to 5-hydroxytryptophan by interfering with the action of the enzyme tryptophan hydroxylase, decreases the raphe concentration of serotonin, because 5-hydroxytryptophan is a serotonin precursor. This group of cats also became insomniac. Subsequent administration of 5-hydroxytryptophan reversed the insomnia, putting the cats to sleep.

Melatonin is formed from serotonin in the pineal gland by acetylization to *n*-acetyl serotonin by 5-hydroxytryptamine-*n*-acetylase. The enzyme 5-hydroxyindole-*o*-methyl transferase then completes the conversion to melatonin. The synthesis of both serotonin and melatonin, as well as the degradation of serotonin, are illustrated in Fig. 17-7.

Amino Acid Neurotransmitters

Several amino acids have been implicated as neurotransmitters in the CNS, including γ-aminobutyric acid (GABA), glutamic acid, glycine, and aspartic acid. Of these, we know the most about the role of GABA. It was the first amino acid to be established as a neurotransmitter in vertebrate and invertebrate nervous systems. GABA is synthesized in nervous tissue by the alpha

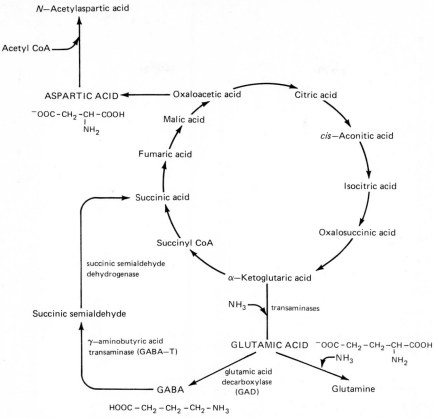

Figure 17-8 The formation of glutamic acid, γ-aminobutyric acid, and aspartic acid from the Krebs tricarboxylic acid (TCA) cycle.

decarboxylation of glutamic acid in the presence of glutamic acid decarboxylase (Fig. 17-8).

GABA has usually been described as an inhibitory neurotransmitter and may function primarily in this role in the CNS. It is unusual among amino acids in that it is produced almost exclusively in the brain and spinal cord. Its importance is evidenced by its wide distribution, which has been estimated to include up to one-third of all CNS synapses. The possibility exists that all of the inhibitory cells of the cerebellar cortex are "GABAergic." This includes the Purkinje, stellate, basket, and granular cells described in Chap. 13. GABA is also suspected to operate as an inhibitory neurotransmitter in the cerebral cortex, lateral vestibular nucleus, and spinal cord. Chemical analysis has also established the presence of GABA in the colliculi, diencephalon, and to a lesser extent, the pons, medulla, and much of the cerebral cortex. GABA produces inhibition by hyperpolarizing membranes through increased Cl^- and K^+ ion conductance. Glycine, another amino acid transmitter, is also suspected to be inhibitory through the same mechanism.

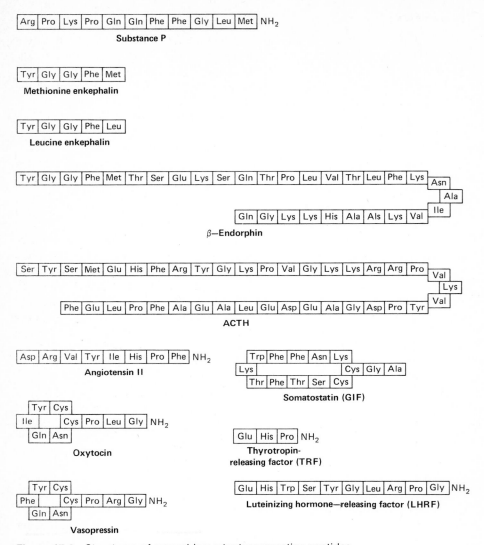

Figure 17-9 Structures of several important neuroactive peptides.

Interestingly enough, glutamic acid, the GABA precursor which chemically differs from it by having two rather than one carboxyl groups, is considered to be an excitatory rather than an inhibitory transmitter. Aspartic acid also appears to be an excitatory transmitter in the spinal cord gray matter. It appears to be associated with interneurons and may oppose the inhibiting action of glycine or GABA-releasing inhibitory interneurons. The formation of these amino acid transmitters from TCA cycle intermediates is illustrated in Fig. 17-8.

Neuropeptides

Over the years, a number of neuropeptides have been identified which play a variety of functional roles in the nervous system (Fig. 17-9). Several have well-known endocrine roles such as ACTH, oxytocin, and vasopressin from the pituitary gland. Also included are the hypothalamic factors which control the release of certain pituitary hormones. These are somatostatin (growth hormone–inhibiting factor), thyrotropin-releasing factor (TRF), and luteinizing hormone–releasing factor (LHRF).

Other neuropeptides appear to function as neurotransmitters. One of these is substance P, found in certain pathways in the brain and in terminal endings of specific primary sensory fibers of spinal nerves. The latter are represented by those fibers which synapse on secondary spinal cord neurons responding most readily to pain. Thus it is hypothesized to operate as a transmitter for painful stimuli from the periphery to the CNS.

Perhaps the most interesting group of neuropeptides are the enkephalins and endorphins. The morphinelike enkephalins have been found in interneurons in the same regions of the spinal cord where substance P is released, and there is evidence to suggest that they inhibit the release of substance P. Thus, enkephalin-containing neurons may work to suppress the transmission of painful information between primary and secondary neurons. Enkephalins probably operate by presynaptically inhibiting the release of substance P from primary neurons, giving them a modulatory role at these synapses.

Enkephalin is also found in several areas of the brain and brainstem, paralleling the distribution of opiate receptors. The highest concentration occurs in the globus pallidus with lesser amounts in the caudate nucleus, hypothalamus, periaqueductal gray matter, and amygdala. The intriguing possibility exists that enkephalins may be naturally occurring analgesics operating as modulating neurotransmitters in various pain-mediating pathways.

REVIEW QUESTIONS

1 All of the following diffuse across the blood-brain barrier, *except*
   a free fatty acids
   b glucose
   c pyruvic acid
   d essential amino acids
   e proteins
2 The blood-brain barrier is conspicuously absent in
   a the median eminence of the hypothalamus
   b the motor cortex
   c the choroid plexus
   d the pineal gland
3 The following is (are) true concerning cerebral blood flow and oxygen consumption:
   a The brain receives 25 percent of the cardiac output.

    b The cerebral blood flow in humans is approximately 55 mL per 100 grams of brain tissue per minute.

    c The arteriovenous O_2 difference in the cerebral blood flow is approximately 19.6 mL per 100 mL.

    d The cerebral oxygen consumption is about 3.5 mL per 100 g per minute.

4 All of the following statements about glucose utilization are true, *except:*

    a Seventy-five percent of the liver's production of glucose is utilized by the brain.

    b The brain's normal glucose consumption is about 10 mg per 100 mL.

    c About 85 percent of the circulating glucose extracted from cerebral arterial blood is converted to CO_2 through the Krebs cycle.

    d Insulin enhances glucose uptake by the brain.

5 Cerebrovascular resistance decreases when

    a the cerebral perfusion pressure decreases

    b the arterial P_{O_2} rises above 96 mmHg

    c a person hyperventilates

    d a person breathes 7 percent CO_2

6 All of the following statements are true concerning the effects of oxygen deprivation, *except:*

    a Loss of consciousness occurs when brain tissue P_{O_2} falls to 40 mmHg.

    b A 50 percent decrease in cerebral blood flow occurs when the P_{O_2} level falls to 30 mmHg.

    c Lactic acid production increases tremendously when the P_{O_2} falls to 15 mmHg.

    d In the absence of oxygen, anerobic glycolysis is insufficient to supply adequate ATP for brain metabolism.

7 All of the following statements are true concerning the effects of glucose deprivation, *except:*

    a Coma commences when glucose levels fall to 8 mg per 100 mL.

    b Blood mannose levels are generally adequate to replace glucose as a metabolic substrate for the brain when blood glucose levels are dangerously low.

    c Mental confusion occurs when blood glucose levels fall to 60 mg per 100 mL.

    d The histological damages associated with hypoglycemia are similar to those associated with hypoxia.

8 Norepinephrinergic fibers in the CNS are heavily concentrated in

    a the locus ceruleus system

    b the raphe nuclei

    c the nigrostriatal system

    d the tuberohypophyseal system

    e all of the above

9 Central nervous system dopaminergic fibers are located in

    a the mesocortical system

    b the periventricular system

    c the lateral tegmental system

    d the pineal gland

10 All of the following statements concerning neuropeptides are true, *except:*

    a Norepinephrine is a neuropeptide.

    b Spinal cord enkephalins are thought to inhibit the release of substance P.

    c Enkephalins are found in high concentration in the globus pallidus.

    d Enkephalins are found in several areas of the brain, paralleling the distribution of opiate receptors.

Answers to Review Questions

Chapter 1

1 a, d   2 a   3 b, c, d, f   4 a, c, d   5 b, d   6 b
7 a, c, d, e   8 b, d   9 c, e   10 a

Chapter 2

1 c   2 b, c, d   3 c, d   4 b   5 b   6 a, b   7 a, c, d
8 a, c, d   9 b, d   10 d

Chapter 3

1 b, e   2 a, c   3 c   4 b, c, e   5 b   6 d   7 c, d, e
8 b   9 c, d   10 a, b, d

Chapter 4

1 b   2 b, c, d   3 a, b   4 a, b, d   5 b, c, d   6 b, d
7 a, b, c   8 b   9 b, c, e   10 e

Chapter 5

1 a   2 c   3 b, d   4 b   5 a, c, d, e   6 a, c, d, e   7 a, e
8 a, d   9 b, c   10 e

Chapter 6

1 a, c, d   2 a   3 e   4 b   5 b, c, d   6 a, c, d   7 a
8 b, c, e   9 c   10 b, c, e

Chapter 7

1 c   2 a   3 d   4 a, d   5 c   6 e   7 a   8 a   9 c, d
10 d

Chapter 8

1 b   2 c   3 a, c   4 a, b, d   5 a   6 a, d   7 d   8 a, c
9 c   10 d

Chapter 9

1 d   2 c, d   3 b, d   4 b, d   5 d, e   6 a   7 b   8 a
9 c   10 a, d

Chapter 10

1 d   2 c   3 b   4 c   5 e   6 b   7 a, c   8 d   9 b
10 e

Chapter 11

1 d   2 a, b   3 c   4 d   5 d   6 c, d   7 c, d   8 d
9 a   10 a

Chapter 12

1 a   2 a, b, c, d   3 b   4 a   5 a   6 a, d   7 b   8 d
9 a   10 d

Chapter 13

1 a, c   2 a, c   3 e   4 a, b   5 b   6 d   7 c   8 e
9 a, b   10 a, c, d

Chapter 14

1 b, c   2 a   3 a   4 d   5 a, b   6 a   7 d, e   8 e
9 c   10 a, b

Chapter 15

1 b   2 a   3 a   4 d   5 a, b   6 e   7 a   8 d   9 b
10 a

Chapter 16

1 a   2 c   3 c   4 a   5 b   6 a   7 c   8 b, d   9 b, c
10 d

Chapter 17

1 a, e   2 a, d   3 b, d   4 d   5 a, d   6 a   7 b, c   8 a
9 a, b   10 a

Suggested Additional Reading

NEUROANATOMY

Clark, Ronald G.: *Manter and Gatz's Essentials of Clinical Neuroanatomy and Neurophysiology,* 5th ed., F. A. Davis Company, Philadelphia, 1975.
House, Earl Lawrence, and Ben Pansky: *A Functional Approach to Neuroanatomy,* 2d ed., McGraw-Hill Book Company, New York, 1967.
Sidman, Richard L., and Murray Sidman: *Neuroanatomy: A Programmed Text,* vol. I, Little, Brown and Company, Boston, 1965.
Tuchmann-Duplessis, H., M. Auroux, and P. Haegel: *Illustrated Human Embryology: Nervous System and Endocrine Glands,* vol. III, Lucille S. Hurley (trans.), Springer-Verlag, New York Inc., New York, 1974.
Williams, Peter L., and Roger Warwick: *Functional Neuroanatomy of Man,* W. B. Saunders Company, Philadelphia, 1975.

NEUROPHYSIOLOGY

Cowan, W. Maxwell, Zach W. Hall, and Eric P. Kandel: *Annual Review of Neuroscience,* vols. 1 and 2, *Annual Reviews Inc.,* Palo Alto, 1978.
Eccles, John C.: *The Understanding of the Brain,* 2d ed., McGraw-Hill Book Company, New York, 1977.

Eyzaguirre, C., and S. Fidone: *Physiology of the Nervous System,* 2d ed., Year Book
    Medical Publishers, Inc., Chicago, 1975.
Hunt, Carlton C.: *MTP International Review of Science,* ser. 1: *Physiology,* vol. 3:
    Neurophysiology, University Park Press, Baltimore, 1975.
Mountcastle, Vernon B.: *Medical Physiology, Volume 1,* 13th ed., The C. V. Mosby
    Company, St. Louis, 1974.
Noback, Charles R., and Robert J. Demarest: *The Nervous System: Introduction and
    Review,* 2d ed., McGraw-Hill Book Company, New York, 1977.
Porter, Robert: *International Review of Physiology,* vol. 10: *Neurophysiology II,* Uni-
    versity Park Press, Baltimore, 1976.
Porter, Robert: *International Review of Physiology,* vol. 17: *Neurophysiology III,* Uni-
    versity Park Press, Baltimore, 1978.
Ruch, Theodore C., and Harry D. Patton: *Physiology and Biophysics I: The Nervous
    System,* 20th ed., W. B. Saunders Company, Philadelphia, 1979.
Shepard, Gordon M.: *The Synaptic Organization of the Brain: An Introduction,* Oxford
    University Press, New York, 1974.

NEUROCHEMISTRY

Lewis, Anthony J: *Mechanisms of Neurological Disease,* Little, Brown and Company,
    Boston, 1976.
Siegel, George J., R. Wayne Albers, Robert Katzman, and Bernard W. Agranoff: *Basic
    Neurochemistry,* Little, Brown and Company, Boston, 1976.

References for Figure Credits

Duane, A.: "Studies in Monocular and Binocular Accommodation with Their Clinical Application," *Amer. J. Ophthal.*, **5**:865, 1922.

Eyzaguirre, C., and S. Fidone: *Physiology of the Nervous System*, 2d ed., Year Book Medical Publishers, Inc., Chicago, 1975.

Eyzaguirre, C., K. Nishi, and S. Fidone: "Chemoreceptor Synapses in the Carotid Body," *Fed. Proc.*, **31**:1385, 1972.

Eyzaguirre, C., and P. Zapata: "Release of Acetylcholine from Carotid Body Tissue, Further Study on the Effects of Acetylcholine and Cholinergic Blocking Agents on the Chemosensory Discharge," *J. Physiol.*, **195**:589, 1968.

Gambaryan, P. P., G. N. Orlovsky, T. G. Protopopova, F. V. Severin, and M. L. Shik: "Work of the Muscles in Various Forms of Progressive Movement of the Cat and Adaptive Changes of the Moving Organs in the Family Felidae," *Tr. Zool. Inst. Akad. Nauk. U.S.S.R.*, **48**:220, 1971, in G. N. Orlovsky and M. L. Shik: "Control of Locomotion: A Neurophysiological Analysis of the Cat Locomotor System," in R. Porter (ed.), *International Review of Physiology*, vol. 10: *Neurophysiology II*, University Park Press, Baltimore, 1976, p. 281.

Goodman, L. S., and A. Gilman: *The Pharmacological Basis of Therapeutics*, 5th ed., The Macmillan Company, New York, 1975.

Guyton, A. C.: *Textbook of Medical Physiology*, 5th ed., W. B. Saunders Company, Philadelphia, 1976.

Henneman, E., and C. B. Olson: "Relations Between Structure and Function in the Design of Skeletal Muscles," *J. Neurophysiol.*, **28**:581, 1965.

Hodgkin, A. L.: "Ionic Movements and Electrical Activity in Giant Nerve Fibers," *Proc. Roy. Soc. Lond. B.,* **148**:1, 1958.

Hodgkin, A. L., and A. F. Huxley: "A Quantitative Description of Membrane Current and its Application to Conduction and Excitation in Nerve," *J. Physiol.,* **117**:500, 1952.

Hunt, C. C., and S. W. Kuffler: "Stretch Receptor Discharge During Muscle Contraction," *J. Physiol.,* **113**:298, 1951.

Katz, B.: "Depolarization of Sensory Terminals and the Initiation of Impulses in the Muscle Spindle," *J. Physiol.,* **111**:261, 1950.

Lloyd, D. P. D.: "Reflex Action in Relation to Pattern and Peripheral Source of Afferent Stimulation," *J. Neurophysiol.,* **6**:111, 1943.

Loewenstein, W.: "Excitation and Inactivation in a Receptor Membrane," *Ann. N.Y. Acad. Sci.,* **94**:510, 1961.

Marks, W., W. Dobelle, and E. MacNichol: "Visual Pigments of Single Primate Cones," *Science,* **143**:1181, 1964.

McPhedran, A. M., R. B. Wuerker, and E. Henneman: "Properties of Motor Units in a Homogenous Red Muscle (Soleus) of the Cat," *J. Neurophysiol.,* **28**:71, 1965.

Pffafmann, C.: "Gustatory Nerve Impulses in Rat, Cat, and Rabbit," *J. Neurophysiol.,* **18**:429, 1955.

Renshaw, B.: "Activity in the Simple Spinal Reflex Pathway," *J. Neurophysiol.,* **3**:373, 1940.

Rose, J. E., N. D. Gross, C. D. Geisler, and J. E. Hind: "Some Neural Mechanisms in the Inferior Colliculus of the Cat Which May Be Relevant to the Localization of a Sound Source," *J. Neurophysiol.,* **29**:288, 1966.

Shik, M. L., F. V. Severin, and G. N. Orlovsky: "Control of Walking and Running by Means of Electrical Stimulation of the Mid-Brain," *Biofisika,* **11**:659, 1966 (Eng. trans., **11**:756, 1966). G. N. Orlovsky and M. L. Shik: "Control of Locomotion: A Neurophysiological Analysis of the Cat Locomotor System," in R. Porter (ed.), *International Review of Physiology,* vol. 10: *Neurophysiology II,* University Park Press, Baltimore, 1976, p. 281.

Tasaki, I.: "Nerve Impulses in Individual Auditory Nerve Fibers of Guinea Pig," *J. Neurophysiol.,* **17**:97, 1954.

Van Bergeiyk, W. A.: "Variation of a Theme of Bekesy: A Model of Binaural Interaction," *J. Acoustic Soc. Am.,* **34**:1431, 1962.

Wersall, J., L. Gleisner, and P. G. Lundquist: "Ultrastructure of the Vestibular End Organs," in A. V. S. De Reuck and J. Knight (eds.), *Myotatic, Kinesthetic and Vestibular Mechanisms,* Little, Brown and Company, 1967.

Wuerker, R. B., A. M. McPhedran, and E. Henneman: "Properties of Motor Units in a Heterogenous Pale Muscle (M. Gastrocnemius) of the Cat," *J. Neurophysiol.,* **28**:85, 1965.

Zotterman, Y.: "Special Senses: Thermal Receptors," *Ann. Rev. Physiol.,* **15**:357, 1953.

Index

Page numbers in *italics* indicate illustrations.

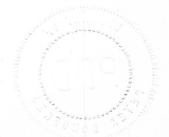

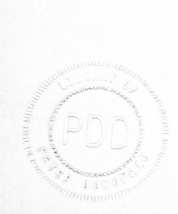